WOMEN'S health & WELLNESS 2004

Real Life Solutions from the Editors of *Health* Magazine

Oxmoor House®

Women's Health and Wellness 2004
©2003 by Oxmoor House, Inc.
Book Division of Southern Progress Corporation
P.O. Box 2463, Birmingham, Alabama 35201

Published by Oxmoor House, Inc.

Hardcover ISBN: 0-8487-2750-9
Softcover ISBN: 0-8487-2751-7
ISSN: 1537-4394
Printed in the United States of America
First Printing 2003

The articles in this book were printed in *Health* magazine and prepared in accordance with the highest standards of journalistic accuracy. Unless otherwise noted, these articles have not been updated since their original publication in 2003. Readers are cautioned not to use information from this book as a substitute for professional health care and advice.

To order additional publications,
call 800-765-6400.

For more books to enrich your life,
visit **oxmoorhouse.com**

Cover: Photography by David Roth

health

Editor/Vice President: Doug Crichton
Executive Editor: Lisa Delaney
Design Director: Paul Carstensen
Managing Editor: Candace H. Schlosser
Deputy Editor: Lisa Davis
Senior Editors: Nichele Hoskins (*Fitness*), Adam J. Martin (*Body*), Susie Quick (*Food/Nutrition*), Abigail M. Walch
Beauty and Fashion Editor: Colleen Sullivan
Editorial Coordinator: Christine O'Connell
Associate Editor: Leah Wyar (*Beauty/Fashion*)
Assistant Editors: Alisa Blackwell (*Food/Nutrition*), Su Reid-St. John (*Fitness*), Eric Steinmehl (*Body*), Molly Taylor (*Beauty/Fashion*)
Associate Art Director: Kevin de Miranda
Graphic Designer: Christen Colvert
Photo Coordinator: Angie Wilson Kelly
Assistant Photo Coordinator: Jeanne Dozier Clayton
Contributing Graphic Designers: Blair Ethridge, Susan Baskin Gray
Copy Chief: John R. Halphen
Copy Editors: Julie H. Bosché, Martha Yeilding Scribner
Research/Copy Assistant: Joseph O. Boone
Production Manager: Faustina S. Williams
Production Assistant: Kristin Lane
Office Manager: Stephanie Wolford
Editorial Assistants: Beth Dreher, Amanda Storey
Contributing Copy Editors: Lisa C. Bailey, Lori C. Pruitt
Contributing Researchers: Deborah L. Gallaway, Carmine Loper, Jason P. Mitchell, Holly Ensor Smith
Health.com Editor: Jerry Gulley II
Health.com Managing Editor: Laurie Herr

OXMOOR HOUSE, INC.
Editor in Chief: Nancy Fitzpatrick Wyatt
Senior Health Editor: Sandy McDowell
Art Director: Cynthia R. Cooper
Copy Chief: Allison Long Lowery

Editor: Suzanne Powell
Copy Editor: L. Amanda Owens
Editorial Assistants: Terri Laschober, McCharen Pratt
Senior Designer: Emily Albright Parrish
Publishing Systems Administrator: Rick Tucker
Director of Production: Phillip Lee
Production Manager: Theresa L. Beste
Production Assistant: Faye Porter Bonner

Contributors
Indexer: Sandy Charles
Editorial Consultant: Bill Gottlieb

Contents at a Glance

Table of Contents

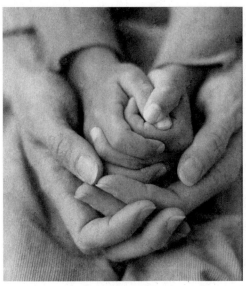

A debate is unfolding in the medical community regarding the healing power of prayer (page 48).

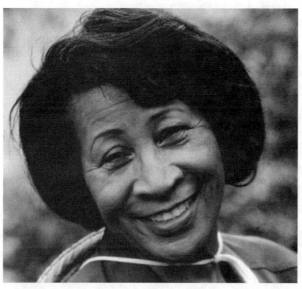

**Menopause is an inevitable part of life for women.
Discover how you can make the best of it (page 128).**

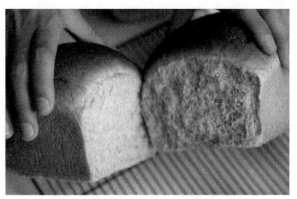

Is the bread you eat as healthy as you think it is (page 196)?

VII. Relationships: The Secrets to Happiness for Work, Love, and Play

Discover how women are learning to enjoy intimacy more than ever (page 318).

VIII. Mind & Spirit: Improve Stress Management and Find More Inner Peace

Editors' Picks

Here's a glance at some of the most intriguing stories appearing in this year's edition of *Women's* Health *& Wellness.*

THE TOP 10 **MEDICAL BREAKTHROUGHS** OF THE YEAR

The year has been full of great advances in medicine—here are the ones that are likely to help you and your family the most.

Whether you are searching for relief from chronic back pain or you are interested in a new form of contraception, the medical community is booming with new developments. Learn about these—and many more—that affect you (page 12).

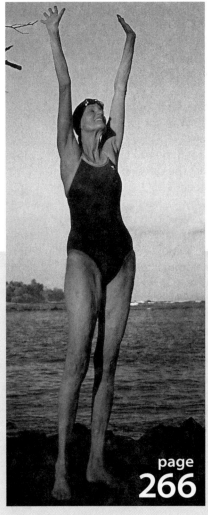

page
266

◀ **LATE BLOOMERS**

Five women realize it's never too late to discover the athlete within.

These women may not have been busy getting their high school letters as teenagers, but that doesn't mean they don't have the hearts of champs now. They prove that learning and mastering a new sport can happen at any age (page 266).

HOW TO **COOK SIMPLE** ▶

Health's Food and Nutrition Editor Susie Quick shares her secrets for creating fast, healthy, and delicious meals at home.

So you're not exactly a gourmet chef. That doesn't mean you're doomed to eating frozen dinners. Enjoy mealtime with these kitchen tips and easy recipes—even on a busy schedule (page 216).

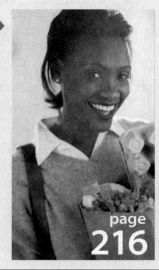

page
216

HOW TO HANDLE THE CURVE BALLS OF
MENOPAUSE

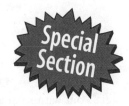

From hormone therapy to alternative care, discover the best ways to stay in control during this time of your life.

Menopause is one of a woman's biggest transitions. At times it may seem overwhelming, but you *can* take charge by learning more about it and the options available to you (page 128).

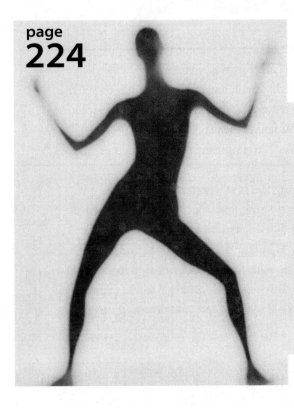

page
224

◀DISCOVER YOUR BODY-SPECIFIC WORKOUT PRESCRIPTION

Experts show you the best exercise plan for your individual fitness profile.

The three-mile run your neighbor takes every morning may work for her—but is it right for you? Not everyone is at the same place when it comes to a fitness plan. You need to find a workout especially for where you are now (page 224).

DON'T BE A VICTIM

Medical mistakes kill thousands of people each year. Here's how to protect yourself.

Everyone's heard about freak accidents that have occurred in hospitals: missed diagnoses, unnecessary operations. Unfortunately, the reality is that these misfortunes *do* happen. Learn the steps to prevent them from happening to you and your loved ones (page 68).

Editor's Note

No woman I know wants her health to take a backseat to other concerns. After all, we all know how important it is to eat right and exercise regularly and that mental well-being is just as crucial. But with so much conflicting information about what is and isn't good for you, it can be awfully tough to figure out those things you really need to pay attention to. That's where *Women's* Health *and Wellness 2004* comes in. The third in the series, this year's book offers you straight-talking advice and the latest on everything from nutrition, fitness, stress management, relationships, medicines, disease, and more.

Health magazine understands the power of living well. In fact, we see our job as inspiring women like you to take charge of your mind and body so you can truly enjoy your life. That's why we've compiled a year's worth of wisdom into this one incredible volume, making it easier to get the health information you want. In our eight comprehensive chapters, you'll find real-life solutions to issues that concern you most: "Breakthroughs in Women's Health," "Everyday Wellness," "Female Body," "Nutrition," "Fitness," "Healthy Looks," "Relationships," and "Mind & Spirit."

This book is packed with get-real advice, from learning the best workout for you (page 224) to finding clothes that really fit (page 298), even discovering how you can improve a bad mood in minutes (page 344). And there's a lot more: For example, you'll discover what's preventing you from shedding those extra pounds in "The Top 5 Diet Types ... and Why They Don't Work" (page 160). You'll learn what could be gnawing at your relationship in "Save Your Marriage Now" (page 320). And don't miss our special bonus section, "How to Handle the Curveballs of Menopause" (page 128); it'll help you deal with the ups and downs of one of the biggest transitions of your life.

So read on, and I hope you enjoy this 2004 edition of *Women's* Health *and Wellness.*

Best regards,

Doug Crichton

Health Editor/Vice President

breakthroughs
in women's health

**the latest in medical news
and alternative care**

The Year's
Top 10 Medical Breakthroughs

The year was full of great advances in medicine—here are the ones that are likely to help you and your family the most.

BY MICHAEL CASTLEMAN AND DOROTHY FOLTZ-GRAY

ADDITIONAL RESEARCH BY ERIC STEINMEHL • PHOTOGRAPHY BY DAVID EMMITE

1

NEW TEST RAISES ODDS OF OVARIAN-CANCER SURVIVAL

One of the deadliest diseases, ovarian cancer is especially difficult to cure because it usually is caught too late: Today, more than 80 percent of cases are detected at an advanced stage of the disease, when a woman has a mere 35-percent chance of surviving for five years. But in February 2002, researchers announced a study in which a computerized test found ovarian cancer in 100 percent of women who had it, with a false-positive rate of only 5 percent. The procedure was able to diagnose the disease at Stage 1, when the chance of surviving for five years is 95 percent.

The new finger-prick blood test was developed by the U.S. Food and Drug Administration (FDA), the National Cancer Institute (NCI), and Correlogic Systems, Inc. Using computers with sophisticated

> **New blood test finds ovarian cancer in its early, most preventable stage.**

programming, researchers analyzed blood samples from 116 women for particular protein patterns that are typical of ovarian-cancer patients. The test correctly identified all 50 who had cancer; three of the 66 women who didn't also received a positive diagnosis, although researchers say the false-positive rate could increase if the test were used on a large scale. (In contrast, the widely used CA-125 test recognizes cancer in only half of women with early disease and in 80 percent of those with advanced stages. Plus, the exam's high false-positive rate makes it an inadequate detection method on its own.)

"The most important subsequent goal is validating these results in large multi-institutional trials," says Lance Liotta, M.D., Ph.D., senior investigator for a study on the test at the NCI's Center for Cancer Research. Studies are already under way on women at high risk for the disease based on family history or genetic mutations. Extensive clinical trials are needed before the test can receive FDA approval and become available nationwide.

In addition to helping prevent 13,900 ovarian-cancer deaths each year, the new test is expected to be just as useful for finding other cancers. To find out how you can participate in a study, contact the NCI at 888-624-1937.

INNOVATION REDUCES EYE-SURGERY RISKS

Now there's a solution for farsighted people who want permanent vision correction without the possible side effects of LASIK surgery. Conductive keratoplasty (CK), a laser-free procedure approved by the FDA in April 2002, is a better option for the 20 percent of Americans who are farsighted.

Nearsighted folks have corneas that peak in the middle; with LASIK, doctors can reshape and correct them by removing tissue. Farsightedness is characterized by flat corneas. In CK, a hair-width probe is inserted into several spots along the outer edge of the cornea, heating them and causing the transparent disk to constrict. "Imagine a half-dozen guys standing on the edges of a waterbed. Their weight makes the center of the bed mound up. With CK, the same thing happens to the cornea," says ophthalmologist Michael Aronsky, M.D., who performs CK at Kremer Laser Eye Center in King of Prussia, Pennsylvania. "When the center rises, light strikes the eye at a different angle, which corrects farsightedness."

With CK, farsighted patients are less likely to experience side effects that are common in LASIK, such as poor night vision, glare, blurriness, and dry eyes (a particular problem among menopausal women who go the laser route). These negatives have caused many people to avoid surgical correction because they didn't think their sight was bad enough to warrant the risks, says Edward Manche, M.D.,

assistant professor of ophthalmology and director of cornea and refractive surgery at Stanford University. "This procedure will open up the possibility of treatment to a lot more people."

Currently, CK is approved only to treat hyperopia, or farsightedness that is unrelated to age. However, current clinical trials may soon earn it approval as a treatment for presbyopia, the more common age-related farsightedness. Recovery time is comparable to that of LASIK. "Most people can drive and return to work one to two days after surgery, but you might need glasses for a short while," Manche says. "However, most people get full CK benefits in two to three weeks." In about 1 percent of cases, people who have CK continue to need corrective lenses.

The 15-minute procedure (including prep time) costs about $1,000 to $2,500 per eye and is covered by some insurance policies.

"CK won't replace glasses, contacts, or LASIK," Aronsky says. "But for many people with farsightedness, especially women, it's great—and it's safe."

To find a physician who performs CK, check the Web site of the company that manufactures the equipment, Refractec (www.refractec.com).

BLOOD SUBS SAVE LIVES IN THE OPERATING ROOM

Bleeding profusely and near death, the shooting victim was rushed to Denver Health Medical Center. Luckily, trauma surgeon Ernest E. Moore, M.D., got the call. Moore was involved in a clinical trial of an experimental blood substitute called PolyHeme. "We started infusing it the moment he arrived," Moore recalls. "There was no need for time-consuming blood typing or running to the refrigerator for whole blood. With massive bleeding from gunshot wounds, every second counts." The patient survived, and Moore says PolyHeme just might have been the reason.

Since blood substitutes first started to attract attention, they've made tentative strides toward acceptance in the OR. PolyHeme and another sub, Hemopure, are currently awaiting FDA approval; a third, Hemolink, is undergoing clinical trials. They all contain hemoglobin (the molecule that carries oxygen) extracted from whole blood and chemically modified to maintain its effectiveness. "It's elegant," Moore says. "The proteins for blood type are on the cell membrane. By using just hemoglobin, there is no cell membrane," meaning the patient's type doesn't matter.

As red as the real thing, blood substitutes appear to be just what the EMT ordered for everything from industrial explosions to terrorist attacks.

Because the substitutes last only about 24 hours inside the body, they're strictly a stopgap. "But with patients stabilized on a blood substitute, you have a day to either bring whole blood to them or transport them to it," Moore says. In rare cases, side effects such as high blood pressure, kidney failure, and allergic reactions can occur.

As red as the real thing, but a little thinner, the substitutes appear to be just what the EMT ordered for everything from industrial explosions to terrorist attacks. But they probably will be most widely used during everyday surgery, Moore explains, saving precious whole blood for the conclusions of procedures. While the products await government approval, the FDA has allowed their "compassionate use" in special cases—for example, with Jehovah's Witnesses, whose religion prohibits whole-blood transfusions.

But blood substitutes won't make the genuine article obsolete. "Eventually, people need whole blood," says Peter Page, M.D., senior medical officer with the American Red Cross in Washington, D.C.

ARTIFICIAL DISKS GIVE BACK-PATIENTS REAL RELIEF

On December 29, 2000, a stranger changed 35-year-old Edna Torres-Ortiz's life. He ran a red light and rammed his car into hers, which flipped onto another vehicle and then bounced upright. The accident damaged a disk in Torres-Ortiz's spine; for the next 19 months, pain became her constant companion. Her life became a round of doctor visits, X-rays, physical therapy, and pain pills. Bike rides near her Peekskill, New York, home with her children, now 5 and 11, were history. Her inline skates gathered dust. On trips to the market, her son would climb into the grocery cart himself, a selfless gesture that reduced Torres-Ortiz to tears. Sex became torturous for her.

This is not what I want for my life, she told herself. But therapy wasn't working, and surgery was far from a sure thing. Searching for alternatives, Torres-Ortiz stumbled onto a revolutionary new device: an implant that replaces the damaged disk and significantly eases pain while preserving range of motion.

Prodisc, made of a plastic ball-bearing core with cobalt-chrome endplates, snaps into place in the spine once the damaged disk is removed. It mimics the movement of natural disks, much as artificial hips and knees mimic those joints.

Designed in the late 1980s by a French orthopedic surgeon, Prodisc is only now being tested in 13 centers in the United States. But in early studies, 93 percent of patients were satisfied or extremely satisfied at their seven-year follow-ups. Back-pain experts have high hopes that the device will help the 200,000 people each year who undergo surgery for disk damage.

Until now, spinal fusion was the standard option, and not a particularly good one: It lessens mobility, stresses other parts of the spine, and relieves pain in only about 80 to 85 percent of cases. But with Prodisc, "we can eradicate the pain from degenerating disks without sacrificing motion," explains Frank P. Cammisa, M.D., chief of spine surgery at the Hospital for Special Surgery in New York City and principal investigator for the multicenter Prodisc study.

Torres-Ortiz, who signed on to take part in the study, says her pain vanished seven weeks after the artificial disk was implanted. She feels pressure in her spine, a sensation Cammisa says should be gone within a year.

The latest implant, Prodisc, can end pain from degenerating disks without sacrificing motion.

The Prodisc study won't be completed until 2005, after which time the device still will have to be vetted by the FDA. If approved, it's expected to have wide applications: Anyone between the ages of 18 and 60 with a painful degenerating disk and no evidence of bone disease, cancer, infections, or spinal deformities could be a candidate for implantation (most potential patients are in their 30s and 40s). Downside: While spinal fusions are permanent, researchers estimate that the artificial disk may have to be replaced after about 25 years. "It may last longer than artificial hip and knee replacements because there's no fluid that could wear away at the plastic," Cammisa says.

If the car accident robbed Torres-Ortiz of her wonderful, active life, the new disk has restored it. She's already thinking about hitting the ski slopes with her children this winter—assuming Cammisa and her physical therapist give their OKs—and she's looking forward to more intimate moments with her husband. She's also searching the closets for her inline skates. These days, she takes nothing for granted, least of all her newly healthy back. "I'm grateful," she says. "I'm thrilled."

HEPATITIS C: CLOSER TO A CURE

Three years ago, Ellen McKee and her husband, Frank, of Huntingdon Valley, Pennsylvania, underwent routine blood tests while applying for lower rates on their life-insurance policy. He sailed through, but her application was denied. An adjuster broke the news: McKee, then 36, had hepatitis C.

A nasty, tenacious virus that untreated can cause liver failure, cancer, and cirrhosis, hepatitis C wasn't discovered until 1989, 10 years after a blood transfusion during surgery had passed the virus into McKee's bloodstream. But the timing of her diagnosis was lucky. New treatments now on the market and in clinical trials offer significantly higher success rates than previous drug regimens.

The new therapies combine the drug ribavirin, previously used with interferon to treat hepatitis C, with pegylated interferon, which binds the chemical polyethylene glycol (PEG) to the standard interferon molecule. "PEG adds a new physical property to the interferon that allows it to stay in the body's circulation for a week," explains Donald M. Jensen, M.D., director of the liver unit at Chicago's Rush-Presbyterian-St. Luke's Medical Center. "So its ability to fight the virus is more sustained than that of standard interferon, which circulates in the body for less than 24 hours."

In one study, 54 percent of patients who took a PEG interferon drug plus ribavirin cleared their bodies of the virus; a study of a newer PEG interferon formulation shows a 61-percent success rate. That's much higher than the average 38-percent success rate for ribavirin plus standard interferon, which was the best remedy until now.

The treatment also halts the liver inflammation caused by hepatitis C and reverses some of the damage. Even sufferers who already have mild cases of cirrhosis see some improvement. Health experts consider this a major advance, since about half of all liver-related deaths are due to hepatitis C infections, and liver failure is now the 10th leading cause of adult death in America.

The PEG interferon regimen is also easier on patients, requiring injections only once a week versus three times a week with standard interferon (the ribavirin is taken orally). But the 48-week treatment is no walk in the park. McKee had her first shot in February 2002. "By week two, I was weak and nauseated," she says. "I couldn't lift my head."

Soon she was unable to run, lift weights, or keep up with her 12-year-old daughter. Her red blood count plummeted, her hair thinned, and she was constantly thirsty—typical side effects of the medication. But after three months, she was virus-free. Her course of treatment ends this month. If she remains in the clear for six months after therapy, she's considered a "sustained viral responder," the closest doctors can come to pronouncing any hepatitis C patient cured.

For McKee, now 39, the experience has been worth it. She knew that without treatment, the virus could catch up with her, even kill her. "I thought, 'I have a kid. I have to be around for her,'" she says.

PILLS PROVIDE REAL HOPE FOR PEOPLE WITH IBS

It's easy to underestimate the pain and embarrassment experienced by people with irritable bowel syndrome (IBS), unless you're one of them. An estimated 20 percent of the population—56 million people—lives with the disease, which is characterized by persistent, painful abdominal cramps and bloating; two-thirds of cases occur in women. About one-third of IBS sufferers have chronic constipation, another third have diarrhea, and the rest alternate between the two.

"Most of us have no idea how miserable this condition makes people feel. And it has a huge economic cost—an estimated $30 billion a year in lost workdays and doctor visits," says gastroenterologist Walter Peterson, M.D., a professor of internal medicine at the University of Texas Southwestern Medical Center in Dallas.

Two new developments may give IBS sufferers better lives: In July 2002, the FDA approved Zelnorm, the first new drug that relieves the symptoms

The new drug, Zelnorm, promises to relieve symptoms of constipation-type IBS. Meanwhile, Lotronex returns to the market to help ease diarrhea.

of constipation-type IBS. It regulates peristalsis, the wavelike muscle contractions that move waste through the colon. It's the first of a new class of medications called 5HT4 agonists, which target specific receptors in the gastrointestinal tract involved in peristalsis. The drug doesn't cure constipation-type IBS; however, in three scientifically rigorous 12-week studies, it relieved symptoms in about 60 percent of cases—significantly better than placebo treatment and with few side effects. "Zelnorm doesn't work for everyone," Peterson says, "but when it does, it can relieve all IBS symptoms."

In June 2002, in the first reversal in the agency's history, the FDA lifted a ban on the IBS medication Lotronex, which was pulled off the market in 2000. Reports had linked it to more than 200 cases of side effects, including dangerous circulatory problems and serious constipation that resulted in hospitalizations, surgeries, and several deaths. After the ban, thousands of Lotronex users implored the FDA to reconsider, saying the drug was the only treatment that helped them. In April 2002, an FDA advisory panel voted 16 to 2 to bring back Lotronex, but at half the initially approved dose and only for the approximately 5 percent of diarrhea-type IBS sufferers with debilitating symptoms. Experts suspect that slashing the dose and limiting use will lower risks and the incidence of side effects.

NEW PROCESS PINPOINTS BEST DRUG, DOSAGE

Figuring out what kind of drug you need—and exactly how much—has been largely a matter of trial and error. But a new test is helping physicians zero in on the best medication and dosing based on your genetic makeup.

Haplotyping, or HAP technology, was developed by scientists at Genaissance Pharmaceuticals, a New Haven, Connecticut, biotechnology company. It allows doctors to screen patients' blood or saliva for subtle genetic variations that affect reactions to common asthma medications and chemotherapy drugs used primarily to treat children with leukemia. Already, the technology is helping protect patients from dangerous, even fatal, drug overdoses.

For instance, the test is being used to identify the single gene that controls absorption of the leukemia drug Purinethol. Most of us produce a protein that deactivates about 90 percent of the substance, making a higher dosage necessary for it to be effective. But a genetic variation in some people creates the potential for a life-threatening situation by rendering this protein inactive, causing 100 percent of the medicine to flood their systems.

With haplotyping—named for the complicated genetic sequences, or haplotypes, that control drug reactions and other physical processes—"kids who can't break down Purinethol are given 10 percent of the standard dose. That prevents them from being exposed to a toxic overdose," says Richard Judson, Ph.D., senior vice president for medical affairs at Genaissance.

"In the not-too-distant future," Judson says, "we envision physicians taking a swab of saliva, running it through a machine, and quickly learning which drug and dosage will work best for that person in treating a broad range of conditions."

While the machine may be a long way off, the process is already making a difference. At the University of Cincinnati, Stephen Liggett, M.D., a professor of medicine and molecular genetics, has used HAP technology to predict asthma patients' reactions to albuterol, a drug commonly prescribed to treat this complex disease.

Before haplotyping, people who did not experience relief from a standard dose of albuterol were often prescribed a higher one, but that can cause heart-rate spikes, tremors, even asthma attacks. "Now we can predict who will and won't respond to albuterol," Liggett says. "Those who won't respond can be given other medications immediately."

HAP technology is still experimental and is currently available only in clinical trials. But evidence is mounting that it has a wide range of possible applications. In April 2002, Genaissance scientists demonstrated its ability to predict which of three familiar cholesterol-lowering medications—Lipitor, Pravachol, or Zocor—works best in different individuals based on variations in 27 genes. Personalizing prescriptions according to a patient's genetic profile, Liggett says, is "the future of drug therapy."

3-D BODY SCAN PUTS PROBLEMS IN SHARPER FOCUS

A new three-dimensional scan lets doctors see the inner workings of your body in precise detail, enabling earlier and more accurate disease diagnoses. The new imaging system combines two tests you have probably heard of, or had, before: the high-tech X-rays of computerized tomography (CT) and the scans of positron-emission tomography (PET).

CT scans detect tiny anatomical abnormalities by generating cross-section pictures of the body, like pieces of bread sliced from a loaf. PET measures concentrations of subatomic particles called positrons in living tissue to create images that highlight areas of increased metabolic activity. Individually, each procedure only catches some early tumors, so patients often must have both scans separately.

The combined technologies use a single new machine to produce state-of-the-art PET and CT scans simultaneously, then fuse them into a single 3-D image using a built-in computer. "Combining PET and CT represents an entirely new dimension in imaging," says PET pioneer James Mountz, M.D., Ph.D., professor of radiology and director of the division of nuclear medicine at the University of Alabama at Birmingham Medical Center. "It can detect cancer, heart disease, and brain disorders earlier and better than ever."

PET-CT scans could help doctors determine whether a particular tumor is malignant or benign; they could also greatly reduce the number of unnecessary biopsies.

PET-CT scans especially hold potential for detecting cancers of the breast, lung, colon, and lymph nodes. "With PET alone, you can see the abnormality, but you can't tell where it is located," Mountz explains. "But with PET-CT, you can see the lesion and determine its position with great accuracy. It can also provide more accurate staging and aid planning of radiation or surgery. That's a major advance."

A PET-CT scan usually takes about 30 minutes. Approximately 45 minutes beforehand, a person is injected with a fluid that contains a very low dose of a radioactive compound, which completely washes out of the body a few hours later. Then the patient lies on a special bed that rolls into a cylindrical opening in the machine. PET-CT is painless, but, as with other scans, some people may experience claustrophobia in the enclosed space.

By the end of 2001, there were about 40 PET-CT setups in operation around the country (to find one, ask your doctor to refer you to a nuclear-medicine facility; call and ask if they use the technology). One caveat: "If you get a PET-CT scan," Mountz advises, "be sure it's read by a physician trained in both radiology and nuclear medicine."

BACK-SURGERY BREAKTHROUGH EASES PAIN FAST

A protein that acts like Miracle-Gro for bone promises to speed healing for back-surgery patients and almost guarantees success. Bone morphogenic protein (BMP) is a natural compound that stimulates bone growth. Twenty-four types of BMP have been identified; one of them can now be produced in bulk using genetic engineering.

The FDA approved recombinant BMP number two (rBMP-2) in July 2002 for connecting vertebrae when a disk is removed during spinal-fusion surgery.

Usually, doctors must use bone harvested from cadavers or from the patient's own body to rejoin vertebrae. But cadaver bone often results in nonunion, or failure to fill the gap; using a bone graft from the patient, usually from the pelvis, requires painful surgery and prolonged recovery time.

rBMP-2 offers a quick alternative. "It's pretty amazing stuff," says Daveed Frazier, M.D., assistant professor of orthopedic surgery at Columbia University and president of Orthopedic Associates of New York City. "New bone grows completely within three months, which is a lot faster than even the best bone graft, and there's virtually no nonunion risk." Depending on the patient's health, bone regeneration with the new process takes about half as long as before.

Soon doctors could also be using rBMP-2 to speed along the healing of bone fractures. "Now, when an elderly woman breaks a hip, it's very serious," says Randall Hendricks, M.D., an orthopedic surgeon at Central States Orthopedic Specialists in Tulsa, Oklahoma. "But with BMP, she might be back on her feet in as little as three weeks." It also has potential as a treatment for osteoporosis. "In the not-too-distant future, we might inject it into women's bones and see strong new bone develop," Frazier says.

Orthopedic surgeons are just beginning to perform spinal fusions using rBMP-2. In follow-up studies over five years, the new bone has stayed strong without causing any significant problems. "I'll feel a lot better when we have 20-year data," Frazier says, "but so far, so good."

SCALPEL-FREE PERMANENT CONTRACEPTION SLASHES RECOVERY TIME

You could say Gabriella Avina and her husband, Robert, of Martinez, California, were meant to have kids—lots of them. After the birth of their second daughter in 1998, Avina considered having her tubes tied to keep the family at a manageable number, but she opted for an intrauterine device (IUD) instead. However, the IUD, one of the most reliable contraceptive methods, failed; six months later, Avina was pregnant. Despite bleeding for 17 weeks and preparing herself for the baby's death with each doctor's visit, she delivered a healthy son. To prevent another pregnancy, Avina's husband had a vasectomy. But lab tests revealed that his procedure, too, was a failure.

Avina, a nurse who specializes in reproductive science, thought she and her husband had run out of permanent contraceptive options. Then she heard about Essure, an experimental, high-tech, noninvasive replacement for tubal ligation.

Essure is a small, springlike coil made of polyester fibers and nickel-titanium alloy, the same material used to make artificial heart valves. It is inserted into the vagina (no incision necessary), then threaded through the cervix and into each fallopian tube, where the coil is released. It expands, anchoring itself in place and irritating the tubes' lining. The resulting inflammation causes scar tissue to form, creating a blockage. After three months, dye is shot through the cervix and uterus to the tubes to make sure they are completely obstructed.

Avina felt she had nothing to lose. "What appealed to me was that I wouldn't have to have surgery that would take me away from my family," she says. "My husband is a firefighter, gone 24 hours a day.

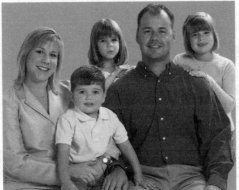

After three kids, the Avinas opted for Essure—an experimental, high-tech, noninvasive replacement for tubal ligation.

I needed something that would let me get right back to my children, something safe and easy." She felt only a tiny cramp during the 45-minute procedure. That evening, she went home, cooked dinner, helped with homework, and gave the children baths. "I felt perfectly fine," she says.

Most women who have used Essure in clinical trials had experiences similar to Avina's. Of 650 women studied in the United States, Europe, and Australia, 92 percent missed only one day of work or less following the procedure, compared to four days after tubal ligation. And 96 percent had blocked tubes after three months. The most common side effect is cramping; some women also complain of vaginal discharge, bloating, and headaches. In a small number of cases, the device is expelled or perforates the fallopian tubes. In the latter instance, the puncture heals without surgery, and the coil can be reinserted.

Essure gained FDA approval in November 2002, so more women like Avina can experience its benefits. When tests confirmed that her tubes were completely blocked, her husband celebrated by tossing out all other forms of birth control. "For so long, all I did was think, 'If I touch him, I might get pregnant again,'" she says. "I didn't have to think that anymore." ▪

New Law Ensures the Validity of Organic Labels

If you want a guarantee that you're soaking in real organic lavender bath oil or applying true organic lip balm, then look to the left coast. As of January 2003, the California Organic Products Act of 2003 is in effect, ensuring that consumers who buy organic makeup and personal-care products get what they're looking for.

New label language will differentiate between products made with at least 95-percent organic ingredients and those made with 70 percent or more. Federal standards for edibles have been in place since fall 2002, but this is the first step toward regulating organic nonfood items. You won't have to head west to reap the benefits, though—it's unlikely that manufacturers will use one label for cosmetics sold in-state and another for the rest of us.

Save Your HEART

with the Latest Blood Test

CRP screening may be the best weapon against heart disease since cholesterol testing.

BY SUSAN FREINKEL

First, the good news: Your cholesterol test came out OK. Now for the bad news: That test is a shockingly imperfect crystal ball. Cardiologists tell countless stories of patients who had no idea they were at risk for a heart attack until they wound up in the emergency room. In fact, every year half of all people who suffer heart attacks have normal cholesterol levels.

The really good news: Another blood test may do a better job of assessing your real risk of heart disease. An improved version of a test that's been around since the mid-1960s, it measures levels of a substance known as C-reactive protein, or CRP. Many experts believe it's the best weapon against heart attack and stroke since cholesterol testing was introduced more than 20 years ago. "It has immense value," says Eric Topol, M.D., chairman of cardiovascular medicine at the Cleveland Clinic. An official stamp of approval for the high-sensitivity CRP (hsCRP) test

> **Women with the highest CRP levels were nearly four times as likely to have a heart attack and three times as likely to suffer a stroke as the women with the lowest levels.**

came in early 2003. In February 2003, the American Heart Association (AHA) and the U.S. Centers for Disease Control and Prevention (CDC) jointly endorsed the test and released guidelines for its use.

CRP screening fits into the new thinking about the cause of heart disease. Doctors used to see it as a plumbing problem: Arteries, like pipes, were clogged by cholesterol deposits. But now doctors think the damage starts when artery walls become inflamed by LDL (bad) cholesterol, as immune cells rush to combat the fatty particles. Those cells knit a sort of scab to contain the cholesterol in the walls. But the immune system is also likely to break up the scab, which can trigger a blood clot that leads to a heart attack.

So inflammation—the body's own defense—could be the real culprit. And because CRP is a marker for inflammation, elevated levels are an alarm bell for heart disease.

Experts have known that CRP, which is produced by the liver, skyrockets when someone is acutely ill. The new hsCRP test measures small changes. "It's like a thermometer for gauging slow, chronic inflammation," says Peter Libby, M.D., chief of cardiovascular medicine at Boston's Brigham and Women's Hospital.

Studies show that tiny increases in CRP levels signify raised risks of heart disease, stroke, and diabetes later in life, according to Harvard University cardiologist Paul Ridker, M.D., who pioneered research in the field.

In a recent study, Ridker and associates reviewed research that had followed nearly 28,000 women for an average of eight years. They found that those with the highest CRP levels were nearly four times as likely to have a heart attack and three times as likely to suffer a stroke as the women with the lowest levels. The women at greatest risk were in danger even if they did not smoke, had no family history of heart disease, and had cholesterol levels that seemed healthy.

That study made a persuasive case for widespread CRP testing, according to Topol. He believes it could easily be added to the standard cholesterol workup. It's relatively inexpensive—as little as $25—and non-invasive. If your CRP is low, your cholesterol is normal, and you have no other risk factors, you've got a clean bill of heart health. If your CRP is high, you can reduce it by improving your diet and exercising.

Still, the test is controversial. The AHA/CDC guidelines pointedly tell most people not to bother with it, warning about a number of unknowns.

False positives are a real possibility. CRP levels not only rise if a person has heart disease but also if someone has, say, bronchitis, cystitis, or an infected tooth. And they can increase slightly in people who are depressed, chronically fatigued, overweight, or on hormone-replacement therapy.

In such cases, the test may generate needless anxiety, says Thomas Pearson, M.D., a cardiologist at the University of Rochester and chairman of the AHA/CDC panel. A misleading read might prompt someone to get more expensive, invasive, and unnecessary tests, such as angiograms (which require inserting a tube into the arteries that feed the heart). "CRP is not a test everyone should have," Pearson contends.

Another concern is the dearth of research. Nearly every study, for instance, has focused on whites; there's little data about normal CRP levels among ethnic groups, such as African-Americans, who have higher rates of heart disease.

The biggest unknown is what to do with the results. Doctors don't know whether high CRP is a separate risk factor for heart disease or just a marker. So they don't know for sure that treating high CRP makes sense. To date, no studies have proved that reducing CRP lowers the odds of a heart attack, for instance, although preventives, such as aspirin and statins, have been shown to lower levels of the protein. Research designed to address such questions is just getting under way. Ridker has begun a study in which 15,000 people with low cholesterol and high CRP levels will be given either a statin drug or a placebo. He'll then compare how the two groups fare over five years.

For now, the AHA/CDC guidelines say that only people who have a 10- to 20-percent chance of a heart attack in the next 10 years should be tested. So if your LDL is a little high (above 130) or your HDL (good cholesterol) is a little low (below 60), your blood pressure is up, you're overweight, or you're showing early signs of diabetes, you're a candidate for the test. In those borderline cases, Pearson says, finding out your CRP level could help a doctor decide whether to treat you, or how aggressively. (You might be put on a statin drug if both your LDL and your CRP are high, for example.) If you're already being treated for heart disease, however, the AHA/CDC panel advises against testing, because the result is unlikely to change a doctor's recommendations.

Still, even if you have seemingly healthy cholesterol, there is one good reason to get the test: Proponents say that learning your CRP level might force you to make smarter choices about your health. "Anything we can do to motivate people to take better care of themselves is important," Topol says.

Susan Freinkel is a freelance writer in San Francisco.

The FAT That Fights FAT

A new kind of oil promises to please your taste buds while helping you lose weight.

BY TIMOTHY GOWER

It sounds way too good to be true: a type of fat that makes you burn fat? That's the claim of a new product called Enova, which is being touted as the first cooking and salad oil that keeps you from packing on pounds. The scientists who developed this chemically altered blend of canola and soybean oils say that it turns into fuel for the body as soon as it's digested—unlike other forms of dietary fat, which are apt to go into long-term storage on your thighs and belly, as often as not. What's more, Enova supposedly accomplishes this feat without any of the gastrointestinal indelicacies caused by such fat substitutes as Olestra.

But does this stuff *really* live up to all the hype?

Enova was developed in Japan, where it went on sale back in 1999 (under a different name) and quickly became one of that country's best-selling cooking oils. It's debuting stateside courtesy of a joint venture between Decatur, Illinois-based Archer Daniels Midland Company (ADM) and the product's creator, Kao Corporation of Japan. ADM Kao is currently test-marketing Enova in

> **Dieters consuming the modified oil lost about 45 percent more weight than those who ate conventional foods.**

Atlanta and Chicago, and plans to make it available nationwide. You can also buy it online.

Tablespoon for tablespoon, Enova contains just as much fat and the same number of calories as the corn or extra-virgin olive oil in your cupboard. Its waist-management potential lies in its ability to perform a bit of metabolic magic. Conventional oils consist almost entirely of triglycerides—molecules that contain three fatty acids attached to a spine of glycerol, forming an E shape. Those oils also contain a tiny percentage of molecules with just two fatty acids, called diglycerides (also known as DAGs), which form a C shape.

Triglycerides in cooking oil must be broken down into smaller pieces by enzymes in order to be digested. Here's where the quirk comes in: The molecules must be reassembled by other enzymes before being pushed into the bloodstream and distributed to cells throughout the body, where they're either burned as fuel or stored as fat.

But the enzymes that facilitate digestion are bewildered by C-shaped DAGs, according to Brent Flickinger, Ph.D., a nutritional-research scientist at ADM. These chemicals can break down DAGs, but they can't put the molecules' weird fatty acids back together. Instead of passing into the blood for distribution, DAGs go to the liver, where they're promptly burned.

Studies suggest that replacing your usual oil with a DAG-based substitute—such as Enova, which consists of about 80-percent DAGs—may help rein in a wayward waistline.

Research published in December 2002 compared two groups of overweight adults who went on moderately low-calorie diets. Scientists at the Chicago Center for Clinical Research asked both groups to incorporate prepackaged muffins, crackers, cookies, soup, and granola bars into their diets—but the foods for one group were prepared with regular cooking oil, while DAG oil was used to make the items fed to the other group. After six months, the first group had lost an average of about 5½ pounds; the group that ate DAG foods had lost nearly 8 pounds overall.

The DAG advantage was clear, says Kevin Maki, Ph.D., an epidemiologist and the study's lead researcher. Dieters consuming the modified oil lost about 45 percent more weight than those who ate conventional foods. A four-month Japanese study of men on controlled (but not low-calorie) diets yielded similar results. The subjects who ate DAG foods lost 5 pounds—twice as much as their counterparts.

Of course, the people in these experiments were substituting DAGs for a large percentage of the fat they normally consumed each day. Simply replacing your usual cooking and salad oil with Enova is unlikely to produce dramatic weight loss. "It might make you lose just a pound or two," Maki says. "But it may also help prevent weight gain." Which is no small feat in a country with rising obesity rates.

In addition, diglycerides appear to cause weight loss where it matters most. In Maki's study, subjects who ate foods made with DAG cooking oil lost a greater percentage of body fat than the control group, much of it from the abdomen. That's good news, because people with spare-tire fat have increased risks of diabetes and heart disease, says Sara Kurlandsky, Ph.D.,

a nutritional biochemist at Syracuse University. Other studies suggest eating DAG foods may cut heart-attack risk by lowering elevated triglyceride levels.

The downside? There doesn't seem to be one so far. But no one knows yet if consuming Enova long-term will produce side effects. The longest human study to date lasted only a year. "Until we have more data, there's always a question," Kurlandsky says. She cautions against feeding Enova to children under age 2, since growing brain cells require extra dietary fat. Otherwise, the existing evidence suggests Enova is safe. "I'd try it," Kurlandsky says.

If she does, she should brace herself for sticker shock: A 20-ounce bottle costs about $5; a 32-ounce bottle of regular canola oil sells for about half that price. On the other hand, while Enova may be rough on the wallet, it's gentle on the palate. In a small and highly unscientific test, the author made raspberry vinaigrette for a salad and fried a few chicken breasts with Enova, then did the same with canola oil. In a blind tasting, his wife was unable to detect any difference in flavor. You probably won't notice any difference, either—except, perhaps, when you step on the bathroom scale. ▪

Timothy Gower is a contributing editor.

How Fat Can Heal You

Talk about good fats: New research suggests that the stem cells in fat removed during liposuction can be banked, according to the American Society for Aesthetic Plastic Surgery. Less controversial than stem cells from embryos, the material may one day be used to regenerate nerves, bone, or muscle, says Peter B. Fodor, M.D., associate clinical professor of plastic surgery at the University of California, Los Angeles. A separate component of bankable fat, its collagen matrix, could be used to enhance lips and cheeks. But don't run out and rent a vault to store your cellulite yet. Large clinical studies are only just beginning (besides, processing and storing harvested fat costs up to $2,000).

PAIN RELIEF
from your fridge

Move over aspirin. Anti-inflammatory foods
are helping not only arthritis patients,
but also those with heart disease, cancer,
Alzheimer's disease, and Type 2 diabetes.

BY ANNE UNDERWOOD

Miriam Nelson, Ph.D., is a runner and hiker, the director of the Center for Physical Activity and Nutrition at Tufts University in Boston, and the author of several best-selling books on the virtues of strength training. But in her latest book, *Strong Women and Men Beat Arthritis*, she touts not only exercise but diet, too. Thanks to the anti-inflammatory effects of certain foods, she's seen arthritis sufferers improve—not enough to eliminate their pain entirely, but enough to reduce their reliance on medication and improve their ability to function. Hoping to prevent arthritis herself, Nelson is busy applying her rules to her own diet. "Unless there's a lot of evidence, I'm slow to change," she says. But there *is* and she *has*, adding flaxseed to her breakfast cereal and eating more cold-water fish, such as tuna and salmon.

Move over, antioxidants. Make room in the pantry for anti-inflammatories, the new kids on the nutritional block. It's not just people with arthritis pain who need them. Researchers now believe that inflammation contributes to heart disease, cancer, Alzheimer's, and Type 2 diabetes—and that anti-inflammatory compounds in your food can counteract it. You don't have to go out of your way to find these substances: Foods rich in anti-inflammatories are in not only your fish market but also your produce bin and even the curries at your favorite Indian restaurant.

Inflammation isn't always bad. When you cut yourself, for example, the body sends in white blood cells to fight infection; it also brings in oxygenated blood to repair the damage, plus other fluids to cushion the injured cells. (That's why a cut looks red and swollen.) But a more insidious form of low-grade inflammation can result from less obvious damage, such as oxidation within blood-vessel walls. Antioxidants can help prevent this type of damage in the first place. But when that fails, you need anti-inflammatories. Otherwise, the body's attempts to repair the harm can lead to chronic inflammation. You don't notice it as it's happening, but over the years, this persistent inflammation slowly attacks healthy tissue in the joints, arteries, and brain.

Among some of the most effective kinds of anti-inflammatory agents are omega-3 fatty acids, found in abundance in fish. This isn't exactly recent news—in 1775, doctors in London began advertising cod-liver oil, a rich source of omega-3s, as a miracle cure for arthritis. In the body, omega-3s are converted into hormonelike substances that reduce inflammation.

Omega-6 polyunsaturates, found in corn and other oils, act in the opposite way, ratcheting up inflammation. Omega-6s and omega-3s form a dietary yin and yang that must be kept in balance. When you consume roughly equal measures of each, inflammation is held in check. But doctors estimate that most people eat as much as 20 times more omega-6s than omega-3s because their diets are heavy on processed foods, many of which abound in omega-6–rich oils, such as corn and sunflower. Conversely, people tend to skimp on omega-3s, also found in flax-seed, canola oil, walnuts, and such dark greens as spinach and kale.

Medications such as aspirin and ibuprofen work by interfering with enzymes that contribute to the inflammatory properties of

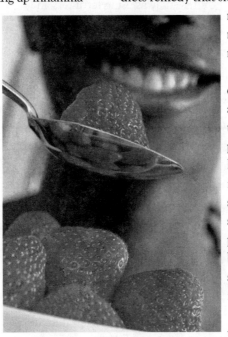

Berries are just one food that may ease pain as well as aspirin does.

omega-6s. But some foods can provide comparable effects. Muraleedharan Nair, Ph.D., professor of natural-products chemistry at Michigan State University, has shown in lab experiments that tart-cherry extract can stop the formation of some inflammatory agents 10 times better than aspirin. His findings have helped fuel a cult of cherry-juice devotees among hundreds of arthritis patients who swear by the stuff: 2 tablespoons of concentrated juice daily. In recent research, Nair found that sweet cherries, blackberries, strawberries, and raspberries produce similar effects.

Another way to reduce inflammatory damage is to boost the body's repair crews. Blueberries appear to be efficient handymen. Rachel Galli, Ph.D., assistant professor of psychology at Simmons College in Boston, has been measuring compounds called heat-shock proteins in the brain. "Think of them as the body's duct tape," she says. "They help cells repair the damage from oxidative stress, inflammation, and toxins." As you age, you produce fewer of these protective proteins. Galli has seen blueberry-fortified diets remedy that situation in the brains of aging rats, who responded to inflammatory challenges as ably as much younger animals.

Fruits and vegetables in general, especially the most colorful ones, appear to fight inflammation, thanks to hundreds of beneficial phytochemicals, such as bromelain in pineapples and quercetin in apples and onions. Even the so-called nightshade vegetables, such as tomatoes and bell peppers—long vilified for exacerbating pain in some arthritis sufferers—contain about 20 anti-inflammatory compounds apiece.

Put it all together, and what do you get? It's the same type of diet nutritionists have been pushing for years: fruits, vegetables, fish, and whole grains. In contrast, diets high in sugar, refined flour, and trans fats (partially hydrogenated vegetable oils) increase inflammation, as does obesity. "You can make your diet work for you or against you," says Ronenn Roubenoff, M.D., a rheumatologist at Tufts New England Medical Center. So why not make it work for you? Eating to fight inflammation could be one of the best things you ever do for yourself. ▪

Anne Underwood writes about health and medical topics for Newsweek *and is co-author of* The Color Code: A Revolutionary Eating Plan for Optimum Health.

Buying Organic Pays Off
More antioxidants help fight disease.

If you find yourself in the produce aisle debating over whether to shell out the extra cash for organic strawberries, a new study might help you make up your mind. Organically grown fruits and vegetables contain higher levels of cancer-fighting antioxidants than conventionally produced foods, according to a recent report in the *Journal of Agricultural and Food Chemistry*.

This study was one of the first to measure the effect of pesticides on levels of certain phytochemicals (aka plant chemicals), and even the researchers were surprised at the results. Organic produce boasted up to 50 percent more antioxidants. "When a plant is attacked by insects, it naturally produces phytochemicals like flavonoids to protect itself," says Alyson Mitchell, Ph.D., a food scientist at the University of California, Davis, and the study's lead author. "If you apply pesticides, you take away the pest pressure, so the plant doesn't need to make these compounds."

Mitchell compared the amount of antioxidants in plants grown conventionally to those in foods grown sustainably (defined in this study as using fertilizers and in some cases herbicides, but no pesticides) or organically (without herbicides, pesticides, or fertilizers). Sustainably grown produce yielded the highest levels of disease-fighting compounds—even higher than the organics. Mitchell suspects that the lack of pesticides, plus the abundance of nutrients from fertilizers, increased antioxidant production.

Mitchell studied corn, strawberries, and a type of blackberry called marionberries, because those plants were in season. Next, she plans to research tomatoes, peppers, and broccoli, among other vegetables.

Three Must-Have Supplements

If it seems like everyone's popping pills these days, you're not far off the mark: 40 percent of Americans take dietary supplements. To help you find the ones that are best for you, we asked two physicians, a traditional one and an alternative practitioner, what they take each day. On both doctors' shopping lists were a multivitamin, calcium, and omega-3 fatty acids. Barrie Cassileth, Ph.D., chief of integrative medicine at Memorial Sloan-Kettering Cancer Center in New York City, says these are the top three supplements for most women. "For a very few, calcium may conflict with some medications," she says, "so talk to your doctor if you have questions. And stick to the recommended dietary allowances for vitamins—in this case, more isn't better.

Drinkable Yogurt Packs More Healthy Bacteria

Relieving such unpleasant conditions as diarrhea and urinary-tract infections might be as simple as choosing the right beverage.

Beneficial bacteria, also known as probiotics, including *Lactobacillus casei* and *Lactobacillus acidophilus,* have long been available in the United States in supplements and in yogurts with the words "live and active cultures" on their labels. But drinkable yogurtlike products containing these good germs have just made their way to mainstream supermarkets. Dannon recently launched a potable called Actimel, a move that could heighten Americans' probiotic awareness.

Sipping your daily helping of microorganisms has definite health benefits. According to Barry Goldin, Ph.D., director of the biochemistry and microbiology lab at Tufts University, Actimel and the like have significantly higher culture contents (up to 10 billion per 8-ounce serving) than regular yogurt (about 10 million per serving). Probiotic drinks, available at natural-food stores and some large supermarket chains, also provide nutritional advantages, such as calcium, protein, and a smattering of vitamins, that capsules and pills don't have.

How to Be Supplement Savvy

Follow these five tips to make sure you get what you pay for.

BY EVA MARER

Fish-oil capsules don't guarantee a healthy heart, and ginkgo biloba may or may not boost your memory, but thanks to new regulations proposed by the U.S. Food and Drug Administration (FDA), supplement manufacturers will have to prove that their products actually contain what the labels claim they do. The catch is that companies still won't have to provide the rigorous proof of safety and effectiveness required before a new drug can get FDA approval.

A 1994 federal law already requires dietary-supplement makers to maintain "good manufacturing practices," but the statute has not been rigorously enforced—and it has several loopholes. One company recalled a niacin supplement that had been tied to heart attacks, vomiting, and liver damage (the product contained almost 10 times the safe amount of this B vitamin). And the FDA reports that in an independent lab test, one-third of foods and supplements containing probiotics were found to contain less than 1 percent of the healthful live bacteria their labels promised. Contaminants, such as harmful bacteria, glass, lead, and even pesticides, have been found in supplements as well. "The new rules will put some teeth in existing regulations and help weed out those fly-by-night operations that have not invested in protecting consumers," says Paul Bolar, vice president of regulatory and legal affairs for supplement maker Pharmavite and chairman of the Council for Responsible Nutrition (CRN), an industry group that promotes stringent manufacturing standards.

The proposed rules might not take effect for a year or more, and they still won't tell you whether a given supplement actually works or is safe. The following tips from the CRN, though, will help you make smarter, safer choices.

1. Look for third-party seals on bottles, indicating that a product has been screened for contaminants and checked for accurate labeling by an independent lab. Icons worthy of your trust include the USP symbol from the United States Pharmacopeia, a nongovernment organization devoted to pharmaceutical safety; the CL seal from the private firm ConsumerLab.com; and the Good Manufacturing Practices (GMP) certification from the National Nutritional Foods Association.

2. Buy at large, well-known health-food shops, vitamin stores, and drugstore chains, which tend to purchase from reputable suppliers. Don't believe the claims of infomercials or unknown online providers, or the too-good-to-be-true scenarios touted by pro-supplement personal trainers.

3. Check the label for a phone number and Web site. No clear contact info? The company's conscience probably isn't clear, either.

4. Educate yourself about the supplements you take. The Web sites of the National Institutes of Health (dietary-supplements.info.nih.gov), the American Botanical Council (www.herbalgram.org), and the Herb Research Foundation (www.herbs.org) all offer primers, safety alerts, and recent supplement research.

5. Talk to your doctor before using supplements, especially if you already take prescription drugs. ■

Is MERCURY Rising in Your Fish?

For years, doctors have touted the health benefits of eating fish. There's just one problem: Fish may be poisonous.

BY BEN RAINES • PHOTOGRAPHY BY SANG AN

Will Smith's life was falling apart. He had worked for years as a geophysicist, analyzing data for companies that hunted oil under the ocean. But lately, he'd begun to have trouble functioning at the most basic levels. He would leave the house for a meeting only to forget where he was going before he reached his car. Though he had lived in San Francisco for decades, he kept getting lost. And after a career spent in highly technical scientific research, the 52-year-old found himself stymied by simple subtraction and unable to string words into coherent sentences.

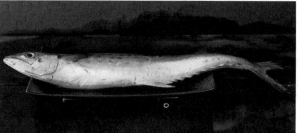

He went to his doctor, but none of the usual diagnostic tools—heart tests, CAT scans, blood work—revealed anything out of the ordinary. He was fit and trim, and yet his doctor told him he might have to trade his current career for a job that would be less mentally demanding.

In hopes of finding clues to his illness, Smith began to write in a journal. In it, he described tremors in his hands and tongue, slurred speech, an ever-present metallic taste in his mouth, numbness in his fingers, crushing fatigue, and even depression. He couldn't concentrate. He couldn't watch television without getting dizzy. He felt high all the time.

"My doctors thought I had encephalitis. Then they thought I had Lou Gehrig's disease," Smith says. "There were four or five months where they were testing, testing, testing, and coming up with wild diseases. I went quite a long time thinking I was going to die."

Then one day his physician, San Francisco internist Jane Hightower, M.D., called. Abruptly, she asked him how much fish he ate.

"It was the weirdest thing," Smith says, "because I ate a lot of fish. Loved it."

Smith told her he ate a can of tuna as a snack three or so days a week. He also enjoyed sushi, especially the ruby-red slices of yellowfin tuna known as ahi. He ate other kinds of fish once or twice a week, sometimes for lunch, sometimes for dinner. He had been eating that way for a long time.

"I think you have mercury poisoning," Hightower said. "Quit eating fish."

For years, doctors have been telling people to eat more fish. Jane Hightower was one of those doctors, and her well-educated, health-conscious patients were apt to follow her advice. But her message isn't so simple anymore. Hightower's research suggests that even moderate consumption of certain kinds of fish—such as eating seared tuna a couple of times a week—can raise mercury levels high enough to cause serious neurological problems. She calls the resulting poor memory and impaired concentration "fish fog."

Hightower's interest in mercury started undramatically in 1999, when a patient came in complaining of hair loss. Hightower sent her to a colleague, dermatologist Kathy Fields, M.D.

During the woman's office visit, Fields remembered a story she'd heard earlier on National Public Radio about research linking hair loss and exposure to heavy metals, such as lead. So she ordered a blood test. The results showed extremely high levels of a heavy metal, but it wasn't lead.

"Her mercury levels were through the roof," Fields says. The patient's daughter was also losing hair, it seemed; her blood-test results showed the same thing.

Fields and Hightower, friends as well as colleagues, routinely talked shop, especially when confronted with a puzzling case. Neither doctor could figure out where the mercury was coming from. The family hired an environmental-testing firm to analyze their water, their home, the dirt surrounding it, even the air. But there was no mercury to be found.

"And then I asked them about their diet, because I knew that some fish were supposed to have mercury in them," Hightower remembers. "They were eating tons of fish. Swordfish, tuna, everything."

Hightower told them to cut it out, all of it. Within a few months, the family's mercury levels returned to normal. Their hair started to grow back, too.

After that, Hightower began running mercury tests on lots of her patients, especially those with persistent symptoms that she couldn't explain or

cure. Test after test came back showing levels higher—many times higher, in some cases—than those deemed safe by the U.S. Environmental Protection Agency (EPA).

A psychiatrist who regularly ate tuna and Chilean sea bass was hospitalized for an irregular heartbeat. His mercury level was twice the EPA's safe limit.

Some patients who ate fish just twice a week had severe memory and concentration problems: "fish fog." ——Jane Hightower, M.D.

A plastic surgeon who ate fresh tuna steaks twice a week was suffering from hair loss, tremors, memory problems, and confusion so intense that she was preparing to give up her medical practice. Her mercury level was six times the EPA's safe limit.

A child who began to eat fresh tuna and king mackerel at age 3 had become profoundly withdrawn by the time he was tested at 5. His mercury level was 15 times the EPA's safe limit.

Many of Hightower's patients ate seafood just twice a week, their choices being some of the most popular fish in America. Apparently, though, that perfectly normal diet caused a host of ills: impaired memory, depression, disorientation, irritability, headaches, shakiness, numbness and tingling in the hands and feet, thinning hair, joint pain, and speech difficulties.

Every time a test came back showing high mercury levels, Hightower told the patient to stop eating fish. And in every one of the cases, she says, those levels came down, and most of the symptoms disappeared. "In medicine, you don't get much better evidence than that," she says.

As the pile of test results grew, Hightower and Fields started spreading the word to local medical groups. Their efforts, while generally well-received, didn't cause a ripple in the wider scientific community. After all, few thought the problems they described could stem from eating fish—not the EPA, which regulates fish caught for sport, and not the U.S. Food and Drug Administration (FDA), which governs seafood sold commercially. According to conventional wisdom, the metal poses a threat only to a fetus, a young child whose brain is still developing, or a woman who plans to conceive. Fish consumption simply isn't cause for concern in most adults.

Hightower is primarily trained in clinical practice. She is quick to admit that her findings need to be followed up with rigorously controlled studies and reviewed by experts. Still, she believes that high mercury levels and illnesses related to them are much more common than they seem and that more people will be diagnosed as doctors become aware of the symptoms. With reports pouring in from all over the nation, an increasing number of scientists and federal health officials are beginning to agree with her.

Scientists have known for centuries that mercury is dangerous. The phrase "mad as a hatter" stems from a psychosis that plagued 18th- and 19th-century hatmakers exposed to the metal in their work. Hundreds of years later, two famous environmental tragedies, one in Japan and the other in Iraq, formed the basis of modern mercury science.

In the 1950s, the small fishing village of Minamata, Japan, was devastated when mercury discharged by a chemical company built up in Minamata Bay. People in the town gradually began to have trouble with rudimentary tasks: walking, buttoning their clothes, even swallowing. Sixty-eight died; mothers exposed during pregnancy gave birth to children who were blind, deformed, or mentally disabled. In 1971, another disaster unfolded when Iraqi villagers made bread out of American grain meant for planting, unaware that the seeds had been treated with a mercury-based fungicide. These episodes made clear that mercury poisoning can be catastrophic. But scientists also took away another lesson: that adults risk neurological damage only when contamination is extreme. On the other hand, studies showed that children exposed in the womb or during their first few years of life are likely to have learning disabilities. So when regulators set limits for mercury in fish, they focused on protecting the young.

The FDA's only warning regarding mercury in fish is directed toward children and women of reproductive age. These people, the organization says, should avoid eating shark, swordfish, tilefish, and king mackerel. Otherwise, the FDA has been relatively unconcerned about the effects of mercury in adults. For years, the agency maintained that men and women could safely harbor levels of about 4 parts per million (ppm), measured in hair. That's four times as high as the EPA's recommended level. Just a couple of months ago, however, the FDA made a sudden about-face. Now, along with the EPA, it uses 1 ppm as the upper safety limit.

If new research is right, even that level might be much closer to the danger zone than previously thought. Many of Hightower's adult patients exhibited symptoms with levels as low as 2 ppm, for instance. And several recent studies appear to support her contention that such levels can cause problems.

Among the most alarming discoveries comes from Finland.

> The FDA publishes what it believes to be average mercury levels for fish, but EPA scientists say the data is fundamentally flawed and essentially useless.

Should You Get a Mercury Test?

If you eat large ocean fish on a regular basis, you might want to consider a mercury test, say experts like Kate Mahaffey, Ph.D., a co-author of the *Environmental Protection Agency's Mercury Study Report to Congress*.

What kind should your doctor order? A hair test is best when long-term exposure is the concern. While the amount of the metal in your blood fluctuates dramatically with meals, hair provides a sort of ticker tape record of a person's average level, possibly going back several months, depending on the length of the hair.

How much mercury is OK? The EPA sets the safe level for mercury, as measured in hair, at 1 part per million. Some studies suggest that a mere doubling of that level increases the risk of heart disease.

What if you test high? Don't panic. Because mercury is excreted in hair, skin, nails, and feces, your levels will begin to decline as soon as you stop exposing yourself to the stuff.

The Good, the Bad, and the Briny

Memory loss, depression, nerve damage: The consequences of mercury poisoning are enough to make you lose your appetite. But you don't have to give up the pleasures of fish or its heart-healthy omega-3s. To be safe:

Think small. Big, boneless fillets may be easy to cook, but they come from large fish that have absorbed mercury from the smaller fish they've eaten. Species that run small, such as flounder and sole, are better choices for frequent consumption than predators, such as tuna and swordfish.

Develop a taste for shellfish. It's generally low in mercury. But beware of scallops: While the genuine article is safe, unscrupulous fishermen create a dangerous ersatz version using a sort of cookie cutter on mercury-rich shark meat. Real scallops have a small "stalk" at one end.

Support your local farms. Tests have shown that farm-raised fish are lower in mercury than their wild cousins. But farm fishing is an imperfect solution, as waste from penned fish can damage the surrounding environment.

Be adventurous. Mercury is not the only danger that lurks in the deep. PCBs (polychlorinated biphenyls), for instance, can also accumulate in fish. To avoid exposure to high levels of any toxin, eat a variety of fish rather than making a habitual meal of any single kind.

Eat All You Want

Pick frequently from this group, especially if you follow the American Heart Association's recommendation to eat fish at least two times a week.

	MERCURY LEVELS	OMEGA-3 LEVELS
CATFISH	low	low
CLAMS	low	low
ORANGE ROUGHY	low	low
OYSTERS (PACIFIC)	low	high
OYSTERS (ELSEWHERE)	low	medium
SALMON	low	high
SARDINES	low	high
SHRIMP	low	low
TILAPIA	low	low

For Occasional Meals

Once a week is safe for men and for women finished with childbearing. Women in their reproductive years and children should limit mahimahi and red snapper (which have the highest mercury levels in this group) to once a month.

	MERCURY LEVELS	OMEGA-3 LEVELS
FLOUNDER	medium	medium
MAHIMAHI	medium	low
RED SNAPPER	medium	low
TROUT	medium	high

Avoid These Fish

A single meal can put you over the Environmental Protection Agency's safe limit for the month.

	MERCURY LEVELS	OMEGA-3 LEVELS
AMBERJACK	high	low
CHILEAN SEA BASS	high	medium
GROUPER	high	low
HALIBUT	high	low
SHARK	high	medium
SWORDFISH	high	medium
TUNA (FRESH)	high	high

Research undertaken there suggests that low levels of mercury can increase heart-disease risk. One study, for example, tracked 1,833 Finnish men for seven years. All the men were healthy to begin with, but those who had mercury levels of 2 ppm or higher were more likely to have suffered heart attacks by the study's end than men who had levels of around 1 ppm.

A married couple in Wisconsin had mercury levels 10 to 12 times as high as the EPA's safe limit. They ate Chilean sea bass once a week.

"They found an increased risk of death from coronary heart disease—and it wasn't small," says Kate Mahaffey, Ph.D., author of the *Mercury Study Report to Congress* and director of the EPA division that sets the agency's mercury policy. "Increased amounts of mercury almost doubled the risk."

But the metal's effect on heart health is still very much an open question, Mahaffey says. In 2002, two other major studies were published: one showing an increase in heart-disease risk in men with elevated mercury levels, and another showing no increase. "We just don't know as much as we should about the health effects of mercury in adults," Mahaffey says.

If mercury does turn out to be more dangerous at lower levels than previously believed, that's just half the bad news. Americans also seem to be getting more mercury from fish than regulators have figured.

That's partly because people are eating more fish than they used to. Between about 1980 and 1991, the amount of seafood caught for market each year nearly doubled, from 6.5 billion to 10 billion pounds a year, according to the National Marine Fisheries Service.

The types of fish favored by consumers have changed, too. The most popular choices used to be small inshore fish, such as flounder and mullet. But these days, people like the big ones: huge predators, such as swordfish and tuna; and hulking, sedentary giants, such as Chilean sea bass, halibut, and grouper. A growing body of evidence shows that these are the very fish most laden with mercury, because of the way the metal moves through the environment.

Most mercury is bound up underground or inside plants. But when it's released into the atmosphere through the burning of fossil fuels, it falls back to Earth and ends up in waterways and oceans. Bacteria make a meal of the metal; then these organisms are eaten by such creatures as snails, which are eaten by small fish, which are eaten by larger fish—each absorbing the mercury from the animals it follows in the chain.

In a little-publicized bulletin from 2001, known internally as the "Do Not Consume" list, the FDA said that children and women of child-bearing age should avoid swordfish, shark, king mackerel, and tilefish (sometimes sold as snapper), because mercury levels in those fish are too high—more than 1 ppm. That's the "action level": According to federal regulations, fish with levels above 1 ppm can't be sold. (Government data shows that many samples of these species contain levels as high as 6 ppm.)

In practice, however, the action level isn't enforced. The FDA simply doesn't know how much mercury is in the high-dollar fish popular in restaurants and seafood markets, agency officials acknowledge. The FDA publishes what it believes to be average mercury levels for many of these fish, but the EPA says the data is fundamentally flawed and essentially useless.

That's because no one recorded the size of the fish when most of the testing was performed. Size is critical, because smaller, younger specimens tend to contain much less mercury than bigger, older ones.

Recent tests conducted by the National Marine Fisheries Service, the state of Florida, and the *Mobile Register*, an Alabama newspaper that has reported extensively on mercury contamination, indicate that such species as Chilean sea bass, fresh tuna, grouper, bluefish, amberjack, cobia, and redfish are often every bit as high in mercury as the swordfish and shark on the FDA's "Do Not Consume" list.

These contamination levels may help explain recent reports of Americans who eat fish once or twice a week but have mercury levels comparable to those of Alaska's Inuit people, who subsist almost entirely on fish.

High levels are being reported all around the country, mostly in upper-middle-class people who eat moderate amounts of fish. In Wisconsin, the state health department was stunned to discover two married lawyers with mercury levels 10 and 12 times as high as the EPA's safe level; they ate Chilean sea bass once a week. In Louisiana, a museum director who ate fresh tuna weekly had levels four times the upper limit.

"People with these high mercury levels are certainly not particularly hard to find," says Mahaffey, who in 2002 won the EPA's highest scientific honor for her research. "We find them every time we start looking. I think it indicates they are much more common nationwide than we thought."

In February 2002, signs started going up at seafood counters all across the state of California, with "warning" in prominent letters, a drawing of a fish, and the names of the four species on the FDA's hit list. The signs were brought in to satisfy Bill Lockyer, the state attorney general, who had filed suit against major grocery chains. He charged that the stores had been violating California's Proposition 65, which requires retailers to warn customers when they sell products containing chemicals known to cause reproductive harm or cancer. "The signs are a step in the right direction," Hightower says. "But we need to tell people how much mercury is in other kinds of fish."

How Much Canned Tuna Is Too Much to Eat?

It's a hotly contested question. The lunchtime staple is generally believed to be low in mercury, but that assumption is based on fairly limited testing. To make things even more complex, many different tuna species go into the can, each with a different mercury profile.

At a recent U.S. Food and Drug Administration (FDA) meeting, H. Vas Aposhian, Ph.D., a scientist on the agency's Food Advisory Committee, announced that he had personally tested 10 cans of tuna for mercury. One contained 1.24 parts

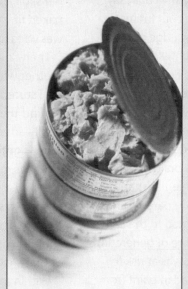

per million, more than 500 percent higher than the FDA's published average for mercury in canned tuna—so high, in fact, that federal rules would prohibit that can from being sold to the public.

The FDA's current standards say that kids and women of childbearing age can safely eat 12 ounces (or two regular cans) of tuna per week. Yet that advice puts a woman over the safety limit set by the Environmental Protection Agency (EPA) says Alan Stern, who served on a National Academy of Sciences panel that studied mercury's health effects. "A woman can safely eat about 8 ounces of canned tuna a week, provided that she eats no other fish high in mercury," he says. Kate Mahaffey, whose EPA division regulates mercury, says a small child should eat no more than one-third of a can per week.

In summer 2002, the FDA assembled an internal panel to examine the canned-tuna issue. That panel was moved to strongly advise that the agency lower its recommended consumption limit for kids and women who might get pregnant to a single can per week. The FDA has yet to act, however.

The Poisoning of Sophie *Mercury and*

BY AYELET WALDMAN

When my daughter Sophie was 4, she was a Jewish mother's dream. Her favorite lunch wasn't Chicken McNuggets, but a tuna sandwich with plenty of celery and pickles. And you should have seen her in a sushi restaurant, gobbling up maki rolls. I, of course, attributed her sophisticated palate to my parenting skills. But all was not as it seemed. Our bright, inquisitive child had lately begun to exhibit some peculiar developmental plateaus. By age 3, she could tie

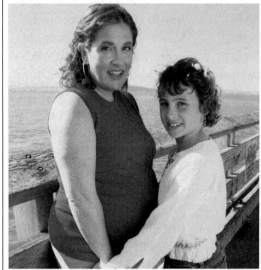

her shoes; at 4, she had inexplicably forgotten how. For a while, she'd been making good, even accelerated, progress in learning to read. More recently, she seemed to slow down or (could it be?) regress.

Don't get me wrong—nothing about her behavior could be described as developmentally delayed. Only we, her parents, were worried, albeit suspicious of that worry. After all, what kind of nut starts fretting not that her child is below average, but that she isn't sufficiently above average? We hesitated to express our fears, even to each other.

I wish I could say it was our intimate knowledge of our daughter that led us to figure out that something was seriously wrong, but only an accidental discovery saved her from permanent brain damage. Sophie, like many kids whose parents are devoted to the architecture of generations past, was at risk for exposure to lead in paint from the walls of our Craftsman bungalow. On our pediatrician's advice, we were all regularly tested for lead. When Sophie was 4, a heavy-metal test revealed something even more

A heavy-metal test revealed that Sophie, at age 4, had high levels of mercury in her body wreaking havoc on her brain.

frightening: Our perfect baby, our darling firstborn, had high levels of mercury—just above the cutoff of what the Federal Drug Administration considered acceptable.

I panicked. I desperately inventoried the contents of our house, snatching up thermometers to ensure they weren't broken. As I watched Sophie sleep that night, I wished I could reach into her skull and tear out with my naked fingers the poison that was wreaking havoc on her brain.

Then I did what any American mother with a computer would do. I surfed the Web, and there I found the person who would finally answer all my questions. Jane Hightower, a physician who has made the dangers of mercury a professional crusade, agreed to see me right away. While we were on the phone, she told me the likely source of Sophie's exposure: canned tuna.

Within a couple of days, I was in Dr. Hightower's office, listening as she assured me that the damage, while serious, was still reversible. In words that seemed designed to strike fear in the hearts of neurotic Yuppie parents

My Daughter

the world over, she said, "Look, if this child ends up going to state college, you'll never know if it was the mercury exposure that kept her out of Harvard."

Out of Harvard? Mentally, and with deep sorrow, I began to unpeel the proud decal from our car's rear window.

Happily, that was a bit premature. We eliminated fish from Sophie's diet, as Dr. Hightower suggested. This resulted in more than a few grocery-store tantrums, Sophie clinging to a can of tuna while I tried enticing her with boxes of cookies. But within a couple of months, her mercury levels dropped. Her reading skills came back on track. One day, she put on her shoes and effortlessly tied two perfect bows.

I had encouraged Sophie to eat fish because I believed it was good for her brain, her heart, and her immune system. But I had poisoned her. For now, my children eat no fish but salmon, and I, pregnant with baby number four, haven't enjoyed a piece of seared ahi in longer than I can remember. As for Sophie? Once a year on her birthday, her father makes her a special dinner: tuna casserole, crumbled potato chips and all.

Right now, no one can give people that information, because nobody knows for sure. But that may be about to change. The National Marine Fisheries Service has started testing 2,500 samples of fish from the Gulf of Mexico and plans to test in the Pacific and Atlantic as well. Results won't be known for at least a year, but if they show that mercury levels in other species top 1 ppm, the FDA will consider adding more fish to its "Do Not Consume" list, says David Acheson, M.D., chief medical officer of that organization's Center for Food Safety and Nutrition.

In the meantime, what are you supposed to eat? Mercury aside, seafood is still good for you, as the American Heart Association has stated. It's low in saturated fat and high in omega-3 fatty acids, which Western diets sorely lack, says Alan Stern, a doctor of public health who served on a National Academy of Sciences panel that studied the mercury issue. Fortunately, he says, you can get the benefits of seafood with minimal risk—if you choose your fish wisely.

In many cases, the large ocean fish with the highest mercury levels also happen to be poor sources of omega-3s, for instance. Conversely, many of the best sources of those beneficial fatty acids, such as salmon, are low in mercury. In addition, relatively small species, such as flounder, sole, mullet, and sardines, are known to be low in the metal, Stern says. Farm-raised fish also tend to have lower levels than their wild counterparts.

Hightower offers some homespun advice: "If the fish you're cooking is too big for your pot, buy a smaller fish, not a bigger pot." If you see a large, boneless hunk of fish at a seafood counter, be wary; she says it could only come from a very large fish. And if you frequent sushi restaurants, be aware that much of the menu is composed of large predators, such as tuna. (Some bluefin tuna has been shown to contain mercury at more than 10 ppm—on par with many of the fish consumed by victims of the Minamata disaster.)

If your levels are high, don't panic, Mahaffey says, especially if you haven't noticed symptoms. Mercury is excreted in hair, skin, nails, and feces, which means that the amount in your body is halved every 40 to 100 days.

That's why the advice Hightower gave years ago to her geophysicist patient Will Smith was so effective. "Change your diet," she'd said. Once so severely debilitated that he couldn't think clearly, Smith is feeling much better these days. He's back at work. He can watch television without getting dizzy, and he can remember where he's going when he gets in the car. The tremors are finally gone, and he can once again manage complex mathematical computations.

As for fish, he won't go near it. ■

Ben Raines, a reporter for the Mobile Register, *has received awards from the National Press Club and the Oakes Fund for Environmental Journalism for investigating the issue of mercury in fish.*

Making Sense of the New Blood-Pressure Guidelines

A surprising thing happened in spring 2003: Thanks to new federal guidelines, millions of healthy Americans were suddenly deemed "prehypertensive," or on their way toward high blood pressure, a major cause of heart attacks, strokes,

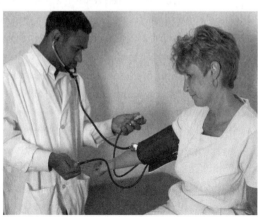

and kidney failure. Now, anyone with a systolic pressure (top number) of 120 to 139 or a diastolic pressure (bottom number) of 80 to 89 is considered prehypertensive. Under the new standard, about 22 percent of Americans fall into this category, according to the National Heart, Lung, and Blood Institute, part of the National Institutes of Health.

Experts changed the guidelines because they now know that artery and kidney damage can begin at fairly low blood pressure levels—those formerly considered normal (everything less than 130/85). Bear in mind, however, that not all doctors agree with the new recommendations. "The notion of prehypertension is irrational," says Lawrence Resnick, M.D., professor of medicine at Weill Medical College of Cornell University. "It is based solely on statistics, not on biology. If you were to call it a disease, the blood vessels would have to be working improperly."

But both critics and proponents agree that any measure meant to help Americans adopt healthier lifestyles is a good thing. "We're not saying you need to start on medication if your blood pressure slants slightly high, but rather that you should be making some lifestyle changes to prevent it from getting worse," explains Sheldon Sheps, M.D., former chairman of the Division of Hypertension at the Mayo Clinic in Rochester, Minnesota, and co-author of the report.

People who are prehypertensive need to watch their diets (more fruits, vegetables, and low-fat dairy foods; less saturated fat and cholesterol), exercise more, drink in moderation, and quit smoking. That's good advice, even for people with normal blood pressure who want to keep it that way.

No More Animal Testing

Over the past 20 years, the practice of animal testing has decreased by more than 90 percent, according to the *Cosmetic Ingredient Review,* an independent organization that reviews safety data on beauty products. And in March 2003, the European Union (EU) announced that by 2009 it will ban the sale and importation of new cosmetics tested on animals. Manufacturers worldwide are under pressure to develop nonanimal tests so that their products will be accepted by the EU. Many American companies, such as Avon, Burt's Bees, and Estée Lauder, already have policies in place against animal testing. Others may be forced to follow suit.

Potatoes: *The Latest in Bloodclotting*

Researchers at the Mayo Clinic in Rochester, Minnesota, have developed a starchy powder made from potatoes that clots blood instantly. It avoids many of the allergy risks commonly linked to coagulants made from human and animal plasma (it costs less, too). Bleed-X, an over-the-counter version for nosebleeds, cuts, and scrapes, has already been approved by the FDA for consumer use and should be in drugstores soon.

New Help for Aging Brains?

Researchers at the University of Utah may have discovered why the mind slows down in old age: a lack of GABA, a chemical that helps neurons be choosy about the signals they respond to. When the scientists injected GABA into the brains of elderly rhesus monkeys, the animals almost immediately became more alert. The researchers speculate that the substance shut down background brain activity so the monkeys could focus better. The findings may lead to new drugs, or new ways to use existing ones, that will increase GABA production and perhaps help slow the aging process in humans.

Thin Bones Linked to High Blood Pressure

You've probably heard about the potential dangers of lead in paint. Now a recent study in the *Journal of the American Medical Association* suggests that the element may even be hiding in a place you wouldn't suspect: your bones. According to the researchers, low levels of lead stored in your bones from previous exposure can leach into your blood, where it can cause damage.

"Lead is taken up by bone and acts as calcium does," says study author Ellen Silbergeld, Ph.D., professor of environmental-health sciences at Johns Hopkins Bloomberg School of Public Health. Both substances, she explains, can enter and leave bones over a lifetime; the difference is that lead is toxic. Leaching can happen when bone density is compromised—during pregnancy and menopause,

prolonged bed rest, or such illnesses as thyroid disease.

The study examined 2,165 women ages 40 to 59 and found that those with the most lead in their blood—about 6.4 micrograms per deciliter (mcg/dl) on average—had the highest blood pressure.

The findings suggest that lead levels well below the government's current occupational-safety limit of 40 mcg/dl could be harmful. Other studies have linked lead exposure to high blood pressure in men, but the Johns Hopkins report is the first to examine how thinning bones can release lead acquired from exposure decades earlier and contribute to hypertension risk in women. Prevent bone loss by eating a calcium-rich diet and performing regular weight-bearing exercises, such as walking and running.

Turn to Your Palm for the Latest Health Info

Does ostrich meat contain more protein than turkey? Just check your Palm. The United States Department of Agriculture's Agricultural Research Service has made its nutrient database available for download to personal digital assistants (PDAs). It contains information on more than 6,000 foods—from alfalfa sprouts to zwieback—listing calories, vitamins, minerals, protein, carbs, and fat grams for each. The free software takes about a minute to download, runs on the Palm OS, and requires about 2 megabytes of memory.

Our tester loaded the database onto her Palm Zire and took it to the grocery store. A quick check of lettuces revealed that romaine is a better source of fiber and folate than Bibb. Knowing that Parmesan has twice the calcium of mozzarella made choosing toppings for pizza easier.

Data was available for almost all grocery items we entered, but it came up short at a Chinese restaurant—ethnic fare like egg rolls and fried rice failed to make the list. Still, having this much info in a portable, easy-to-search format could be a boon to people with nutritional concerns. See www.nal.usda.gov/fnic/foodcomp. (For the PDA-less, a publication called *Nutritive Value of Foods* can be printed from the site.)

Beware of This

DANGEROUS DETOX

Chelation therapy promises to rid your body of mercury and other poisons. But could the procedure damage your health?

BY MICHELLE DALLY

In 1998, Jana Nestlerode, a 49-year-old criminal-justice professor at West Chester University in Pennsylvania, was seeking a permanent cure for her sluggish thyroid. After two years of taking daily medication, she visited Byron Braid, M.D., a physician her dentist had recommended for his "cutting edge" treatments. After an initial exam, she recalls, Braid said he suspected that her disorder was caused by mercury poisoning—specifically, her metal dental fillings. The doctor injected her with a chelator, a drug that binds with heavy metals like mercury and ushers them out of the body through the kidneys. Within 10 minutes of receiving the shot, which Braid had told her would reveal mercury in her urine, Nestlerode experienced severe nausea, dizziness, and a racing heart. After a few weeks, she began to suffer joint pain, exhaustion, disorientation, and memory lapses. "I got up one morning, and I couldn't remember where I worked," Nestlerode says. "Telephone numbers were out of the question." Many of the side effects went away on their

> **People will mortgage their houses and take out loans for chelation ... they will do ANYTHING to feel better.**
> —Jeffrey Brent, M.D.

own, but five years later, she still grits her teeth in pain when she has to climb stairs, and she has not yet regained enough energy to work out regularly. (Braid did not respond to *Health*'s repeated attempts to contact him.)

Nestlerode has since joined a small but vocal collection of patients and experts who are determined to stop a growing number of doctors from using chelation therapy as a cure-all for conditions such as chronic fatigue syndrome (CFS), Alzheimer's, heart disease, thyroid disorders, and autism.

"Some doctors will say to their patients, 'Your aches and pains, your fatigue, and your memory problems are all caused by mercury.' People will mortgage their houses and take out loans for chelation therapy, because they will do anything to feel better," says Jeffrey Brent, M.D., Ph.D., clinical professor of medicine at the University of Colorado Health Sciences Center and immediate past president of the American Academy of Clinical Toxicology. There is no scientific proof, though, that mercury contributes to these ills or that chelators are a safe or effective way to treat them. The U.S. Food and Drug Administration has approved chelation only to counteract severe heavy-metal poisoning, such as that caused by prolonged exposure to lead-based paint. Because all other uses are considered off-label, doctors are free to prescribe it for whatever ailment they want.

No one disputes that chelators rid the body of toxins, but critics say that isn't tantamount to treating disease.

Physicians who are pro-chelation argue that more and more people are being exposed to toxic levels of mercury and other heavy metals in dental amalgams, vaccines preserved with thimerosal (a mercury derivative), and fish harvested from mercury-contaminated waters. But multiple reports published in mainstream medical journals have exonerated dental fillings and vaccines. (Even so, manufacturers began eliminating thimerosal from children's vaccines in 1999, because of pressure from pending lawsuits and public fear. In addition, a joint statement issued in 2000 by the U.S. Public Health Service and the American Academy of Pediatricians suggested a theoretical, although unproven, risk of harm from cumulative exposure to the additive.)

Opening the door for further debate, two studies published in November 2002 in the *New England Journal of Medicine* present contradictory findings about the health risks of mercury in fish. One found no link between mercury levels and heart disease; the other concluded that men who'd had heart attacks showed higher levels than those who had not. The American Heart Association (AHA) reiterates that the health benefits of eating fish outweigh the risks and stands by its recommendation that adults eat at least two weekly servings, especially of salmon, canned tuna, and shellfish, which contain relatively low levels of mercury. (Pregnant and nursing women should watch their fish consumption to reduce the risk of brain damage in their babies.) The fundamental point is that mercury, though undeniably

toxic at high levels, is not known with any certainty to be harmful in low doses.

But for people who haven't found relief from intractable diseases through conventional medicine, even the smallest possibility that mercury poisoning could be the cause—and chelation the cure—can give them enough hope to try it. An estimated 800,000 Americans a year seek out the therapy for purposes other than its officially sanctioned one. Some of these people are even satisfied customers. Martin Dayton, M.D., a physician in North Miami Beach, Florida, who has performed chelation for 30 years, says it's useful in treating arthritis, scleroderma, psoriasis, and CFS. (After several attempts, we were unable to find patients treated successfully for these diseases who would talk to us on the record.) Furthermore, the remedy's grassroots popularity has thwarted some states' efforts to regulate it. In New Jersey and California, medical-board hearings have been deluged by citizens claiming the practice saved their lives, ending attempts in both states to limit chelation to its FDA-approved use.

No one disputes that chelators rid the body of toxins. Critics contend, however, that this isn't tantamount to treating disease; they also dispute the accuracy of the examinations some doctors use to determine whether people need these drugs in the first place. At best, detractors say, a patient may spend thousands of dollars and have nothing to show for it. At worst, they warn, this therapy can kill—you could have a fatal reaction to the medicine, or you could die of an illness that it failed to cure.

"The evidence that chelation therapy actually works is based on personal, not clinical, anecdotes," says Robert S. Baratz, M.D., Ph.D., D.D.S, president of the National Council Against Health Fraud (NCAHF). *The Journal of the American Medical Association* has published studies showing that chelation is ineffective for treating anything but heavy-metal poisoning. The AHA has found no scientific evidence of any other benefit from it and warns of possible kidney damage and other harm from its use. The U.S. Federal Trade Commission has filed suit against chelation's primary advocacy organization, the American College for the Advancement of Medicine, for false advertising. And Stephen Barrett, M.D., an NCAHF board member and chairman of Quackwatch, another group that investigates spurious health claims, describes it as "the most dangerous health scam around."

A $30 million study recently launched by the National Institutes of Health (NIH) to investigate the effect of chelation on heart disease should offer some answers. Drew Carlson, director of communications for the Federation of State Medical Boards, says his group encouraged the NIH to fund this study, hoping it will prove conclusively that chelation is quackery. But proponents like Dayton point to the same research as a sign that mainstream medicine is finally waking up to the practice's worth.

For now, chelation therapy remains a lucrative enterprise. Physicians who perform it charge anywhere between $90 and $180 per intravenous treatment. A patient usually undergoes between 10 and 30 sessions, which can add up to more than $5,000 in all—not counting the initial visit and the cost of dietary supplements that are also typically prescribed. "Doctors will have 20 to 30 patients in their office every day. Add up all the numbers, and you're talking $600,000 a year, maybe more. And remember, insurance doesn't cover off-label use. It's a cash business," says Baratz, who has testified before the U.S. Senate Special Committee on Aging about chelation's hazards.

Jana Nestlerode feels robbed of more than just cash. A former attorney, she sums up her experience this way: "Some of the people I prosecuted for violent crimes did less damage than these guys." ▪

Michelle Dally was part of the Denver Post *team that won a 2000 Pulitzer Prize for its coverage of the Columbine shootings.*

Keep an Emergency Room in Your Closet
A device for restarting hearts is now available for home use.

You might have recently noticed defibrillators—contraptions used to jump-start the heart after sudden cardiac arrest—mounted on a wall at the gym or mall. Now the U.S. Food and Drug Administration (FDA) has approved a simpler, smaller version for home use. (They've also just OK'd a pediatric model for children under age 8.) That's good news, because cardiac arrest, which happens when the heart starts to flutter wildly, kills more than 250,000 people each year—often without warning and usually at home. Without defibrillation, which shocks the heart back into a normal rhythm, a person's chance of recovery drops 10 percent with every passing minute. In fact, 95 percent of all victims die before reaching the hospital. A home defibrillator can buy a victim six to seven minutes of critical time.

The American Heart Association is still reviewing data before recommending the home model, but many doctors are already touting its benefits. "We've been waiting for a device that's approved for home use," says P.K. Shah, M.D., director of cardiology at Cedars-Sinai Medical Center in Los Angeles. "The home is where there is the greatest opportunity to save lives." The FDA-approved Philips model, about the size of a laptop, features simple voice prompts that guide even the least medically inclined through every step "It's idiot-proof," Shah says. Those who may need it most: people who have had heart attacks or have clogged coronary arteries, two of the biggest risk factors for cardiac arrest. At $2,300, the device is pricey, but your insurance company may partially cover the cost. It is available by prescription.

Rx Precautions:
Newer Pills May Pose More Risks

When you're sick, you want relief—and fast. But before you swallow the latest miracle cure, consider this: Adverse drug reactions are a leading cause of death in the United States, and a recent study suggests that new drugs may pose a greater risk than older ones.

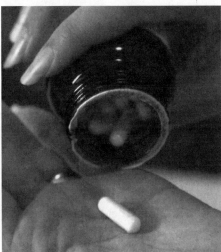

Harvard researchers examined 548 drugs approved between 1975 and 1999, and found that 8 percent of the meds had since acquired "black boxes," or warnings about the potential for serious reactions, such as heart or liver problems. "Half of all drug recalls take place within two years, and half of all adverse reactions arise in the first seven years of the drug's approval," says lead study author Karen Lasser, M.D., of Harvard Medical School.

Sometimes a new remedy is the best choice—for example, if it's a breakthrough medication or the only one that's available for your condition. But if that's not the case, here's how to avoid the pitfalls of new drugs.

Press your doctor. "Ask, 'Why this drug?' Find out if there's an older alternative that's been proven safe," Lasser says. If given a choice between a new medication and an older one, pick the one that has been around the longest.

Pay attention to new symptoms. They may be a reaction to the drug. Though this is sage advice for any medicine, it's especially important for new ones, which might have some unforeseen side effects.

Ask about generic alternatives. They're not just older than newfangled drugs, they're usually much cheaper.

Zoloft Approved for Anxiety Treatment

The antidepressant Zoloft could help the nearly 5.3 million Americans who suffer from social-anxiety disorder. A study of more than six hundred people found that 53 percent had fewer symptoms with Zoloft, compared with the 29 percent who took placebos. The drug does have possible side effects, including upset stomach, insomnia, and low libido, so talk to your doctor to see if it's right for you.

FDA Approves New Drug for Joint Pain

If you suffer from rheumatoid arthritis, ask your doctor about Humira. The Federal Drug Administration (FDA) recently approved the drug, which not only relieves pain but also slowed the destructive damage of arthritis in more than half the people studied. If you want to try natural remedies, new findings also suggest eating fruits, veggies, beans, and fiber to ease the pain.

PROZAC

Good for the Head *and* the Heart

New research reveals that certain depression medications have an added benefit—they may prevent heart attacks.

BY ALICE LESCH KELLY

The metaphorical heartache of depression, it turns out, has a basis in physiological reality. A growing body of scientific and epidemiological evidence shows that the condition may be as great a contributor to heart disease as smoking, high cholesterol, or high blood pressure. Understanding the link could yield new treatments for people who are at risk for heart problems—whether they're depressed or not.

In 2002 a team led by Stephen E. Kimmel, M.D., assistant professor of medicine and epidemiology at the University of Pennsylvania, studied 653 male and female smokers ages 30 to 65 who were hospitalized for their first heart attack (a control group of 2,990 randomly selected smokers had never had one before). The scientists were investigating whether nicotine patches caused heart attacks, but they also collected detailed information on other medications the subjects were taking at the time, including antidepressants.

People who took such medications as Prozac, Luvox, Paxil, or Zoloft—selective serotonin reuptake inhibitors (SSRIs)—reduced their risk of a second heart attack by 65 percent. "We think there's something unique about SSRIs above and beyond treatment of depression," Kimmel says.

His research is the latest, and perhaps the strongest, in a series of studies that demonstrate a connection between depression and heart disease. Recent evidence shows that a person who is clinically depressed is nearly four times more likely to develop coronary heart disease than a person who isn't. Other studies suggest that depressed people who undergo heart transplants are five times as likely to die in the first few years after surgery as patients in good mental health. Depression can also significantly increase a heart-attack survivor's chances of a second episode, according to studies.

Scientists say it's not just that depressed people are more likely than their emotionally stable peers to be sedentary, to smoke, to be overweight, and to ignore their doctors' medical advice. Depressive disorders could be independent risk factors for heart disease, says Reiner Rugulies, Ph.D., a researcher at the University of California, San Francisco, who has studied the correlation. One theory suggests that depression alters cardiac rhythms, increases blood pressure, and raises insulin levels.

Another, says Robert Carney, M.D., professor of psychiatry at Washington University School of Medicine in St. Louis, is that depression promotes inflammation, which has recently been linked to heart disease. Depression triggers the release of glucocorticoid hormones, which help control inflammation; however, a glut of these chemicals has a negative effect, lowering the body's anti-inflammatory defenses.

Platelet activity could also play a part. Scientists have long known that platelet clumping and blood clotting contribute to heart disease; in fact, the majority of heart attacks are caused by blood clots. "Studies show that platelets are more activated in depressed patients—though we're not quite sure why—and platelets are more likely to clot when they're more active," explains Andree Stoves, M.D., assistant professor of psychiatry at the University of Alabama at Birmingham (UAB).

One possible remedy: SSRIs, which have been shown in the lab to decrease platelet activity. Does this mean they could reduce cardiovascular disease in nondepressed people?

A team led by Stoves at UAB hopes to find out soon. They are in the final stages of a four-year, $1.25 million National Institutes of Health study that examines the links among depression, platelet activity, and heart disease. Stoves says preliminary findings suggest that SSRIs may make platelets less sticky and less likely to clump into artery-blocking clots.

Whether lowered platelet activity translates to reduced heart disease rates remains to be seen. Stoves is optimistic and predicts that SSRIs may someday be prescribed as preventive medicine for people at high risk, even if they're not depressed. "I won't be surprised if that happens," Stoves says. "This could have a major impact on the health of many people."

Rugulies is more cautious, however. "I think it's too early to come to a conclusion," he says. "These drugs are much too powerful to give to healthy people." Though SSRIs are easier on the body than previous generations of antidepressant medications, they do pose such potential side effects as diminished sexual desire, dry mouth, headache, and insomnia. That's why Stoves is also interested in looking into whether treating depression with nonpharmacological methods, such as psychological counseling, might reduce

heart disease risk as well. "My guess is that therapy may help. We know from scans and studies that brain chemistry differs before and after treatment," Stoves says. Until researchers have more answers, the best prevention plan is to maintain healthy habits and talk to your doctor if you feel depressed. ◾

Alice Lesch Kelly is the co-author of Conquering Infertility: Dr. Alice Domar's Mind/Body Guide to Enhancing Fertility and Coping with Infertility.

Lower Your Heart-Disease Risk Today

Concerned about depression's possible effect on your heart? Try these steps.

1. See a doctor if you're depressed. Treatment can alleviate symptoms in more than 80 percent of cases.

2. If you've ever had a heart attack or been treated for cardiovascular disease, get screened for depression. One in three people who have survived a heart attack becomes depressed. Medication and therapy can help.

3. Be heart-healthy. Stop smoking, eat less saturated fat, and drop a few pounds if you're overweight. Have your blood pressure and cholesterol checked; if they're high, work with your doctor to control them.

4. Get moving. Exercise can improve your mood and strengthen your heart.

5. Practice mind/body relaxation strategies. Meditation, visual imagery, Tai Chi, yoga, and other techniques can reduce your blood pressure, heart rate, and levels of stress hormones in your blood.

6. If your therapist prescribes an antidepressant, tell your cardiologist. Make sure your doctors work together on your treatment plan to prevent dangerous drug interactions. For example, some antidepressants can magnify the action of such blood-thinning drugs as Coumadin, which can lead to uncontrolled bleeding.

The New Field of "Medical Intuitives"

Some swear by this new twist that adds a bit of mysticism to conventional medicine. But can you trust it?

BY NANCY ROSS-FLANIGAN

I trust my own intuition, but at times I've been disappointed in other people's. Like the time a New Orleans fortune-teller assured me that a particular loved one was "doing really well," when, in fact, he was dead. Since then, I haven't put much stock in psychics, but while watching a TV program about Mona Lisa Schulz, a bona fide M.D. and Ph.D. who is also a self-described medical intuitive, I started to reconsider. Knowing only the name and age of a woman she's never met face-to-face, Schulz claims she can do a head-to-toe rundown of her physical condition over the phone, zeroing in on whatever's ailing her.

With Web sites and newspaper ads touting the powers of medical intuitives, this field appears to be the latest twist on the conventional checkup. Some practitioners work by phone; others perform readings in person and use touch to pick up on pain; a few are physicians themselves, and others work with doctors. The common denominator is their belief that they can divine a person's state of health and its emotional underpinnings.

> Some practitioners work by phone. Others perform readings in person. They all believe they can divine a person's state of health and emotional underpinnings.

Intrigued by the idea, I schedule a $235, half-hour consultation with Schulz. (Before our appointment, I sign a consent form stating that I understand this is not for diagnosis but is informational only, and that our conversation does not constitute a doctor-patient relationship.)

From the start, this meeting goes nothing like I'd expected. Crisp and clipped, my intuitive sounds more like Miss Manners than Miss Cleo. We briefly exchange pleasantries, and then she asks if she can put me on hold for a couple of minutes while she looks at the emotional setting of my life. Several minutes pass. I start to wonder what she's doing: checking her E-mail? Googling me?

Back on the phone again, Schulz tells me that I'm a "human wire for empathy," and she wonders whether I often end up mothering people who have relationship problems. "Uh, not really," I tell her. But she's pretty sure I do.

Moving on to my physical health, she zips through my organs like a Harley down a highway: heart, left lung, right lung, left breast, right breast, digestive tract, kidneys, and so on. To my amazement, every place she comments on is a medical hot spot. She notices redness in my upper GI tract (I have heartburn), pauses at my liver and asks if addiction runs in my family (oh, yeah), notes something funny about my upper spine (I broke it in a fall), and says there's also something different about my neck and thyroid gland (cancer treatment 12 years ago made a mess of that whole area).

I'm impressed, and I take Schulz's commentary along when I visit my internist a few weeks later. Michael J. Dionne, M.D., is an open-minded type—he even admits to trusting gut feelings—but the notion of intuiting a patient's ills sight unseen strikes him as "totally ridiculous," he says.

What about Schulz's analysis? My doctor concedes that her reading jibes with my medical chart. However, he says, the broad statements she made would probably fit many woman in my age group. Heartburn, neck problems, thyroid imbalances, even a family history of addiction are not unusual. Schulz's intuition may just be educated guessing, Dionne says.

How to Find a Medical Intuitive

Because the field is unregulated, locating a reliable practitioner is a challenge. These suggestions can help guide your search.

1. Check with local hospitals that have complementary- and alternative-medicine departments. They may have medical intuitives working with regular medical staff.
2. Ask someone you know who's had a reading from an intuitive. What recommendations did she make? "If an intuitive is telling people to do wild and possibly dangerous things, stay away," says James Dillard, M.D., author of *Alternative Medicine for Dummies*.
3. If you're having a face-to-face reading with an intuitive who works from home, take someone with you. If touch is involved, ask how, and if you don't feel comfortable with what will be done, find another healer.

As for my own conclusion? This foray into mystical medicine was entertaining and thought-provoking, kind of like my New Orleans psychic encounter. But I'm not about to ditch my own doctor and put a medical intuitive on speed dial. If anything, the experience made me trust my doctor's hunches and wisdom more than ever. He has repeatedly made sense of weird symptoms, and he always seems to know, even before my test results come back, if something's really wrong. What's more—and I'm grateful for this—he's never referred to me as a "human wire." ■

Michigan-based writer Nancy Ross-Flanigan has covered health and science for 20 years.

Zap Away Your Phobia

Researchers in Puerto Rico recently found they could zap fear out of rats through electronic stimulation. By pinpointing the part of the brain that controls fright, scientists hope to find new (and, thankfully, voltage-free) ways to disconnect the panic button in humans.

Acupuncture Sticks It to UTIs

Acupuncture may keep pesky urinary-tract infections (UTIs) from coming back, according to a recent Norwegian study. Women who went under the needle two times a week for four weeks reduced their risk of reinfection by 50 percent during the six-month follow-up.

Not Your *Typical* Detox

BY STEPHANIE JO KLEIN

My friends have tried nearly every diet and fitness trend—underwater Spinning classes, raw foodism, and yoga boxing. I used to scoff at them. But with my jogging-and-bagels routine failing to help me lose those 10 pounds, I decided to join the trendoids.

The idea of the moment is detox—not the Betty Ford Center type, but the kind that promises to rid your body of impurities and leave you trimmer, energized, and more focused. Just what I needed. So I signed up for a five-week cleansing diet offered by Universal Force Healing Center, a Manhattan yoga and wellness studio. It sounded too good to be true, so I took notes at the sessions, and I asked a nutritionist and a fitness expert to evaluate the program.

WEEK 1

Mission: Start cleansing my colon with an 11-day diet.
Class notes: "Can't have it" seems to be the theme. For homework, I eliminate foods deemed toxic. The rationale? The nutritionist (actually a local pharmacist) tells us that processed foods cause rotting matter and other wastes to build up in the intestines. These toxins supposedly overload your liver and keep your digestive system from functioning properly. The diet clears out the intestines, she says, and helps prevent common ills, such as irritable bowel syndrome. Each day I nix a food: the first is meat (but eating fish is OK); on day two, I give up caffeine and refined sugar. Then I quit dairy, soy, and wheat to reduce "harmful" mucus in my gastrointestinal tract. By week's end, I am eating mostly fruits, vegetables, legumes, and assorted nuts and seeds. I can't find suggested alternative grains, such as spelt or quinoa, easily, so I end up eating mounds of string beans and brown rice that keep me in the bathroom all day. For once, though, I can locate my cheekbones, which are visible because I am probably losing water weight, but I could do without the gas.
Expert's take: Your colon doesn't need cleansing. "Food does not rot in intestines, and protective mucus is not an evil the body must rid," says Audrey Cross, Ph.D., a professor of nutrition at Columbia and Rutgers universities. "The body expels harmful things naturally." Eliminating food groups and drastically cutting calories will not translate into lasting weight loss, Cross says. Without enough calories, your body will begin to leach protein from muscles for fuel, which lowers metabolism, she says.

WEEK 2

Mission: Energize with a three-day liquid-only diet: five or more glasses of juice and as much vegetable broth as I can stomach.
Class notes: I am so drained from the first week's regimen that I fall asleep before class and miss it all. I call for instructions and spend the next day downing apple, mango, and strawberry juices, which are tasty but not filling. By evening I'm so cranky and hungry that I decide I deserve a break. I order a Chinese feast of brown rice and chicken with vegetables. I try juicing again the next morning, but after one sip of the spirulina concoction, I realize that if I had wanted to drink algae, I'd have swallowed the lake water at summer camp. So I give up on the juice fast and eat a tuna sandwich for lunch.

My stomach churns for the rest of the week, and I feel exhausted even though I am sleeping. I am also feeling very manic. I learned I had manic depression five years ago, but my illness usually stays in check; later, our experts tell me my stomach was too empty to absorb my medicine. Though I had signed a liability form and briefly discussed my medical history with the staff, no one warned me about this possibility. **Expert's take:** I discover what I wish I'd known before: Antianxiety drugs, birth control pills, and antibiotics, among other medications, don't pair well with detox diets, says Hilary Horton-Brown, a registered dietitian and fitness consultant at Idaho State University who uses yoga in her treatment for eating disorders. Many prescription medicines need to be taken with food or milk—not juice—for effective absorption and reduced stomach irritation.

WEEK 3

Mission: Create a calming personal yoga routine. **Class notes:** The hour-and-a-half session focuses on stretching and upper-body work, supposedly increasing my lung capacity. More oxygen, the instructor tells us, means less stress. I have never consistently practiced yoga, but stretched into the cobra position, I begin to appreciate the calm it gives me. Outside of class, I continue bouncing between restraint and excess to make up for lost calories. I polish off whole boxes of cookies and packs of cold cuts, behavior that runs completely counter to everything I know about healthy eating. I gain 5 pounds. The closest I get to practicing my new moves is talking about them with my friends. **Expert's take:** Cross isn't surprised about my feeding frenzies. "Eliminating meat and drinking spirulina juice are major changes," she says. "They drive you to seek things that are familiar." The yoga workout is more sensible: Studies suggest that certain poses may increase lung capacity, helping you calm down.

WEEK 4

Mission: Reduce stress with breathing and meditation. **Class notes:** As a nonsmoker and jogger, I've always believed that my lungs were healthy. But the "breath of fire" exercise shows me that they can use a little extra toning. I rapidly breathe in and out for three minutes, tightening my abdominal muscles with each exhalation. This technique lives up to its name, as it initially makes me feel as if I'm hyperventilating.

When the class begins to chant together, I feel silly repeating *"wahe guru"* and other mantras, but later, focusing on the sounds helps me stop worrying about everyday matters. I try to repeat the routine at home, but I get the directions wrong and mostly just huff and puff. Even so, taking moments for reflection is a soothing way to start my day. **Expert's take:** "The mind/body connection is everything," Horton-Brown says. "Whether you're meditating by emptying your mind of thoughts or by focusing on one positive thought, it's very healthy."

WEEK 5

Mission: Heal minor aches and pains using yoga poses. **Class notes:** I walk into the last session with a headache that feels like a dance club has exploded in my brain. But I am pleasantly surprised that this week's yoga lesson works better than a dose of Advil. In a pose intended to be restorative, I lie supported by blankets under my spine and shoulders, with a foam block beneath my head. Within 10 minutes, the pain is gone. I am so impressed that I buy the block. **Expert's take:** "This class was a wonderful idea, since it addresses healing your body without the medicine cabinet," Horton-Brown says. Studies in India and at universities in the United States indicate that certain yoga poses can help relieve pain caused by PMS, carpal tunnel syndrome, and other conditions.

COURSE EVALUATION

Horton-Brown and Cross agree that though this detox plan was a little extreme, adopting some of its more sensible aspects can be better than keeping bad habits forever. Sure enough, I eat more fish and grains, and I've cut back on coffee. My breakfast bagel seems massive, so I substitute an English muffin. While my energy is back to where it was before, I'm not as charged up as the instructors claimed I'd be. And I still haven't lost those 10 pounds.

If someone offered me money to try a detox diet again, or even just to sip a spirulina smoothie, I'd say no. However, I'd pay for a yoga class anytime. I can live with my toxins—it's the stress I can't stand. ∎

The Prayer Prescription

Can prayer really heal? Scientists set out to discover exactly how effective it can be.

BY ALICE LESCH KELLY

God is making headlines—and not just in the religion section of the newspaper: A debate is unfolding in the medical community regarding the healing power of prayer. In a Columbia University study of South Korean women who were undergoing in vitro fertilization, those who had been prayed for were twice as likely to get pregnant as those who had not. Recent Mayo Clinic findings, on the other hand, concluded that prayer on behalf of cardiac patients had no statistically significant effect on their medical outcomes. Meanwhile, the National Institutes of Health (NIH) has announced that it will fund a four-year study at Johns Hopkins University to investigate whether prayer benefits African-American women with breast cancer. And a group of top prayer researchers in the United States is guarding the outcome of a major new study as closely as the Academy guards Oscar nominations.

Can science prove that prayer really heals? Most medical investigation is pretty straightforward—give this group a pill, give that group no pill, and see who gets better. For the most part, prayer is receiving the same approach: One group gets prayed for, one doesn't. But evaluating how prayer affects a person's medical condition is much more complex than measuring the effects of drugs.

Researchers have known for years that participatory prayer, particularly such repetitive variations as saying the rosary or chanting a mantra, can lower stress and blood pressure. But a growing interest in intercessory prayer, or praying for others, has raised new questions. Scientists admit that even designing studies of it can be an enormous challenge. In the Mayo Clinic study, for example, just deciding what "dosage" of prayer to use sparked debate: Should the patients be prayed for once a week? Once a day? Should specific prayers be prescribed? And what should people pray for—a particular result or just a "good outcome" for the patient? "If someone had a stroke and is a vegetable, maybe the best outcome is for that person just to pass on," says Stephen L. Kopecky, M.D., a

> **Research is tricky. Evaluating how prayer affects a person's medical condition is more complex than measuring the effects of drugs.**

Mayo Clinic cardiologist and co-author of the study. "Sometimes what we're saying is a bad outcome could actually be a good outcome."

Another challenge is deciding what, if anything, patients, caregivers, and even the people doing the praying should be told. A hallmark of good research is keeping study participants from finding out information that would bias the outcome. For instance, in a double-blind drug study, neither the subjects nor the health-care providers know who is receiving medication and who is getting a placebo. Because the very nature of prayer requires those praying to know something about

Ninety-six percent of hospital patients use prayer to aid their recovery. When that many patients believe in a source of healing, doctors should know as much about it as they can.

the people for whom they are sending good vibes, double blindness can be tricky, though not impossible. In the Mayo Clinic study, neither the researchers nor the patients knew who was being prayed for, and the people praying had only the most basic information—a patient's first name, age, diagnosis, condition, and gender. The Columbia study took blindness a step further: None of the women knew they were being prayed for. They didn't even know they were part of the study, nor did their caregivers.

An even larger question looms: Can science be applied to such a metaphysical phenomenon? "Many physicians question the appropriateness of addressing religious or spiritual issues within a medical setting, and almost all are uncertain on how to go about this," says Harold G. Koenig, M.D., associate professor in the department of psychiatry and behavioral science at Duke University Medical Center.

But the medical debate hasn't stopped patients from believing. Some 96 percent of hospital patients acknowledge using prayer to aid their recovery, Kopecky notes. When that many patients believe in a source of healing, he says, doctors should know as much about it as they can. And, he adds, "a study where we put the personal interface back into the mix would be very enlightening." ■

Alice Lesch Kelly is the co-author of Conquering Infertility: Dr. Alice Domar's Mind/Body Guide to Enhancing Fertility and Coping with Infertility.

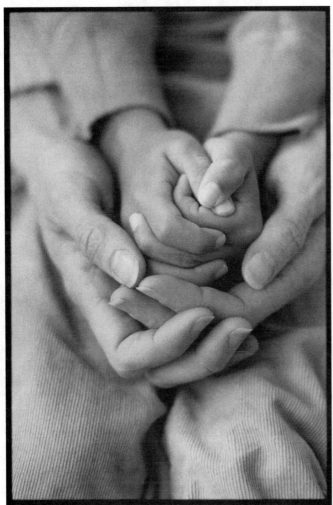

vital *stats*

75
Percentage of hospital
JOB OPENINGS
posted for NURSES

126,000
Number of NURSES
CURRENTLY NEEDED to fill
vacancies at hospitals

68,759
Number of
NURSING-SCHOOL
GRADUATES in 2001

88
Percentage of FEMALE
doctors who wash their hands
after patient contact

54
Percentage of
MALE doctors who do

490,000
Number of CAR CRASHES
caused by animals
each year

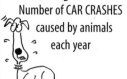

10,000
Number of HUMAN INJURIES
caused by animal-related
crashes

$2,000
Average insurance claim
for repairs and injuries in a
DEER-car collision

11
Percentage of Americans who
say they've had sex
with only ONE person

11.3
Average number of sexual
partners among people in
the MIDWEST

11.6
Average number of sexual
partners among people in the
NORTHEAST

14.9
Average number of sexual
partners among people in the
SOUTH

18.9
Average number of sexual
partners among people in the
WEST

15
Percentage of Americans who
never use CONTRACEPTION
(including condoms)

15.3
Number of new STD
INFECTIONS, in millions,
diagnosed each year in the
United States

1
Rank of the United Stated
among industrialized nations
with the highest per capita
incidence of STDs

41
Percentage of MEN who
report increased tension in their
relationships when
their partners
have PMS

31
Percentage of WOMEN who
report increased tension in their
friendships when their
friends have PMS

15.6
Pounds of SEAFOOD the average
American ate in 2000

11.8
Pounds eaten in 1970

66
Pounds of BEEF the average
American ate in 1999

89
Pounds eaten in 1976

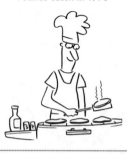

44
Percentage of women who
think LIVING WITH A SPOUSE
before marriage increases the
likelihood of divorce

36
Percentage of MEN who
think so

37
Percentage of Americans
who lived with their spouses
BEFORE MARRIAGE

20
Percent chance a
FIRST MARRIAGE WILL END
in separation or divorce within
five years

49
Percent chance that couples
WHO LIVE TOGETHER before
marriage will break up within
five years

7.2
Median LENGTH of
marriage, in years

Sources: American Association of Colleges of Nursing, Insurance
Information Institute, *American Journal of Infection Control*,
Durex Global Sex Survey, *International Journal of Eating Disorders*,
SkyGuide, National Association of Nurse Practitioners in Women's
Health, CDC National Prevention Information Network, National
Marine Fisheries Service, American Meat Institute, Gallup Poll,
Divorce Magazine   —Reported by Laura Riccobono

chapter 2

everyday wellness

**practical advice for healthy
living and disease prevention**

The 7 Ironclad Health Rules

you don't have to follow

With the demands of work, family, and play, who has time to live up to the health ideal? Maybe you don't have to: Top health experts break down what's really necessary and what's not. As it turns out, healthy living isn't as big a chore as you might think.

BY DARYN ELLER

EAT THREE SQUARE MEALS A DAY

The real deal: You don't always need to sit down to meals with utensils, but you shouldn't run on empty for too long, even if that means snacking on the go.

The rationale: "Your body needs energy all day, and if you don't supply it with fuel, it will burn fewer calories and even eat away at muscle tissue for energy," says Cynthia Sass, R.D., a spokeswoman for the American Dietetic Association. So if you think skipping lunch will help you drop pounds, think again. According to the Calorie Control Council's last poll in 2000, 28 percent of dieters skip meals for weight loss, down 12 percent from 1986. But that's still too large a number, Sass says. Then there are the mealtime truants who think they simply don't have time to eat. If that's you, get through the day without breaking your stride by throwing bags of whole-grain cereal, unsalted nuts, or dried fruit into your purse for on-the-go snacking. Or stop at a drive-through and order one of the healthier options—a bean burrito or chicken soft taco from Taco Bell, for instance. "Even a latte with skim or soy milk from Starbucks is better than nothing," Sass says.

TAKE A DAILY MULTIVITAMIN

The real deal: No need to pop a pill if you fuel up on fortified foods.

The rationale: If you eat a fairly balanced diet, you're most likely getting enough nutrients to keep all your body's systems functioning and free from such deficiency-related illnesses as anemia. But for maximum protection against cancer and heart disease, Harvard Medical School researchers recommend a daily multivitamin supplement. Can't remember or don't like the idea of swallowing a pill every day?

52

Fortified foods are a good alternative. "If a fortified cereal offers 100 percent of the major vitamins, there really is no need to take an additional multivitamin," says Kathleen Fairfield, M.D., co-author of the Harvard study. But you'll have to eat a serving of the cereal every day, she says, or fill up on other fortified foods. Unfortunately, loading up on extra vitamins one day doesn't mean that you're off the hook the next. Because some essentials (such as vitamin C and all the B vitamins) are water-soluble and aren't stored in the body, you need to get your vitamins in some form every day.

STRETCH AFTER EVERY WORKOUT

The real deal: You don't have to commit to regular total-body stretch sessions, but a few key moves could ward off the kinks.

The rationale: According to the American College of Sports Medicine, you should make time for stretching—if not after every workout, at least a couple of times a week—to increase your flexibility and prevent future injury. But if you're worried about waking up tight and achy the next day, stretching might not be the antidote. A recent review of published studies by Australian researchers found no evidence that stretching either before or after a workout helps prevent muscle soreness. The scientists suggest that a better way to ward off aches is to build up resistance through regular exercise.

But even though stretching may not prevent soreness, it can relieve tightness. "Muscle tightness can be caused by prolonged sitting and computer work," says occupational physiologist Mike Bracko, director of the Occupational Performance Institute in Calgary, Alberta. The following two moves, which take less than two minutes to complete, target the most troublesome areas: the shoulders and lower back.

• Shoulder/chest stretch: Stand with your feet hip-width apart and hold your arms out to your sides, parallel to the floor. Move your arms backward until you feel a good stretch in your shoulders.

• Hamstring/lower-back stretch: Stand with your back against a wall. Raise your right knee and pull it toward your chest. Hold for 10 to 20 seconds. Repeat on the other side.

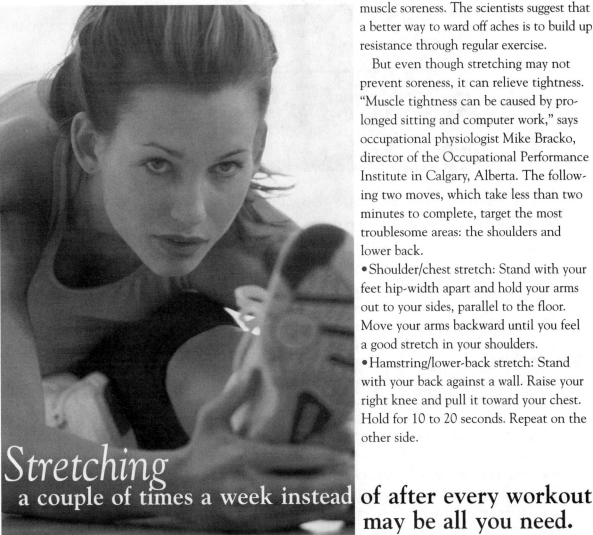

Stretching a couple of times a week instead of after every workout may be all you need.

4 DRINK EIGHT GLASSES OF WATER A DAY

The real deal: Unless you live in a very warm climate or you're doing heavy aerobic exercise, you can probably get by with six or seven glasses of water—or another type of beverage—a day.

The rationale: Heinz Valtin, M.D., professor emeritus of physiology at Dartmouth Medical School, recently published a review of hydration studies that found no evidence supporting the eight-glasses-a-day rule. "Some people have told me that their skin looks better, they have less

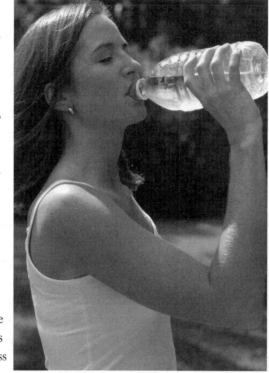

A recent study found that subjects who consumed caffeinated drinks were just as hydrated as those who drank water.

pain from arthritis, and they have fewer migraines when they drink eight glasses a day," he says. "If that works for you, then do it, but most healthy adults probably don't need quite that much water every day."

That's good news, since most people get only about 4.6 servings of water daily, according to a survey conducted by the Nutrition Information Center at Weill Medical College of Cornell University in New York City. And although you might have heard differently in the past, even beverages containing caffeine count. A 2000 study conducted by researchers at the Center for Human Nutrition at the University of Nebraska Medical Center in Omaha found that subjects who consumed caffeinated drinks were just as hydrated as those who drank water. "It's well-known that pure caffeine given in pharmacological doses is a diuretic, but the lesser doses in drinks don't have the same effect on people who drink them regularly," Valtin says. If six to seven beverages is still hard for you to swallow, at least drink when you're thirsty. Valtin says that cotton-mouthed feeling generally kicks in before your body gets significantly dehydrated.

5 WASH AND MOISTURIZE YOUR FACE BEFORE BED

The real deal: You don't have to go through the whole routine every night, but going to bed without removing your makeup can have some unsightly side effects.

The rationale: "If you're acne-prone, sleeping with foundation on can cause whiteheads and blackheads," explains Debra Jaliman, M.D., a clinical instructor of dermatology at Mount Sinai School of Medicine in New York City. Slumbering in your eye makeup can cause trouble, too: Worst case, you may develop tiny cysts under your eyes or in the lids that can only be removed by inserting a needle

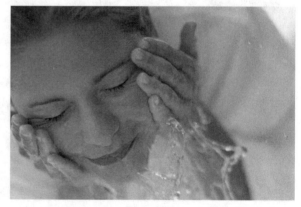

containing an electric current into the bumps. At the very least, you may wake up with puffy, irritated eyes.

But even Jaliman confesses to being lax about taking off her makeup sometimes. Her solution: She keeps cleansing wipes and lotions on her bedside table so that she can freshen and moisturize before nodding off. "Another thing you can do is wash your face when you get home, so you don't have to deal with it before bed," Jaliman says.

FLOSS AFTER EVERY MEAL

The real deal: Flossing even just a couple of times a week will help fight off harmful bacteria.
The rationale: Unfortunately, no high-tech toothbrush can take the place of old-fashioned floss. "Floss gets into nooks and crannies where a toothbrush can't," says Richard H. Price, D.M.D., consumer adviser for the American Dental Association (ADA). It removes food debris, which prevents the formation of plaque, a sticky substance that keeps bacteria tight against the tooth, where it can cause decay. But if you're like nearly half of Americans, who can only get it together to floss once a day (a mere 4 percent floss after each meal, as the ADA recommends), do it at night since that's when bacteria really build up. "When you're asleep, your mouth is like a petri dish," Price says.

EAT FIVE SERVINGS OF FRUITS AND VEGETABLES DAILY

The real deal: Ok, so you really do need to get your five a day—well, most of the time.
The rationale: Hundreds of studies suggest that people who load up on fruits and veggies have significantly lower risks of cancer and heart disease than people who don't. But only about 26 percent of people reach the quota set by the National Cancer Institute (NCI). If you miss the mark every so often, relax. "It's how you eat on average over the long term that's important," says NCI researcher Gloria J. Stables, R.D., Ph.D.

To sneak more produce into your life, think strategically. Have a piece of fruit and a glass of juice at breakfast, and you're almost halfway there. Put some carrots, grape tomatoes, or other vegetables in a bag and bring it to work with you. "We should change the stereotype that only fruit is a good snack," Stables says. Also, try keeping produce in a bowl at eye level in the fridge instead of tucked away in the crisper. Or when you come home from the market, make a list of the fruits and vegetables you've bought, and stick it on the refrigerator door. Cross each item off the list as you eat it. ■

Daryn Eller lives in Los Angeles and has written for O *and* Parenting.

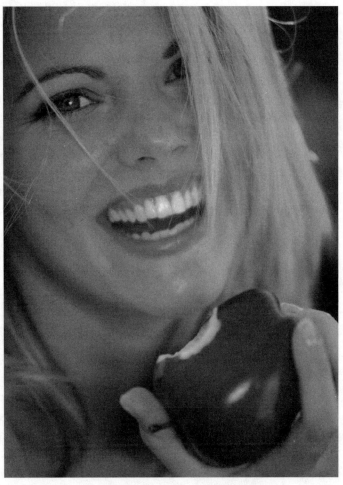

6 Health Habits You *Can't* Shrug Off

1. Get Regular Breast Exams.
Even though a recent study showed that breast self-exams do not reduce the risk of death, the American Cancer Society (ACS) still recommends that all women perform them monthly. Women between ages 20 and 39 should be examined by a doctor every three years, then each year starting at age 40. The ACS also continues to recommend yearly mammograms for women age 40 and older.

2. Quit smoking.
This is the number-one way to improve your health. The ACS estimates that more than 65,000 women died from lung cancer in 2003; about 90 percent of those cases were smoking-related. That's not to mention all the additional ills smoking contributes to, including other cancers, heart disease, and stroke.

3. Have protected sex.
Women are biologically more susceptible to sexually transmitted diseases (STDs) than men. Condoms, which are 98 percent effective in preventing AIDS and many other STDs when they are used consistently and correctly, are your best defense.

4. Wear a bicycle helmet.
Stop fussing over helmet hair, and worry about this: In 1997, around 800 bicyclists were killed in collisions with motor vehicles. Ninety-seven percent of the victims were not wearing helmets. The Centers for Disease Control and Prevention estimates that if every rider wore a helmet, 500 bicycle-related fatalities and 151,000 head injuries would be prevented each year.

5. Screen out the sun.
Melanoma, the deadliest of skin cancers, is on the rise, increasing at a rate of 3 percent each year. The ACS predicted 53,600 new cases in 2003 alone. Limiting your time in the sun is your best defense against skin cancer (both melanoma and non-melanoma, which together are the most common kinds of cancer). But when you do get exposure, wear a broad-spectrum sunscreen with at least SPF 15—all year 'round.

6. Get regular Pap smears.
Cervical cancer is rarely deadly, but that's only because it's usually caught early: The advent of the Pap smear marked a 70 to 80 percent decline in death from the disease. Most of the invasive, lethal forms of cervical cancer occur in women who haven't had regular Pap smears, so make certain that you get one as often as your doctor recommends.

Q + A

WHY YOU SHOULD STICK TO THE BASICS FOR HAND WASHING

I've heard that some hospitals are switching from soap and water to waterless sanitizing gels (like the ones you find at the drugstore) for hand washing. Should I be using them at home?

That's like using a fire hose to put out a match. Soap and water do the job just fine (they're cheaper, too). It's true that hand sanitizers kill microbes rather than just wash them away, but this extra cleaning power is most important in hospitals, where it's essential to get rid of germs that could infect patients.

Gels are fine to use when you're traveling and can't get to a sink. Be aware, though, that all they do is disinfect: To get rid of stubborn newsprint smudges or a sticky glob of peanut butter, you'll still need running water.

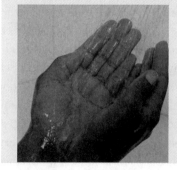

The New (and **Dangerous**) Addiction: <u>Health Fads</u>

These seemingly good-for-you habits may need a reality check.

BY SARAH SCHMIDT

Incessant cell-phone chattering is replacing Joe Camel puffing as a more "positive" addiction, according to a recent British study. In a survey of 110 students, researchers found that people view cell-phone talkers as "fun, cool, confident, fashionable, and playful"—characteristics that were once attributed to cigarette smokers. Here's our thumbnail diagnosis of the addictions currently in vogue among the health-conscious in-crowd.

CELL-PHONE CRAZE

Though there's no conclusive evidence linking cell-phone use to brain cancer, most doctors recommend using a headset, which puts more space between your brain and the radiation from the phone. And since driving while "celling" has been linked to increased crash risk (even if you're using a hands-free phone), calls should be a strictly off-road pastime.

THIRST FOR VITAMIN WATER

It's tempting to believe that gulping fruity fortified waters is as good as chomping on an apple. But while the added nutrients may be helpful, the extra sugar isn't. The Center for Science in the Public Interest, a nutrition- and health-advocacy group, recently named the popular designer water Glacéau as one of its "Health Foods That Aren't" because it's loaded with sugar. A fresh-fruit fetish would be healthier—not to mention cheaper.

DOWNWARD-DOG DEVOTION

First Madonna and Gwyneth began raving about it. Now masses of fanatics are bent on yoga. A penchant for posing can't hurt, as long as you don't indulge in lieu of aerobic activity and weight training. True fitness balance calls for variety.

STUCK ON BREATH STRIPS

With packaging that suggests you "use a second strip immediately after the first one dissolves," it's no wonder these minty antibacterial fresheners are attracting a fastidious following. There's probably no harm done if you do get the Listerine monkey on your back. If sweet breath helps your social life, it could help your body, too: Research has shown that people with close-knit circles of friends tend to have fewer health problems than loners.

IBUPROFEN DEPENDENCY

If you overindulge on weekends, ibuprofen, nicknamed "vitamin I" by devotees, could be your supplement of choice. But instead of reaching for fast relief, "you need to be putting more time into conditioning throughout the week and get chronic pain checked out by a doctor," says Nick DiNubile, M.D., orthopedic consultant for the Pennsylvania Ballet. ■

Sarah Schmidt has also written for the New York Times.

The Top 10 Healthiest Companies for Women

Discover the way office life could—and should—be. These employers are helping women keep their lives in balance.

BY LAMBETH HOCHWALD • PHOTOGRAPHY BY ANGELA WYANT

Some working women accomplish more between the time they switch off their alarms and switch on their computers than you might think possible. They drop off their kids at day care, stretch away stress in a yoga class, or eat a made-to-order veggie omelette—all within minutes of their desks, and all courtesy of their bosses. "The best companies are learning that if they can help their employees balance home and work, family and job, they will be healthy individuals and happy workers," says Gail L. Choate, president of Synergies, a company specializing in corporate and community wellness programs.

Our report on the healthiest companies for women honors 10 employers, chosen by Choate and a panel of health, nutrition, and fitness experts, that are revolutionizing workplaces. Each is creating flexible, accessible programs to help women accomplish the ultimate multitasking feat: balancing professional and personal responsibilities. If your company didn't make the list, tell your boss about the perks outlined here to spur change in your office.

1 BUILDING COMMUNITY TIES ON COMPANY TIME

Clif Bar Inc.; Berkeley, California
Total employees: 117 (65-percent female)
Clif Bar, the company behind the Luna nutrition bar, inspires its workers to make a difference in other people's lives. The 2080 Community Service Program encourages employees to get involved in volunteer activities during working hours (the project is named for the number of hours one full-time employee logs in a year). In 2002, almost everyone (106 people) participated, donating a total of 2,237 paid hours to build a house for Habitat for

Humanity or coach athletics through Sports for Kids. The program recently expanded to include international volunteer opportunities.

Other perks:

- Stressed-out staffers can seek calm in a meditation tent equipped with reclining seats, stereo headsets, CDs, and reading lights. There are also massage tents, where two therapists deliver about 40 rubs a month.

- Eight trainers teach 26 kinds of fitness classes (including Pilates, hip-hop dance, and kickboxing) every week before, during, and after business hours; they also offer one-on-one instruction.

- The company reimburses travel expenses for competitive runners and triathletes.

- Employees can save time at the supermarket, thanks to the Organic Veggie Bucks program ($56 for four weeks). Every week, a local organic farm drops off boxes of produce at company headquarters.

- An aesthetician comes to the office twice a month to provide facials and waxing.

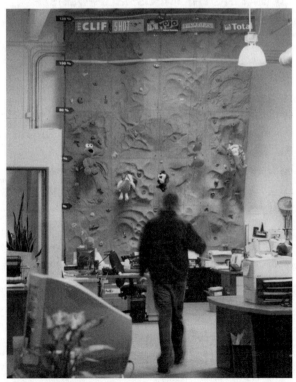

This climbing wall tracks Clif Bar's sales; as numbers climb, so do the stuffed animals.

Our Top Ten List

1. Clif Bar Inc.
2. Bristol-Myers Squibb
3. SC Johnson
4. ARUP Laboratories
5. Genentech
6. New York Life Insurance Co.
7. Roche
8. Verizon Wireless
9. Green Mountain College
10. Guidant Corp.

2 TAKING CARE OF BABIES (AND BUSINESS)

Bristol-Myers Squibb; Princeton, New Jersey
Total employees: 18,290 (49-percent female)

The makers of Excedrin help working moms stay headache-free naturally by keeping their children in close proximity. The company subsidizes 40 percent of the operating costs of three on-site child-care centers (a fourth opened in June 2003). Nearly 400 preschool- and kindergarten-age children are enrolled. Extended hours—from 6:30 a.m. to 7 p.m.—take the pressure off moms when meetings start early or run late. For executives like Judianne Hare, 42, director of operations, the accessibility is reassuring. She nurses her 6-month-old daughter at lunch, and she can get from her desk to the center in only three minutes. "They really treat my kids like their own," says Hare, whose 2½-year-old son also attends.

Other perks:

- Chefs in the corporate cafeterias cook any dish to order and maintain profiles of all staffers with food allergies.

- Expectant parents are given free pagers through the company's Baby Beep program. In 2002, 470 workers used beepers to stay in touch with spouses and child-care providers. Bristol-Myers also offers free baby formula (like Enfamil, which is manufactured by a division of the company) to all parents throughout a child's first year;

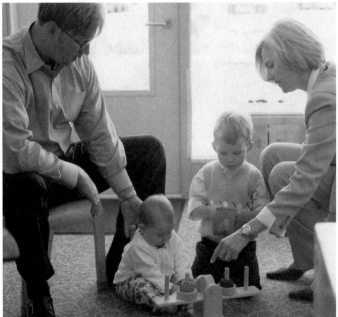

Judianne Hare with husband, Tom, and children Charlotte (left) and Cole in one of Bristol-Myers Squibb's corporate day-care centers.

lactation rooms are available as well for breast-feeding moms.

•The company's fitness center provides T-shirts, shorts, and tube socks so that employees don't have to lug sweaty gear to and from work.

3 MAKING FITNESS FUN, NOT WORK
SC Johnson; Racine, Wisconsin
Total employees: 3,364 (37-percent female)
One of the world's leading makers of housecleaning products, such as Pledge and Windex, this 117-year-old family company reminds employees that a workout doesn't have to feel like work. For $9.25 a month, they can shoot hoops, play softball, or enjoy miniature golf at the corporate-owned, 146-acre Charles Armstrong Park, seven miles from SC Johnson's main and satellite campuses. To further encourage workers to be active, the annual Bike to Work Week, held each July, rewards those who commute on two wheels with a healthy breakfast and gift certificates to a local bike shop. "I'm usually energized after riding to work," says Shemiele Da'Briel, 25, a senior financial analyst. "This week of exercise really motivates me to stay in shape for the summer."

Other perks:
•The on-site Herbert J. Louis Medical Center offers free cancer screenings, blood profiles, and psychological counseling, among other preventive-health services. The clinic also covers up to $200 per year for acupuncture and up to $10,000 for infertility treatments, including artificial insemination, in vitro fertilization, and embryo transfer.
•The company's Sick Child Care program provides parents up to $500 per child each year to go toward inpatient hospital care.
•To help employees who do not work on the main campus stay in shape, the company will pay up to $230 per year for either in-home exercise equipment or membership at a local health club.

4 MAKING THE IMPOSSIBLE POSSIBLE
ARUP Laboratories; Salt Lake City
Total employees: 1,471 (59-percent female)
When Kathi Jones, 45, a projects specialist who has worked at this national medical laboratory for two years, was nominated by her family to be a torch-bearer at the Salt Lake City Olympics in 2001, she was more stressed-out than excited. After all, she hadn't broken a sweat since 1997 because of chronic back trouble, and she was 20 pounds overweight. But ARUP's two part-time wellness coordinators prepped her for the challenge. One of them put together an after-work exercise plan for Jones combining strength-training workouts and stationary-bike sessions at the company gym. In addition, a weight-management class held in a conference room helped her make more sensible diet choices. "We met weekly and brainstormed menus and recipes," Jones says. She completed the two-mile Olympic run, lost the 20 pounds (and has kept them off), and continues to work out regularly.

Other perks:

- A corporate health clinic handles routine physicals, well-child checkups, vaccinations, Pap smears, blood work, allergy shots, and more, all free. Nearly 600 people, including workers, dependents, and retirees, visit the center each month. A separate on-site pharmacy cuts back on drugstore runs, too.
- Project 0, an annual six-week program, helps employees work toward the goal of zero weight gain during the holidays. In 2002, 234 people participated; 163 of them maintained their weight, and some even lost a couple of pounds.

5 GIVING WORKERS TIME (LOTS OF IT) TO RECHARGE

Genentech; South San Francisco, California
Total employees: 5,400 (51-percent female)
This biotech company encourages its employees to develop professional skills and take time for personal reflection. To that end, Genentech offers a six-week sabbatical, with full pay and benefits, to workers who've been on the job for six years or

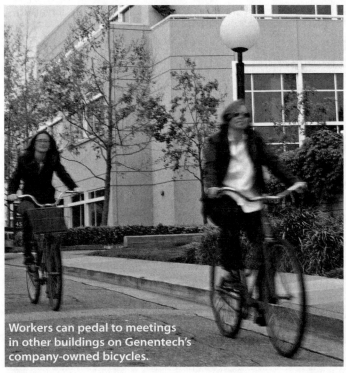

Workers can pedal to meetings in other buildings on Genentech's company-owned bicycles.

longer. Margaret Corkery, 45, a senior financial analyst, recently used her sabbatical to travel around Europe with her husband and two teenagers. They spent much of the trip in Ireland, visiting with relatives for the first time and researching the family's Irish ancestors. "I wouldn't have been able to leave a job and go without a paycheck to do this," Corkery says. "Also, someone replaces you at the office, so you don't have the worry of coming back and facing an overflowing in-box."

Other perks:

- Once a week, a dental van pulls up and offers free cleanings, X-rays, fillings, and whitening. Over the last two years, about 450 employees have visited the traveling dentist.
- To reduce traffic and conserve energy—and to make getting from one building to another quick and easy—staffers can ride one of at least 15 company-owned bikes around the office complex. Started in 1996 by an employee, the GenenClunker/Blue Bike program transforms old donated bicycles into worthy wheels.

6 "SUPPORT STAFF" TAKES ON NEW MEANING

New York Life Insurance Co., New York City
Total employees: 7,512 (54-percent female)
At New York Life, one of the largest insurance companies in the world (and one of *Health*'s top 10 companies in 2002), a continually expanding roster of support groups helps staff deal with personal challenges. Topics include elder care, parenting special-needs children, and infertility. Director of marketing Anna Evangelista, 42, relied on this support network to help her when she and her husband were trying to start a family eight years ago. After attempting unsuccessfully to conceive naturally and enduring three years of in vitro fertilization treatments, Evangelista eventually got some good news; today, she's the mother of a

5-year-old daughter. "When I think back to that time, I think of despair," says Evangelista, who has now been at New York Life for 24 years. "The company stood by me and arranged for me to go on medical leave. I was also lucky to have counseling available on-site."

Other perks:

- An on-premises health center staffed by four full-time physicians offers free physiotherapy, X rays, mental-health care, fertility injections, and oncological blood work.
- The Maternity Transition Program provides new moms three weeks of low-cost child care ($30 per day) at the company day-care center, giving parents some time to investigate and select long-term options.
- Workers can learn how to make healthy lifestyle changes in the four-week Active for Life program. To kick off the course, the instructor measures participants' body fat, weight, and blood pressure, then helps them set realistic goals. Each week, the class focuses on a particular issue, such as stress, nutrition, or fitness. During the final week, vital stats are measured again to track employees' progress.

7 FROM THE CONFERENCE ROOM TO THE EXAMINATION TABLE

Roche; Nutley, New Jersey
Total employees: 4,992 (51-percent female)

In 2002, the Employee Health Services center at this pharmaceutical company logged nearly 12,000 visits, and women made over half of those appointments. The center, staffed by three full-time physicians, four registered nurses, a lab technician, and an X-ray technician, offers a wide range of services, including estrogen-replacement therapy and menopause counseling, pelvic and breast exams, and Pap smears.

Other perks:

- Each day, the 785-seat cafeteria serves a variety of "Health Entrées" that contain fewer than 500 calories and under 15 grams of fat. After you order five healthy meals, you get one free.
- The low cost ($22 per month) and central location of the 10,000-square-foot fitness center lets employees squeeze in a midday or after-5 workout.
- Company-sponsored child care has been available since 1977, when Roche opened one of the first such facilities in the country. The Child Care Center includes a certified full-day kindergarten.

How We Selected the Winners

Health insurance and generous maternity, vacation, and sick leave policies are standards at good companies. But we weren't simply looking for good; we were looking for *great*—corporations that are truly helping women cope with the most pressing challenge in their lives: balance. So, with the help of Gail L. Choate, president of Synergies, along with a panel of the nation's top work/life experts, we created a six-page questionnaire. The document evaluated each company's benefits in six key areas: preventive health, fitness, weight management, career mobility, work/life balance, and office culture. We solicited nominations at Health.com and the Web site for the Society for Human Resources, as well as through newspapers and other media outlets nationwide. Candidates were also asked to submit supporting materials demonstrating the effectiveness of programs and policies. Based on the questionnaire, we assigned each company a score out of a possible 100. Our panel evaluated the top contenders anonymously, highlighting the initiatives they believe had the most impact, and whittled down the list to the top 10. Then we did some digging and on-site reporting, talking to employees to find out the real story. The final ranking combines the questionnaire score, the judges' input, and our take on what's *really* helping women balance their lives.

8 HELPING EMPLOYEES BREATHE EASIER

Verizon Wireless; Bedminster, New Jersey
Total employees: 41,670 (52-percent female)
In 2002, this national wireless company became the first corporation to offer FreshStart, the American Cancer Society's smoking-cessation program. So far, 140 employees have taken the class; Jennifer Swinson, 31, a former 2½-pack-a-day smoker who started her habit at 13, vouches for its success. "I used to sneak smokes—I'd tell people I'd quit, but would keep smoking," Swinson says. In 2002, a coach at one of Verizon's fitness centers encouraged Swinson, who also suffered from asthma and relied on three different inhalers to get through the day, to take the class. "Now that I've quit, I never have to use my inhaler," says Swinson, a lead coordinator in the credit department who has been at Verizon for four years. "The company saved my life."

Other perks:

- Verizon eases the financial strain of starting—or adding on to—a family by covering all prenatal care (except the first $10 co-pay) and delivery expenses.
- For $15 a month, employees can work out at one of the company's 13 fully equipped fitness centers nationwide. At locations too small for a center, Verizon offers discounted memberships at local fitness clubs. Each time an employee uses the gym, she earns points that go toward incentives, such as massages and free gym memberships.
- Regular seminars, such as "How to Cope with Stress Through Laughter" and "How to Develop Your Sense of Humor," help keep the office vibe on the lighter side.

9 TEACHING BY EXAMPLE

Green Mountain; College, Poultney, Vermont
Total employees: 160 (53-percent female)
At this environmentally minded liberal arts college, a two-year-old wellness center offers professors and staff an array of alternative tension-taming treatments and classes at bargain prices. In addition to the usual roster of yoga and massage,

Our Panelists

Pamela M. Ballo, founder of Juxtapose, an organization dedicated to helping companies establish successful work/life initiatives

Peter G. Burki, co-founder and CEO of LifeCare, Inc., a firm that offers work/life programs nationwide

Gail L. Choate, president of Synergies, a health-promotion company specializing in corporate and community wellness programs

Alice D. Domar, Ph.D., Health Relationships columnist, assistant professor at Harvard Medical School, and director of the Mind/Body Center for Women's Health at Boston IVF, Department of Obstetrics and Gynecology, Beth Israel Deaconess Medical Center

Jackie Newgent, R.D., New York City-based dietitian, chef, and food-industry consultant specializing in nutrition communications

Sarah Nichols, national director of program development at Health Fitness Corporation, a provider of corporate health, fitness, and wellness services based in Minneapolis

Robert Rosen, Ph.D., founder and CEO of Healthy Companies International, a research and consulting company based in Washington, D.C.

Stephanie Trapp, executive director of the Alliance for Work-Life Progress, an Alexandria, Virginia–based organization that promotes work/family balance

Neil Treister, M.D., cardiologist and co-founder/medical director of Salus Heart and Wellness, a San Diego firm that provides work/life programs focusing on heart health and stress management

employees can try out such stress busters as reiki ($20 an hour); acupuncture ($5 a session); and the New Age dancers' workout, Neuromuscular Integrative Action, commonly known as Nia ($5 a session). "We may work hard, but one of our jobs is also to demonstrate balance to our students," says environmental-studies professor Rebecca Purdom, 33, who has been at Green Mountain full-time for three years. "We can be intense professionals, but we can also take the time to attend a yoga session during lunch."

Other perks:

- Picking up fresh vegetables for a dinner is as easy as visiting the campus co-op, which sells produce from the school's 10,000-square-foot garden.
- The only doctor in town works at the college's health clinic, which offers such services as blood work, pregnancy tests, Pap tests, and UTI screenings. Walk-ins are always welcome.

10 A TRUE FAMILY FOCUS
Guidant Corp.; Indianapolis
Total employees: 11,029 (47-percent female)
The managers at Guidant Corp. know that a large part of taking care of its workforce means watching out for their entire families. The company, which manufactures medical devices—such as heart pacemakers and defibrillators—offers employees up to 40 hours of paid leave per calendar month to care for ill or injured family members. The office culture is also very kid-friendly—children are welcome at all times, and families get together for monthly movie nights in on-site auditoriums. "My kids get really excited when I tell them it's movie night at work," says Wendy Freeberg, a 33-year-old mother of three who has been with the company for 12 years. "It's always a really easy, relaxing, and cheap outing for all of us."

Other perks:

- Guidant Reaches Out to Women (GROW), a company-sponsored educational program, spreads the latest word on heart disease to its employees through regular seminars and free cholesterol screenings.
- To help make shopping for healthy foods easy and fun, once a week the company van shuttles staffers to a local farmers' market where they can pick from fresh produce. ■

Passive Smoke: Killer or Not?

If you're the type who asks to be moved when you're seated next to a smoker in a restaurant, you might be surprised by a recent study in the *British Medical Journal.* Years of solid data have shown the health dangers of secondhand smoke, but this controversial report found that the nonsmoking spouses of smokers were at no greater risk of tobacco-related illness and death than non-smokers whose partners also abstained.

But before you stop worrying about being around all that smoke, consider this: Tobacco companies funded the research. "I would feel more comfortable if there was no conflict of interest," says Norman H. Edelman, M.D., scientific-affairs consultant to the American Lung Association. Most importantly, he says, the study was flawed. "The definition of secondhand smoke was very simplistic, putting people who got minimal exposure in the same category as those with high exposure," he says. The annoying puffer next to you at dinner probably won't affect your health, but you can still be assured that living with a smoker will.

Sobering Up May Take Longer Than You Think

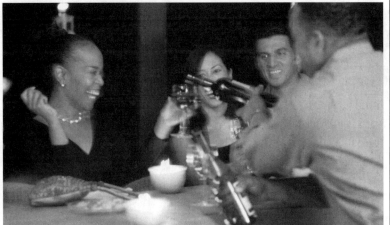

Researchers at McGill University in Montreal have found that drinking heavily may impair people's thinking even after they no longer feel drunk. Scientists gave volunteers either placebos or enough booze—the equivalent of three screwdrivers—to make them legally intoxicated. Then they tested the subjects' ability to reason, plan, and make decisions while tipsy, drunk, and sober. The participants performed poorly even after they said they felt clear-headed. The researchers suggest that after drinking, people should wait up to six hours before they get behind the wheel or make any big decisions.

Weight—Not Sugar—Increases Risk of Diabetes

You've probably heard that your love of sweets could increase your risk of diabetes. But contrary to expectations, women who reported eating the least sugar (less than 35 grams a day—approximately 2^1/$_2$ tablespoons sugar, or about one 12-ounce cola) were no less likely to develop Type 2 diabetes, the most common form of the disease, than those who ate the most (up to 100 grams daily, 7 tablespoons, or four candy bars), according to Harvard University's ongoing Women's Health Study. The researchers reviewed the daily food logs of 38,480 female health professionals ages 45 and older, and tallied the women's sugar intake from such sweet treats as candy bars, as well as from fruits, vegetables, and milk. The conclusion: The real key to preventing diabetes is maintaining a healthy weight, not shunning sugar, the study authors say.

Q + A

SMOG CONCERNS

If I'm healthy and don't have any lung problems, do I need to worry about ozone alerts and Air Quality Index reports?

Listen up when you hear these announcements on the radio. On high-ozone days (which usually occur in the summer, because heat and sunlight speed up ozone formation), anyone can have breathing problems. If you live in a big city, you may also hear the Air Quality Index, or AQI, which measures pollutants in the air. (The federal government requires these daily reports for cities of 350,000 people or more.) If the AQI is predicted to be higher than 150, which is "code red," even healthy people should be extra careful outdoors. Exercising outside can make your airways tighten, leaving you wheezing, or irritate your nostrils, making you more vulnerable to colds and viruses. It can also inflame the lining of your lungs, causing scarring over time and breathing problems later in life. Even if you feel fine when ozone and pollution levels are high, you don't want to make the situation worse for other people by driving more than you have to, filling your gas tank during the day, or grilling outdoors.

10 Questions You Must Ask Before Choosing

Health Insurance

Discover how you can save money (and time) with your bills.

BY KAREN J. BANNAN

A recent gallup poll found that 62 percent of Americans surveyed think the federal government should ensure health-care coverage for everyone. Until that becomes the case (and it probably won't happen anytime soon), ask these questions, which can help you choose the best plan for your needs—and your wallet—from Jim Walsh, editor of *Hassle-Free Health Coverage: How to Buy the Right Medical Insurance Cheaply and Effectively.*

1 HOW OFTEN DO YOU GO TO THE DOCTOR?

If you are under age 45, have a healthy family history, and see the doctor only once a year for a checkup, elect traditional (non-HMO) coverage. "It's usually the cheaper option for young, healthy people, even though you'll probably incur more out-of-pocket expenses for doctor visits," Walsh says. "But if you visit the doctor often because you're older or have a chronic condition, co-payments and diagnostic-test fees, which are often only partially covered, can add up."

2 ARE YOU GETTING MARRIED, STARTING A FAMILY, OR TAKING CARE OF AN ELDERLY PARENT?

Find out how much it costs to add a dependent. If you're thinking about having a baby, make sure your preferred hospital is covered. Also, look into the insurance company's well-child policy. Some offer free or low-cost exams and vaccinations.

3 DO YOU HAVE A CHRONIC CONDITION, SUCH AS ASTHMA, DIABETES, OR CANCER?

Some plans won't pick up any charges related to pre-existing conditions for at least six months from the date you sign up. Also ask about the procedure for covering genetic diseases in case a need arises.

4 DO YOU TAKE PRESCRIPTIONS DAILY?

If so, stick with a managed-care plan that has low co-pays, offers a bulk discount, or includes a medicine-by-mail program. If you fill only one or two prescriptions each year, opt for a plan that has less extensive—and expensive—coverage.

5 IS YOUR DOCTOR REALLY ON THE PLAN YOU'RE CONSIDERING?

Don't trust the provider directory. Ask her if she accepts the plan and if she intends to stick with it. Doctors often drop plans if their compensation changes or paperwork starts weighing them down.

6 DOES THE PLAN MONITOR ITS DOCTORS?

Ask a customer-service representative if physicians are rated and whether or not the company records complaints. A reputable firm will use this information to drop doctors who fail to meet minimum requirements or who have multiple complaints against them.

7 HOW MUCH DOES THE PLAN COST YOUR EMPLOYER?

The answer doesn't matter that much when you're on staff, but if you get laid off and pick up COBRA coverage, it definitely will. When you elect a COBRA plan, which most employers legally must offer, you pay the entire premium plus a small administration fee.

8 WOULD YOU RATHER INK IT, OR POINT AND CLICK?

Many companies are adding online components that can eliminate paperwork completely. If you hate filling out forms of any kind, look for a plan that requires little or no input from consumers (such as an HMO or PPO).

9 HOW FAST DOES THE INSURANCE COMPANY PAY ITS BILLS?

If the plan doesn't pay your physician within 60 days, she can ask you to pay her out-of-pocket. Slow-paying companies are also more likely to deny valid charges in hopes that you'll pick up the tab, Walsh says. Ask your doctor how quickly she's paid.

10 DO YOU WANT ACCESS TO THE MOST ADVANCED MEDICINES?

Ask about the company's position on experimental or alternative therapies. Some insurance providers limit coverage of unproven drugs or the latest cancer treatments, which are often extremely expensive.

Split Pills, Cut Costs

Even doctors know prescriptions cost too much. Now they're helping people do something about it. More and more docs are doubling drug dosages, allowing patients to split each pill in half and make their prescriptions last longer. For example, suppose you take 10 milligrams a day of the blood pressure medicine Zestril. A monthly supply of 30 tablets might cost you $340 a year. If your doctor prescribed the 20-milligram pills instead, you could take half a tablet each day.

Your stash would last twice as long, and you'd save up to $170.

Still, "pill splitting shouldn't be a universal policy," cautions Randall Stafford, M.D., Ph.D., a Stanford University researcher who headed a study listing 11 common meds that can be safely halved. Talking to your doctor is a must—and so is investing in a tablet cutter, a small, guillotine-like device that helps ensure accuracy and is available at drugstores for less than $5.

The Uninsured Aren't Always Poor

If you think only poor people aren't insured, consider these figures from the latest U.S. Census: From 2000 to 2001, the number of Americans without health coverage grew by 1.4 million people, most of whom lived in households with incomes of $75,000 or more. The survey didn't ask participants why they lost coverage, but we'd wager that the faltering economy was partially to blame. What is clear: These days, being uninsured is a problem no one can afford to ignore.

67

Don't Be a Victim

Medical mistakes kill thousands of people each year. Here's how to protect yourself.

BY FRAN SMITH

A 39-year-old health journalist in Boston receives a massive overdose of a breast-cancer drug and dies. A 46-year-old Wisconsin woman is mistakenly diagnosed with cancer and undergoes an unnecessary double mastectomy. A desperately ill 17-year-old girl from Mexico gets a heart-lung transplant at Duke University Medical Center in Durham, North Carolina, one of America's finest hospitals—but the new organs do not match her blood type. Two weeks later, Jesica Santillán is dead.

Every few years, a medical fiasco makes headlines, and people quietly wonder: Could it happen to me?

The question is reasonable, and that makes it all the more frightening. You're more likely to die from a medical mistake than in a car wreck. In hospitals

Mistakes happen when a patient feels too shy or silly to talk about a symptom, the doctor dismisses a complaint that turns out to be serious, or the patient is confused about the doctor's instructions.

alone, errors kill 44,000 to 98,000 patients a year and injure hundreds of thousands more, according to a 1999 report by the Institute of Medicine (IOM). (In comparison, roughly 42,000 people die on the roads annually.) But the mishaps most likely to harm you are not the kind that land on the front page. They're often pedestrian—a misfiled test result, a bungled prescription.

"These things may seem trivial, but they're important," says Susan Dovey, Ph.D., M.P.H., an analyst at the Robert Graham Center: Policy Studies in Family Practice and Primary Care in Washington, D.C.

Fortunately, you can protect yourself. What are the errors you're most likely to encounter, and how can you avoid them? Read on.

MEDICATION MIX-UPS

About 7,000 people die a year because they receive the wrong medicine, the wrong dose, a drug they're allergic to, or one that reacts badly with others they're taking, according to the IOM. This is a big problem not only in hospitals but also doctors' offices. To keep it from happening to you:

Tell your doctor what you're taking. Include over-the-counter (OTC) medications, herbs, and nutritional supplements. Better yet, make a list at home and bring it with you, advises the National Quality Forum (NQF), a coalition of leading hospital, physician, consumer, and research organizations.

Make sure you can read the drug name and dose on the prescription your doctor gives you. Studies show that 10 to 20 percent of prescriptions are illegible. Also ask your doctor to include the medication's purpose. Few physicians are in the habit, but it's a simple precaution against a common problem: mixing up similarly named products designed for different conditions. Such sound-alikes number in the hundreds.

Check the label on the bottle when you pick up your pills. Talk to the pharmacist if the name, dose, or instructions aren't what you expected. Dispensing errors are common, says a May 2003 report by the NQF. Here's one example, reported by the Institute for Safe Medication Practices, a nonprofit organization that collects anonymous reports of medication errors from doctors, hospitals, and pharmacies: A doctor called in a prescription for Zetia to lower a patient's cholesterol. The pharmacist misread the order and gave the patient Zestril, which lowers blood pressure. He repeated the mistake on three refills as her cholesterol rose to dangerous levels.

Look closely at drug patches. They come in many varieties, along with a wide range of instructions about where and how to apply them. Clear ones are particularly hazardous, because they're hard to find when you need to replace or remove them. The U.S. Food and Drug Administration recommends avoiding clear patches altogether.

Pay special attention to OTC cold, allergy, and pain medications. A top seller may come in drops, liquid, pills, capsules, daytime and nighttime formulations, and strengths for infants, children, and adults. You could easily pluck the wrong stuff off the store shelf or grab the wrong bottle out of the medicine chest in the middle of the night. Failing to check labels carefully can be dangerous to adults and kids alike. (About 27,000 children a year accidentally overdose on acetaminophen, the main ingredient in Tylenol.)

TROUBLE WITH TESTS

Lab slips labeled with the wrong patient's name, lost test reports, abnormal results the patient never hears about: Mistakes such as these happen routinely because so many opportunities for error exist. The doctor orders the test, a nurse draws your blood, the technician analyzes it, the clerk mails the report to your doctor, the receptionist opens the envelope—and information can be lost or mishandled at any step. So be sure to:

Follow up. If you don't hear back after a blood test, scan, or routine screening, such as a Pap smear or

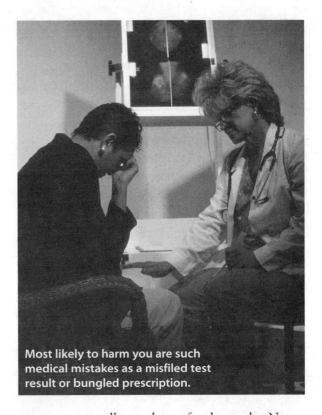

Most likely to harm you are such medical mistakes as a misfiled test result or bungled prescription.

mammogram, call your doctor for the results. No news isn't necessarily good news; it might mean the results were lost, says Dovey, whose study of errors in family practice was published in 2002 in the journal *Quality and Safety in Health Care.* Dovey asked 42 physicians to anonymously record errors in their offices for 20 weeks. One doctor couldn't find an address or phone number for a patient whose skin biopsy showed melanoma. In another case, a biopsy of a breast lump revealed cancer, but the clerk misfiled the report. "It wasn't discovered until eight months later, by which time the cancer had progressed," Dovey says. "That is, unfortunately, not an uncommon scenario."

Get it in writing. Even if you do receive the call or postcard confirming you're in the clear, ask for a copy of the full report. You'll have a record if the doctor loses his copy. You'll read it even if the doctor doesn't because of a clerical foul-up. And with annual cancer-screening tests, you may notice a change worth discussing with your doctor, despite a normal result.

Marie Savard, M.D., a Philadelphia internist and author of *How to Save Your Own Life: The Savard System for Managing and Controlling Your Health Care*, tells the story of a friend who tracked her husband's PSA (prostate-specific antigen) count. It doubled within a year to the high end of normal. She called the doctor, who agreed that the increase warranted more tests. They confirmed prostate cancer, catching it a year earlier than they likely would have without the wife's vigilance, Savard says. "Sometimes, borderline readings really matter."

Have your mammogram double-checked. Skilled mammographers detect tumors in only 70 to 75 percent of cases. The best way to ensure an accurate reading is to visit a center that uses computer-aided

Trust your instincts. Most people don't worry without reason. When a doctor tells you not to worry, it means either "I'm busy" or "I don't know." Push for attention until you're satisfied.

detection (CAD), explains Daniel Sullivan, M.D., associate director of the National Cancer Institute's Biomedical Imaging Program. This technology, in which a computer flags any suspicious spots for the radiologist, increases accuracy by 5 to 20 percent, studies show. Because CAD isn't widely used yet, though, you may have trouble finding a facility that offers it. In that case, go to a center where two radiologists independently review each film—double reading increases cancer detection by at least 5 percent.

A Brother's Legacy
How the loss of one child helped a mother save another.

When Ilene Corina looks back on her firstborn son's final days—the routine tonsillectomy, the recurrent bleeding, the doctors who told her to stop worrying, almost until the moment he died—one thing is clear. "They just didn't take me seriously," she says.

Michael's death in 1990, at age 3, taught Corina more than anyone should ever have to know about medical fallibility. But through her loss, she learned a lesson about her own strength—and how to use it to obtain lifesaving medical care.

Three years later, when Corina was 22 weeks pregnant with her third child, her womb began leaking fluid. Doctors said the

baby couldn't be saved and recommended that she deliver a dead fetus. But she refused. The obstetricians suggested a risky procedure to push back the fetus. Corina agreed, but she insisted that a senior physician do it.

It worked temporarily, but a week later she went into labor. Matthew weighed 1 pound, 7 ounces at birth. The neonatal specialists urged Corina and her husband to let him die peacefully. Corina wanted all-out care, and she virtually moved into the newborn intensive care unit to make sure he got it.

The baby spent 145 days in the hospital. Corina tracked the doctors' every move. When she saw

residents poke around her son's eyes to see whether weeks on oxygen had damaged them, she asked what they would do if they found a problem. "Nothing," they said. "So stop," she replied. She also taped notes to his incubator ordering no eye testing. Friendly nurses whispered advice: Don't let first-year residents touch the baby; some third-years are OK.

Matthew is 10 now. The only signs of his ordeal are the scars on his face and body. "I call them his 'love marks,'" Corina says. "He wouldn't be here if we didn't love him." And he wouldn't be here if his mother hadn't turned her own painful scar tissue into muscle and found the courage to flex it.

WRONG DIAGNOSIS OR TREATMENT

Patients must be able to trust their doctors. But even the best physician can miss a diagnosis or recommend the wrong treatment, says Ilene Corina, founder of the New York chapter of PULSE (Persons United Limiting Substandards and Errors in Health Care), an advocacy organization. In Dovey's study, 13 percent of mistakes involved misdiagnosis, incorrect treatment, or botched procedures. To protect yourself:

<u>Make sure any doctor</u> you're considering is board-certified. Contact the American Board of Medical Specialties (866-275-2267 or www.abms.org; click on "Who's Certified"). As an extra precaution, find out whether the doctor has ever been disciplined by the state in which he practices. Generally, only egregious negligence or misconduct merits disciplinary action—as with the Virginia fertility specialist who impregnated patients with his own sperm, for instance—so if you find sanctions on a physician's record, go elsewhere. An excellent online resource is the Federation of State Medical Boards' Web site (www.fsmb.org; click on "State Medical Board Info," then "Board Directory" to connect to local sites).

<u>Choose a practitioner who listens,</u> respects your concerns, and answers questions in language you understand. Mistakes happen when a patient feels too shy or silly to talk about a symptom, the doctor dismisses a complaint that turns out to be serious, or the patient is confused about the doctor's instructions.

<u>Bring a pal to your appointment.</u> When faced with anything but the simplest illness, people often feel so overwhelmed or frightened that they forget what they planned to ask and what the doctor advised. Susan Love, M.D., the well-known breast-cancer expert, suggests bringing your most obnoxious friend—the one who's never afraid to speak her mind.

<u>Don't settle for the answering service.</u> If you feel sick (or worried) enough to call your doctor at night or on a weekend, make sure you actually speak to him or

In the Hospital

These easy research tips can help ensure a safe stay.

Everyone is likely to stay in a hospital someday or have a loved one there. When that time comes, go where the experience is. Years of research show that for a range of surgical procedures, including angioplasty and many cancer operations, patients find the best results at hospitals that perform them often. The National Quality Forum urges doctors to refer high-risk surgery patients to centers with "intensivists" on staff. Johns Hopkins University researchers found that patients undergoing complicated abdominal surgery were up to three times as likely to survive if the intensive-care unit employed one of these doctors—who are specifically trained in intensive care—as patients in hospitals without this benefit. Only 1 in 10 hospitals has these specialists, though the proportion is likely to grow.

Accreditation is also a crucial indicator of hospital safety. Quality Check, the consumer Web site of the Joint Commission on Accreditation of Healthcare Organizations, is simple to use. Go to www.jcaho.org/qualitycheck/directry/directry.asp; type in the hospital's name to see whether it comes up.

Teaching hospitals have the greatest expertise in surgery and intensive care. But they also have doctors in training, fresh out of medical school. If you have reservations about anything a resident does, ask to talk to the attending physician. Each new class of residents starts July 1. If you have a choice, schedule your surgery from January through June.

Finally, having a friend or relative stay by your side tremendously lowers the risk of a mistake, says internist Marie Savard, M.D., author of a book on avoiding medical errors. Many people have trouble asking someone to sit with them when they're sick. But those same people likely wouldn't think twice about dropping everything to be with someone they care about. So don't be afraid to ask—if you're facing a hospital stay yourself—or to organize shifts of friends and family to visit the person you love.

her. A study published in March 2003 in *The Journal of Family Practice* found that 10 percent of calls picked up by an answering service never got through to doctors. At least half of those callers reported serious symptoms, including chest pain, recurring vomiting, and labor contractions. Americans make 50 to 100 million after-hours calls a year; even a small percentage who don't get the attention they require translates to millions of potentially dangerous delays in care.

If your diagnosis is serious, use the Internet. The National Guideline Clearinghouse (www.guideline.gov) lists treatment recommendations based on the latest scientific evidence. That site is geared to health professionals; if you want reliable, accessible information that's easier to digest, check the Web sites of medical-specialty organizations. A *New England Journal of Medicine* study underscores the importance of being armed with all the facts: Researchers at Rand Corporation found that, on average, patients receive only about half the care called for in guidelines for diagnosing, treating, and preventing 30 common conditions.

If your physician refers you to a specialist, ask why she singled out that particular doctor. Referrals are made for all sorts of reasons, including some that

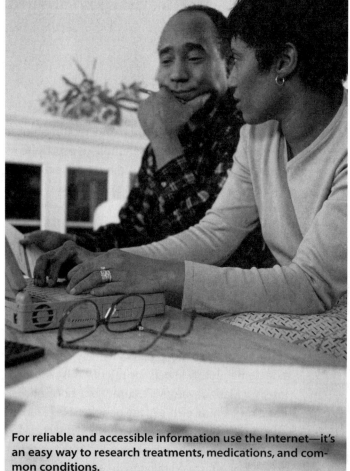

For reliable and accessible information use the Internet—it's an easy way to research treatments, medications, and common conditions.

have nothing to do with your condition, such as pressures from the hospital or HMO. You want a specialist with experience in cases such as yours and who performs the procedure you need.

Request a second opinion before any major treatment. Doctors are sometimes reluctant to second-guess their colleagues, so for a truly independent evaluation, see a specialist who practices in another community or is affiliated with a different hospital.

THE **FINAL** WORD

Whether you're dealing with a chronic complaint or a life-threatening emergency, trust your instincts. If the voice in your head insists something's not right, it probably isn't. Push for attention until you're satisfied.

"I've often heard the words 'don't worry,'" says Corina, whose 3-year-old son bled to death after a tonsillectomy though four doctors at three hospitals insisted he was fine. "I don't just worry for no reason. Most people don't. When a doctor tells me not to worry, it means one of two things: 'I'm busy' or 'I don't know.'" ▪

New Treatment Offers Relief from Hay Fever

When ragweed is at its peak in mid-August, that means hay fever, with its sneezing and itchy eyes, for many of the 40 million Americans who have allergies. For those who take allergy shots, ragweed season means another round of injections. But a medicine being tested in clinical trials could offer relief for several years—or even indefinitely.

In a study sponsored by the Immune Tolerance Network, people who received a single course (six shots in six weeks) of an experimental vaccine called AIC prior to the 2001 ragweed season reported markedly fewer allergy symptoms than the group receiving placebo injections. Relief lasted through the entire 2002 season as well, with no booster treatments required.

Unlike conventional treatments, in which doctors inject people with whatever they are allergic to and hope they develop tolerance, the vaccine consists of Amb a 1, the main protein and allergy trigger in ragweed, to which small pieces of synthetic DNA have been added to reduce inflammation. This combination bolsters the immune response and turns off allergic reactions. "What's exciting is that with a brief regimen, we induced long-term tolerance," says the principal investigator for the trial, Peter Creticos, M.D., clinical director of Johns Hopkins University's Division of Allergy and Clinical Immunology.

The shots won't be available for a few years, but Creticos eventually hopes to reach more allergy sufferers—as well as asthmatics—with vaccines for allergies to grass, dust mites, and cats.

Dogs Cause More Allergy Misery Than Cats

Cats make more people sneeze than dogs do, but the sniffling and wheezing are likely to be more intense for those allergic to canines, according to new research from Penn State College of Medicine. The scientists exposed 809 people with asthma to dog or cat dander, among other substances; the former triggered the greatest release of nitric oxide in subjects' lungs and caused the most immune cells to appear in phlegm—two signs of inflammation. To make breathing less of a chore, the researchers recommend trying such allergy medicines as Allegra and Claritin, changing your sheets often, and kicking Fido out of bed, where allergens can get trapped and worsen symptoms.

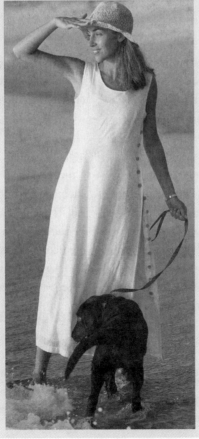

Fighting Hay Fever with Nasal Filters?

Researchers in Australia have come up with a novel way to fight hay fever: nose plugs. Allergy sufferers place a plastic device in each nostril, and a sticky filter keeps out pollen. The contraptions do their job well, but we wonder who on earth would wear these in public.

How to
SHOP
the Drugstore

Try these aisle-by-aisle instructions for finding the best products.

BY LAMBETH HOCHWALD

If a simple trip to your local drugstore leaves you feeling dizzier than if you'd spent all night at a '70s disco party, it's no wonder. The aisles are stocked with more than 600 over-the-counter (OTC) products. All of them promise to help you feel better fast, and Americans are buying into the claims. According to a recent survey conducted by the Consumer Healthcare Products Association, a Washington, D.C.-based trade organization representing manufacturers and distributors of OTC medications, nearly 80 percent of Americans reported using one of these remedies to get rid of aches or pains—almost twice the number who talked with a doctor or took a prescription drug.

To separate the best buys from the duds, we asked 10 health experts from all over the country what they look for when they visit the drugstore. In this article, we examine the best products on the allergy-and-sinus, women's health, and first-aid aisles.

ALLERGY & SINUS

your problem: **Itchy, watery eyes; runny nose; rashes; or sneezing caused by allergies**

what to look for: Antihistamines, which block the chemicals that trigger allergic reactions

best buys: Claritin is the most effective treatment for a runny nose or congestion; it can also help control sneezing fits and relieve nose, throat, eye, and ear itches. For rashes, choose Chlor-Trimeton or Benadryl. "Everyone should have Benadryl in their medicine chests," says Marjorie L. Slankard, M.D., associate attending physician and co-director of the Allergy Clinic at New York-Presbyterian Hospital

cold or allergy? Do you experience itchy eyes, a runny nose, and nonstop sneezing during certain times of the year? Do you have clear phlegm (yellow usually indicates a virus, green a bacterial infection)? If these symptoms linger more than a week, allergies are probably to blame.

in New York City. "It's excellent for acute, severe reactions."

<u>keep in mind:</u> Benadryl and other antihistamines that contain diphenhydramine will make you drowsy. Add a glass of wine to the mix, and you might be out before dinner makes it to the table.

<u>your problem:</u> **A stuffy nose due to the common cold**

<u>what to look for:</u> Decongestants with pseudoephedrine reduce the nasal swelling that can make breathing a chore.

<u>best buys:</u> Sudafed 12 Hour for lasting relief. "The shorter-acting formula is a good option," Slankard says. "You'll get less medicine, but if you need relief right away, it works faster." To avoid the jitters that some of these products cause, try Vicks VapoRub or Afrin Saline Extra-Moisturizing Nasal Spray, a nonmedicated spray with moisturizers that soothe a dry, irritated nose.

<u>keep in mind:</u> Many OTC decongestants contain pseudoephedrine hydrochloride, which makes some people feel hyper. Doctors suggest that you take these medicines first thing in the morning; otherwise, you may be up all night. Other potential side effects include nervousness, dizziness, and headache.

> **be wary: nasal sprays** Medicated nasal sprays (used for three to five days at a time) will temporarily relieve congestion, but you can easily become dependent on them.

If you have a history of glaucoma, high blood pressure, diabetes, thyroid problems, or any type of heart problem, talk with your doctor before using decongestants, as they can speed up your heart rate. For a drug-free solution, try steaming your sinuses before you go to bed. Vicks' Personal Steam Inhaler can help you breathe easy while you sleep.

<u>your problem:</u> **Pressure and pain around forehead, eyes, or cheeks caused by sinus headache**

<u>what to look for:</u> Ibuprofen or acetaminophen to relieve your pain

<u>best buys:</u> Advil (ibuprofen) helps sinus inflammation as well as pain; Tylenol (acetaminophen) works only on your headache.

<u>keep in mind:</u> If you're already taking a decongestant for your sinus stuffiness, avoid two-in-one remedies, such as Tylenol Sinus, if your head hurts. These products contain the same active ingredient (pseudoephedrine), and a double dose of it can make you feel shaky. Stick with plain old acetaminophen or ibuprofen.

WOMEN'S HEALTH

<u>your problem:</u> **Panty protection**

<u>what to look for:</u> Unscented sanitary pads, tampons, and panty liners. "The vagina was never meant to smell like strawberries," says Sharon Hillier, Ph.D., director of the Center of Excellence in Women's Health at Magee-Womens Hospital in Pittsburgh. Using scented feminine-hygiene products and toilet paper can lead to allergic reactions or irritation.

<u>best buys:</u> Tampax Pearl's innovative design fits the flat shape of the vagina, and it expands widthwise to prevent leaking.

<u>keep in mind:</u> Don't rely too heavily on tampons and pads. "You should never use panty liners for minimal discharge," says Suzanne Trupin, M.D., a clinical professor in the obstetrics and gynecology department at the University of Illinois College of Medicine. "Constant contact with liners is more irritating compared to a cotton panty. If you have sensitive skin, you want to avoid wearing panty liners for more than two days in a row."

<u>your problem:</u> **PMS**

<u>what to look for:</u> Nonsteroidal anti-inflammatory drugs (NSAIDs), such as ibuprofen, which stop the production of hormonelike substances (prostaglandins) that cause cramps

<u>best buys:</u> Advil, Motrin, and Nuprin. If ibuprofen alone is hard on your stomach, "alternating between Advil and Tylenol can keep it feeling better during this time of the month," Trupin says.

Try all-in-one remedies if you consistently suffer other symptoms in addition to cramps, she says. Midol PMS and Women's Tylenol Menstrual Relief combine diuretics and acetaminophen to combat breast tenderness, bloating, and cramps.

keep in mind: Diuretics (water pills) can cause dehydration, and NSAIDs can wreak havoc on your stomach, so keep refilling your water glass.

expert tip If you're tripled over with cramps, here's your license to defy label instructions: For fast relief, take three Advil or Tylenol at once—as long as you're not taking them on an empty stomach.

your problem: Vaginal itching

what to look for: Products containing benzocaine, a local anesthetic that soothes pain and itching

best buy: The experts choose Vagisil to relieve discomfort caused by using a new soap, soaking in scented baths, taking antibiotics, or even wearing jeans that are too tight.

keep in mind: It's easy to misdiagnose—as well as mistreat—the cause of itch. "You need to target a general discomfort, not a skin condition," Trupin says. "Look at yourself in the mirror. If you see a patch of red skin or a sore, see your doctor. You might have psoriasis, a wart, or something more serious, like herpes."

your problem: Vaginal dryness

what to look for: A lubricant that stays slick

best buys: K-Y, now in Liquid and UltraGel forms, is ideal for short-term use. But if you're coping with chronic dryness (which can set in after you've given birth, if you're on a low-dose birth-control pill, or if you're past menopause), Vagisil's Intimate Lubricant works well for daily use.

keep in mind: Oral contraceptives, breast-feeding, dehydration, or allergic reactions to soaps can all cause dryness. "If it doesn't improve after two to three applications, see a doctor to get to the root of the problem," Trupin says.

your problem: Yeast infections

what to look for: Once you know you have an infection (and your doctor has confirmed that you've had one before), it's really a matter of shopping around to find the product that works best for you.

best buys: Our experts reach for Monistat, which contains miconazole nitrate. "I would also suggest the dual pack with the external cream. It's extremely soothing," Trupin says. Gyne-Lotrimin, which contains clotrimazole, and Vagistat, which contains tioconazole, are close runners-up. All three products work similarly and help relieve the itching and discharge that come with yeast infections. Choosing among one-, three-, or seven-dose treatments is up to you. "The three- and seven-dose regimens have a lower initial dose, which you might find less irritating," Trupin says.

keep in mind: Some remedies call themselves drugs but are actually cosmetic products that won't clear up the infection. For example, yeast cures that contain pulsatilla, a homeopathic drug, may promise to soothe, cleanse, and eliminate discharge, but they won't stop the growth of yeast cells. Nor have these products been studied as well as Monistat and the like. If you're treating your second infection and it's not getting better or if you have a new partner and a new itch, see your doctor to make sure you don't have a sexually transmitted disease.

your problems: Tracking fertility and testing for pregnancy

what to look for: Kits that measure hormone levels in your urine

best buys: To check your fertility, Clearblue Easy Fertility Monitor is a reliable and hassle-free way to test your urine for one of two hormones (luteinizing or follicle-stimulating) that indicate when you're

be wary Frequent douching can lead to such infections as bacterial vaginosis, and pregnant women who douche are more likely to give birth prematurely or develop pelvic inflammatory disease.

ovulating and most likely to conceive. "If you've done the let's-see-what-happens thing for a couple of months and haven't gotten pregnant, at-home fertility kits are really helpful," Trupin says. The newest pregnancy tests are accurate any time of day, measuring the amount of HCG, or pregnancy hormone, in your urine. (The old tests required you to use the first urine of the day.) Our experts trust the E.P.T Pregnancy Test to be as accurate as what you'd find at your doctor's office.

keep in mind: These kits are rather expensive. The Clearblue monitor costs about $200 (not including the test sticks), and few insurance companies cover such purchases. Home pregnancy tests typically cost about $12 each. "Also, you need to wait until you've missed a period before taking the test; otherwise, you may have a false negative," says Adelaide G. Nardone, M.D., an OB-GYN at Women and Infants' Hospital in Providence, Rhode Island.

your problem: Menopause symptoms

what to look for: Products containing phytoestrogens like soy extracts, which may relieve night sweats and other complaints

best buys: Most of the 70 or so OTC menopause formulas and herbs on the market have not been well-researched and aren't proven to work. But if you want to try one anyway, our experts suggest Soy Menopause by Healthy Woman. Other options include Promensil, a widely available dietary supplement derived from red clover. Clinical studies have shown that red clover reduces the frequency and severity of hot flashes and night sweats in some women. "My patients have gotten some relief from taking this," Trupin says. "I'd say it's only worth spending your money on if it's quickly relieving your hot flashes. If not, I'd skip it."

keep in mind: If you experience such symptoms as breast soreness, unusual discharge, or irregular bleeding while taking one of these treatments, it's possible your dose is too high. "Also, if you're already on a hormone supplement, ask your

physician how much additional phytoestrogen you can safely take," Trupin says. Phytoestrogen products can be costly, too (Promensil, for example, costs $19.99 for 30 tablets).

FIRST AID

your problem: Cuts and scrapes

what to look for: Antibiotic ointments to prevent and treat minor infections

best buys: Cover cuts with Bacitracin, a topical antibacterial cream that is favored by our experts. Top with a bandage to keep the wound as clean as possible.

keep in mind: Avoid iodine and alcohol, which tend to exacerbate cuts and scrapes.

your problem: Blisters or burns

what to look for: Products that seal out contaminants, create a moist environment to speed healing, and cushion the wound

best buys: Band-Aid Brand Advanced Healing Blister stays put, thanks to its two adhesives—one that absorbs blister fluids and another that sticks firmly to skin. If you've burned your finger, run cool water over it (don't apply ice; it can cause further damage), apply a topical antibiotic cream, such as Bacitracin, and top with gauze and tape.

keep in mind: If your grandmother told you to dress a burn with butter, she was—sorry to say—all wrong. This can make the injury worse.

first-aid shopping list

Our experts keep these items on hand:

- ❏ Sterile gauze
- ❏ Surgical tape
- ❏ Bandages
- ❏ Cloth pads
- ❏ An elastic bandage for wrapping sprained joints or making a sling
- ❏ A topical antibiotic ointment for cuts and scrapes
- ❏ Hydrocortisone cream for bug bites
- ❏ Reusable hot/cold compresses
- ❏ Syrup of ipecac, which induces vomiting (Use only if someone in your household has ingested poison by accident.)

your problem: **Scars**

what to look for: Silicone-based dressings to protect and minimize visible scarring

best buys: Our experts pick Curad Scar Therapy and Band-Aid Brand Scar Healing Strips. These may help flatten and fade raised red scars by applying constant pressure.

keep in mind: In order for these scar-minimizing products to work, you have to use them daily for as long as eight weeks. And forget the much-hyped vitamin E—it has actually been found to increase redness over time.

❖

your problem: **Bug bites**

what to look for: Creams or sprays containing hydrocortisone or antihistamines, which can help keep you from scratching till your skin is raw

best buys: Try Cortaid, a 1-percent hydrocortisone itch cream; calamine lotion; or Aveeno Soothing Bath Treatment to reduce itching. A histamine-blocking topical cream, such as Benadryl Itch Stopping Cream, also provides fast relief, according to Robert M. Schiller, M.D., chairman of the department of family medicine at Beth Israel Medical Center and Long Island College Hospital in New York City.

keep in mind: If you experience significant redness and swelling, call your doctor immediately. You may need a prescription-strength antihistamine. ▪

OUR PANELISTS

ALLERGY & SINUS
David Edelstein, M.D., chairman of the department of otolaryngology at Manhattan Eye, Ear, and Throat Hospital
Janet P. Engle, Pharm.D., FAPHA, clinical professor of pharmacy and associate dean for academic affairs, College of Pharmacy, University of Illinois at Chicago
Marjorie L. Slankard, M.D., associate attending physician and co-director of the Allergy Clinic at NewYork-Presbyterian Hospital

WOMEN'S HEALTH
Sharon Hillier, Ph.D., director of the Center of Excellence in Women's Health, Magee-Womens Hospital, Pittsburgh
Adelaide G. Nardone, M.D., an OB-GYN affiliated with Women and Infants' Hospital, Providence, Rhode Island
Suzanne Trupin, M.D., clinical professor of obstetrics and gynecology, University of Illinois College of Medicine

FIRST AID
M.J. Henderson, G.N.P., chairwoman of Nurse Practitioners: Rx for America's Health
Robert M. Schiller, M.D., chairman of the department of family medicine, Beth Israel Medical Center and Long Island College Hospital, New York City
Adam J. Singer, M.D., associate professor of clinical emergency medicine, Stony Brook University Health Sciences Center
Ann R. Skopek, M.D., assistant clinical professor of medicine, Yale University School of Medicine

Q+A   SAY GOODBYE TO OTC ADDICTIONS

I pop a "p.m." cold or headache pill a couple of times a week when I'm having trouble falling asleep. Can I get addicted?

Any sedative, including over-the-counter (OTC) drugs, could cause problems. Taking a nighttime pill as directed when you need to rest up for a big project at work the next day won't land you in rehab. But popping OTCs regularly to help you sleep (rather than to nix a headache or stuffy nose) is a bad idea. The longer you take them, the harder it is to stop. They can also leave you feeling groggy.

When it comes to getting good shut-eye without a pill, you know the drill: Avoid caffeine before you turn in, use the bed just for sleeping and sex, and go to another room if you don't fall asleep within 15 minutes. If you've used OTCs for more than 10 nights in a row, talk to your doctor.

Q + A — CALM YOUR NEEDLE NERVES

I hate getting blood drawn and nearly faint every time. Is there anything I can do to make this easier?

First, ask for the smallest-gauge needle available. With a pediatric needle, for instance, you'll hardly feel a thing, but these are usually used only in hospitals and in offices that treat children. Next best is a butterfly needle, which has a silicone tip that pinches less than the standard kind. Second, stop thinking about what's going on. Close your eyes and imagine you're in a place you love: Trying to see the sights, hear the sounds, and smell the scents can ease your pounding heart. On the flip side, two things don't work: deep breathing (you can hyperventilate or even faint) and anesthetic creams for kids—they could skew your test results, and you'd have to go through the whole ordeal again.

Preventing Blood Clots: Low Dose Is Better

National Heart, Lung, and Blood Institute scientists recently found that low doses of the drug warfarin are extremely effective in treating deep-vein thrombosis (DVT), a condition in which life-threatening blood clots form in the legs and can travel to the lungs. High-dose warfarin is the standard DVT treatment, which also carries a substantial risk of major bleeding; the lower amount reduces this risk.

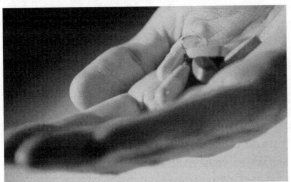

An Aspirin a Day Keeps Colon Cancer Away

The New England Journal of Medicine reports that one baby aspirin a day may cut the risk of colon polyps, which can lead to cancer, by nearly 20 percent. For colon-cancer survivors, a daily adult aspirin may lower the chance of developing new polyps by 35 percent. These results could mean a big decline in colon-cancer deaths, but don't race to the drugstore yet—overusing aspirin can cause strokes and ulcers, so talk to your doctor first. You still need a regular screening, too; current guidelines recommend starting at age 50 (earlier if cancer or polyps run in your family).

Q + A — HELP FOR HANGOVERS

Sometimes I accidentally drink too much at parties. What's the best hangover cure?

As long as you aren't slugging back three or more drinks a day and you don't suffer from ulcers or other bleeding problems, go ahead and pop aspirin, acetaminophen, or ibuprofen. Just don't go overboard: Because many people overdose on over-the-counter painkillers, the U.S. Food and Drug Administration is calling for tighter label warnings.

If you'd rather skip a trip to the medicine cabinet, have fruit juice instead of coffee in the morning (the caffeine could make you feel worse) and spread some honey on your toast—its fructose may help your body burn off the alcohol faster. Finally, remember that it's easier to prevent a hangover than cure one. Sip a glass of water between each cocktail; don't drink on an empty stomach; and watch out for red wine, brandy, scotch, and bourbon. They contain the largest number of congeners, by-products of fermentation that are bound to make your head pound.

How to Prevent Summer Sickness

Experts determine your real risks—and offer practical advice to avoid these disasters before they strike.

BY DIANA KAPP

With a spate of handbooks that spelled out instructions for escaping a bad date or delivering a baby in a taxi, 2002's fad of conjuring worst-case scenarios seemed somewhat entertaining. But in 2003, with the threats of SARS, anthrax, and biological warfare looming, disaster didn't seem as far-fetched—or nearly as amusing. While there's no accounting for world affairs, you can take measures to lower your risks of encountering hazards in your own backyard. We polled experts about four summer health predicaments and asked for their advice to help you sail through the season unscathed.

WEST NILE VIRUS

You're boating on the lake when a mosquito bites you. You think nothing of it until you start to feel disoriented, shaky, and weak. Then you go into convulsions, slip into a coma, and die.

likelihood: Low. While concern may be contagious, the total number of reported West Nile cases in the United States is just slightly more than 4,000. Only 1 out of every 150 people who are bitten by an infected mosquito contracts the potentially fatal diseases caused by the virus, West Nile meningitis and West Nile encephalitis. "We're seeing the fatal forms primarily in people over age 50," says Roy Campbell, M.D., a medical epidemiologist with the Centers for Disease Control and Prevention. The South and Midwest have reported the highest incidences of the virus.

worth knowing: Roughly 80 percent of people infected with West Nile have no symptoms and require no medical attention. "Most people clear the virus within two weeks and develop permanent immunity," Campbell says.

avoid disaster: Cover up when you're outside. Spray exposed skin with repellents containing DEET, which, contrary to popular belief, is safe (for more information, see the box on page 82). If you do get bitten and notice neck stiffness, fatigue, or disorientation, see your doctor. "When there's reason to worry, you'll know," Campbell says. "If West Nile virus invades your central nervous system, you won't confuse it with a garden-variety viral infection."

Only 1 out of 150 people who are bitten by an infected mosquito contracts the fatal disease caused by West Nile virus and about 80 percent of those infected have no symptoms at all.

HEAT-RELATED ILLNESSES

You're jogging on a sweltering day when suddenly you feel nauseated and confused, then you collapse. Ten minutes later, you go into cardiac arrest and die.

likelihood: Low. While cases of athletes dying during practice have made headlines in recent years, heatstroke is actually pretty rare among recreational-sports buffs. Heat exhaustion, a less serious condition, is more common.

worth knowing:
High humidity can be just as dangerous as soaring temperatures. The National Weather Service Heat Index (www.crh.noaa.gov/arx/heatindex.html) determines your risk by assessing heat and humidity in combination. If the index is greater than 105, turn your power-walk into a leisurely stroll or work out in an air-conditioned gym instead.

avoid disaster: Acclimate yourself to the heat. Decrease the intensity and length of your workouts for 7 to 10 days when temperatures spike for the first time of the season. Also, load up on water. The American College of Sports Medicine says you should down 17 ounces two hours before you exercise and stop for more at regular intervals during a routine. Listen to your body: If you feel nauseated or exhausted, or have trouble walking, get out of the heat and drink water right away. To chill out fast, place ice packs on your neck, groin, and underarms. If you still slip into the realm of heatstroke—whose signs include confusion, dizziness, and inability to sweat—hope that someone is around to call for help immediately, because you probably won't be thinking clearly enough to reach for the phone. In severe cases, CPR may be necessary.

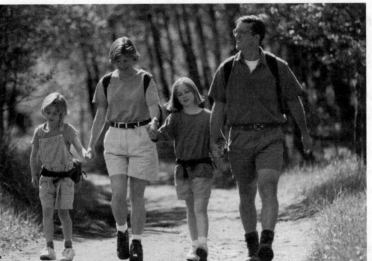

KILLER BEE STING

You're sipping a frozen chai latte at a sidewalk café when a bee stings you. You experience a severe allergic reaction, collapse, and die.

likelihood: Low. The odds are just 1 in 6 million, according to the National Safety Council, a nonprofit public service organization. The risk is about a third lower than that of death by lightning (1 in 4.2 million) and 20 times lower than that of being killed in a bicycle spill (1 in 341,000).

worth knowing:
"If you've experienced a systemic allergic reaction before, you must carry a bee-sting kit," says Leonard Altman, M.D., of the Northwest Asthma and Allergy Center in Seattle. These doctor-prescribed safeguards include shots of epinephrine, which reduces swelling in your throat and controls lung spasms, hives, and blood pressure. If you're not extremely allergic, you can use a simpler tool: a credit card. Scraping out the stinger with your Visa is much more effective than using tweezers or fingers, which can actually squeeze more venom into your body.

avoid disaster: When you are lunching outdoors, don't wear perfume or brightly colored clothes, which attract bees and wasps, and place a plate of scraps five picnic-table lengths (50 feet) away to divert the pests' attention. If you find yourself face-to-face with a bee, ignore it, or at least shoo it calmly—wild waving will only provoke it. Call 911 immediately if you start having a reaction to a sting—marked by hives, swelling that occurs away from the site, difficulty breathing, or confusion. While you wait for help to arrive, lie down and elevate your legs to increase blood flow to your head.

LYME DISEASE

A few weeks after going on a long hike, you can't seem to drag yourself out of bed. You're running a fever, virtually every muscle in your body (not just your thighs) aches, and you have a headache that just won't go away. Your doctor says you're suffering from Lyme disease, so you'd better prepare yourself for the possibility of chronic memory problems and arthritis.

likelihood: Medium. If you summer on the Eastern seaboard, or in Minnesota or Wisconsin, some squeamishness about ticks makes sense—92 percent of the 16,000 annual cases occur in those parts of the country. Otherwise, your risk is much lower.

worth knowing: An infected tick must stay attached for 24 hours to transmit the disease.

avoid disaster: Survey your body, head to toe, each day for these sesame-seed–sized critters. If you find one, remove it completely by holding its body with tweezers and pulling it away from your skin. And watch for the telltale sign of disease: a bull's-eye rash, which appears in 50 to 70 percent of cases. Joint stiffness, headache, and fatigue also signal infection. Caught within three weeks, Lyme disease is almost always treatable with antibiotics and is rarely fatal.

Is DEET Safe?

To fend off mosquitoes and ticks, insect repellents containing DEET are the most effective products that you can buy. And despite reports of the compound causing seizures and other health problems in children, it is actually safe to use, says Mark S. Fradin, M.D., clinical associate professor of dermatology at the University of North Carolina at Chapel Hill and author of a recent *New England Journal of Medicine* study comparing various repellents. Still, don't exceed the dose recommendations on the label. And reapply only when you begin to see bugs landing on you. Products with high percentages of DEET don't work better than those with low concentrations, but they last longer. Formulas made with 23.8-percent DEET last for about five hours, depending on how much you sweat; those with 6.65 percent protect you about two hours. Repellents containing 100-percent DEET are overkill for the average person. Apply the lowest percentage you need for the time you're in a mosquito- or tick-infested area. Don't see DEET on the label? It's often listed by its formal names: N,N-diethyl-m-toluamide or N,N-diethyl-3-methylbenzamide.

Q + A
HOW OFTEN DO YOU NEED TO VISIT THE DENTIST—*REALLY*

My dental insurance recently ran out. Will I wreck my teeth if I put off checkups for a little while?

Probably not, because the every-six-months rule isn't a rule at all. In fact, the American Dental Association doesn't even make this blanket recommendation (another urban legend put to rest). How often you should see your dentist depends on your history of cavities or gum disease. If you've been problem-free for the past two years, you can possibly wait up to a year between cleanings and checkups, as long as you keep up with the brush-and-floss routine. Don't go much longer than a year, though. Catching tooth decay early may help you avoid the dreaded drill, and regular professional cleanings are crucial in preventing gum disease. If you've had cavities or gum problems in the past two years, you should be examined more regularly. Exactly how often can vary from person to person, so ask your dentist how long you can safely go without a checkup.

What's NEW at Your Dentist's Office

The latest pampering perks at dentists' offices will make you do a double take. Masseuses, aestheticians, even plastic surgeons are helping patients fight their fear of drills, needles, etc. Here's what some practices around the country offer. (Most of these treatments are performed before or after your dental procedure.)

CLIMB IN THE CHAIR FOR	WHERE	COST	DENTIST SAYS ...	WE SAY ...
Facial micro-dermabrasion (performed by an aesthetician)	Dr. Berland's Dental Spa for Adult Dentistry, Dallas	First treatment: free; follow-ups: $110 each or $500 for a package of five	"The focus of my practice is cosmetic dentistry," says Lorin Berland, D.D.S. "So microdermabrasion, which improves the skin, is a natural fit."	Although microdermabrasion can be done by an aesthetician, we prefer a dermatologist's expertise. Use your best judgment.
Paraffin-wax hand treatment	Atlanta Center for Cosmetic Dentistry	Free	"Half of Americans don't even go to the dentist on a regular basis, and those who do treat it like a necessary evil," says Debra Gray King, D.D.S. "My mission is to make dental visits a more pleasant experience."	Softer hands for nothing? Go ahead and wax us.
Botox injections	The Rosenthal Group, New York City	$500	"We call our office a 'rejuvenation center,'" says Larry Rosenthal, D.D.S. "You can have a dermatologist do a consultation while you're sitting in the chair. We want patients to like their looks—not just their teeth."	On the plus side, at least it's a dermatologist who performs the procedure. On the other hand, if you get Botox before your dental work, your face may not register any pain you might feel.
A one-hour facial	Dental Spa, Pacific Palisades, California	$75 for dental patients, $85 for nonpatients (Yes, some people go solely for a facial.)	"People schedule regular dental cleanings, but they don't schedule regular skin cleanings," says Lynn Watanabe, D.D.S. "This helps them do so."	If you've got the extra time to spare, we're all for one-stop shopping.
Foot, shoulder, or neck massage	The Dental Spa, Fayetteville, Arkansas	Free	"Massage relaxes patients," says Robert G. Hodous, D.D.S. "And if they're relaxed, they often find their dental procedures more comfortable."	Yes to anything that might take our minds off the drill.
Collagen injections	Paul Tanners, D.D.S., New York City	$400 per injection	"Patients were complaining to me about their wrinkles," Tanners says. "Having an on-site plastic surgeon was an easy way to help do something about them."	If you're the collagen type, this might be cool. As for us, we prefer to spit and split.

6 Secrets to Better Sleep

Having trouble getting your snooze time? Discover how these tips can help.

BY LAURIE HERR

Everyone tosses and turns at night now and then, especially women. "Sleep complaints are about twice as prevalent in women when compared to men," says Amy R. Blanchard, M.D., director of the Georgia Sleep Center. And lack of rest won't just give you under-eye circles. Some experts say that being chronically deprived of enough sleep to wake up refreshed may lead to more than stress and irritability. It can also cause gastrointestinal problems, menstrual irregularities, and even heart disease.

To get into the REM zone, we turned to a variety of sleep specialists: doctors and researchers, as well as nurses who work night shifts and pilots who zigzag across time zones. We asked them what they do when they're tired of counting sheep. After all, even experts pound the pillows sometimes.

1. When I'm lying in bed awake, I don't look at the clock. Instead, I tell myself to get up and do something sensible, such as scrubbing the kitchen floor. Just the idea makes me think, "You're better off staying in bed." Next thing I know, it's morning.
—*Joyce Walsleben, Ph.D., director of New York University's Sleep Disorder Center and co-author of* A Woman's Guide to Sleep

2. I think of famous people whose first and last names begin with the same initial: Alan Alda, Brigitte Bardot, Charlie Chaplin, Danny DeVito ... by the time I reach the Ks, I'm out.
—*Helen Sullivan, spokeswoman for the Better Sleep Council*

3. I visualize colors blending together. I also keep a notepad by my bed so I can write down what's on my mind.
—*Beth A. Malow, M.D., associate professor of neurology and sleep researcher, University of Michigan Medical School*

4. To wind down, I put on headphones, go outside, and look at the stars. If I wake up during the night, I listen to children's lullabies.
—*Janet Kinosian, author of* The Well-Rested Woman: 60 Soothing Suggestions for Getting a Good Night's Sleep

5. When I fly, I keep my watch set on my home time zone, and I try to stick to my normal hours for eating and sleeping. —*Chris Fair, airline pilot*

6. I turn on my sound machine. Instead of outside noise, I hear gentle rain.
—*Patti Kelley, a registered nurse who regularly works from 7 p.m. to 7 a.m.* ■

Stop Working, Start Sleeping

We've heard of working under-cover before, but working under the covers is a different story. A recent British survey found that one in six people works in bed. A third make job-related phone calls, while others catch up on E-mail or use their laptops to do spreadsheets between the sheets. All this overtime adds up to tired employees: More than a third of survey participants get by on six or fewer hours of sleep each night.

To find out what's happening in American bedrooms, we took our own poll at Health.com. More than half of you admitted to working in bed at least once a month, and one-quarter of you said that doing so made you feel tired and stressed. To get the sleep you need, move the laptop, the papers—the TV, too—to another room. Keep the bedroom a sanctuary for sleep (and sex).

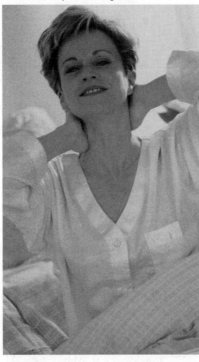

Q + A

NIX NIGHTTIME BATHROOM VISITS

Since my last pregnancy, I have to get up and pee in the middle of the night. What's gone wrong, and how can I fix it?

Having a baby did trigger changes in your body, but your ability to "hold it" shouldn't be among them. Nocturia, or frequent urinating at night, often comes with getting older: As early as age 30, your bladder starts to hold less, so you have to go more often. In fact, the average American gets up to use the bathroom once or more a night.

If your nightly visits seem to have come out of the blue, it's worth a trip to your doctor to rule out a urinary-tract infection or over-active bladder (which makes you go more during the day, too, but usually is most noticeable at night). Otherwise, let common sense prevail—avoid drinking too many liquids after dinner and make sure that what's waking you really is a call from nature. Alcohol, caffeine, or stress could be the actual cause.

Q + A

HOW TO MAKE WAKING UP EASIER

I've read tons of suggestions for falling asleep at night. How about some help for those of us who have a hard time getting out of bed?

Sleep experts (and maybe your mother) will tell you to go to bed earlier. But until an alternate reality comes along in which you don't have to help the kids with their homework, fold laundry, clean up after dinner, and look over your notes for tomorrow's breakfast meeting, you're probably going to have to rely on some other strategies.

Researchers agree that light helps you wake up, so flip a switch or open the curtains to let the sunshine pour in. (Don't hit the snooze button; dozing won't leave you well-rested.) Set your coffeemaker so you'll awaken to the smell of a fresh pot and make sure you have something good on hand for breakfast. You could also time the thermostat so that it's too hot to stay under the covers. Then there's the pet clock: Feed Spot in the early evening, and he'll wake you up for his breakfast.

Diabetes Strikes Surprising Victims

More and more unsuspecting women are discovering that they have diabetes. Find out if you could be one of them.

BY MICHELLE KATLAN

Maria Pia DePasquale was not your usual suspect. Born in Italy, DePasquale followed a sensible, low-fat Mediterranean diet for most of her life. She stayed active by walking and biking. At 5 feet tall, the 127-pound, 38-year-old Vanderbilt University professor might have wanted to drop a dress size, but she never considered a few extra pounds to be a health issue. She was mistaken: Three years ago, while taking advantage of a free screening sponsored by Massachusetts General Hospital, she was diagnosed with pre-diabetes. This potentially life-threatening condition is marked by higher-than-normal blood-glucose levels dangerously close to those associated with adult-onset diabetes.

Twenty years ago, if you asked your doctor who was typically at risk for this disease, she probably would have described an obese, inactive, middle-aged person more likely to indulge in fast food than fruits and vegetables. While that high-risk profile is still valid, a surprising group of younger and, on the surface, healthier candidates like DePasquale have

The number of 30-somethings diagnosed with diabetes has increased nearly 76 percent in the past 10 years.

joined the ranks. The number of 30-somethings diagnosed with diabetes has increased nearly 76 percent in the past 10 years. An estimated 17 million Americans, more than half of them women, live with the disease today; as many as 6 million don't even realize they have it.

The expanding American waistline is partially to blame for the upward trend. A recent study found that every 5 to 8 pounds of extra weight increases your chance of becoming diabetic by 6 percent. "If you are very obese, your odds of developing diabetes are high. But even if you are only slightly overweight you are still not in the clear," explains lead study author Teresa Hillier, M.D., a researcher at Kaiser Permanente Center for Health Research in Portland, Oregon.

The insidious nature of diabetes means that catching it early is especially important. Left unchecked, elevated blood-sugar levels can damage almost every part of the body as many as 10 to 15 years before obvious symptoms appear. "Often you don't even realize you have the disease until the harm is done," says Rhoda H. Cobin, M.D., clinical professor of medicine at Mount Sinai School of Medicine in New York City. Complications of delayed detection can include blindness, kidney failure, and neuropathy (damage to nerves in the extremities that can cause pain and loss of sensation, possibly leading to amputation). Diabetes is the fifth leading cause of death by disease in the United States, with more than half a million adult mortalities each year, the majority from cardiovascular conditions. Roughly five times as many women die from diabetes-related diseases as from breast cancer.

The younger you are when you develop diabetes, the higher your risk of having a heart attack. In a recent study, Hillier found that diabetics over age 45 were three times more likely to suffer heart attacks than other people of the same age. Diabetics ages 18 to 44 were 11 times more likely to experience a heart attack than their nondiabetic peers. Similar research has shown that even having blood-sugar levels in the pre-diabetic range puts a person of any age at a 50-percent greater risk of having a heart attack or stroke. An estimated 16 million Americans are considered pre-diabetic.

The heart threat appears to be especially high for women. "Normally, premenopausal women are somewhat protected from heart disease by estrogen. With diabetes, they seem to lose that protective effect and reach the same risk of heart attack, stroke, and arteriosclerosis as men," says James Rosenzweig, M.D., director of the diabetes-management program at Joslin Diabetes Center in Massachusetts.

Health-care experts recommend that high-risk individuals get screened for diabetes beginning at age 30. Early-screening candidates include anyone who has a diabetic family member; is overweight, which is defined as having a body-mass index over 25; has heart disease, high blood pressure, high triglycerides, or low HDL (good) cholesterol; has had gestational diabetes or delivered a baby weighing more than 9 pounds; or has polycystic ovarian syndrome (a hormonal disorder linked to irregular periods). People in certain ethnic groups, including

Lower Your Risks

Here are five ways that you can prevent diabetes today.

Lose weight. In the Diabetes Prevention Program (DPP), an average weight loss of 15 pounds (for a 200-pound individual) was enough to help pre-diabetics reverse their diagnoses.

Sleep tight. Some studies have shown that sleep deprivation can have a harmful impact on carbohydrate metabolism and endocrine function, lowering the body's glucose tolerance.

Adjust your diet. A 2001 study published in the *New England Journal of Medicine* found that a diet high in cereal fiber and low in saturated and trans fats reduced the risk of developing diabetes. On the flip side, a Harvard University study in February 2002 found that a typical Western diet (packed with red or processed meats, French fries, high-fat dairy products, refined grains, and sweets) increased the risk by nearly 60 percent.

Have a drink. Several studies have shown a connection between moderate alcohol intake and insulin resistance. One recent study published in the *Journal of the American Medical Association* found that consuming two drinks a day had a positive effect on glucose levels in nondiabetic postmenopausal women.

Get moving. As little as 30 minutes of moderate aerobic exercise (in which you break a sweat) five times a week can reduce blood-sugar levels, according to the DPP. Add regular strength-training sessions to further improve your body's insulin resistance.

calculate your BMI A body-mass index (BMI) over 25 is a risk factor for diabetes. To figure out your BMI, divide your weight by your height in inches squared and multiply by 703. For example, 140 ÷ (66 x 66) x 703 = 23. Or find your BMI on Health.com; just click on "Fitness," then on "Are You Overweight?" under "Charts & Guides."

African-Americans, Hispanics, Asian-Americans, and Native Americans, are also considered at high risk. If you experience any of the classic symptoms of diabetes, such as excessive thirst and urination or blurry vision, get tested. Even if you don't fall into one of these groups, ask your doctor about being screened by age 40. "Not everyone who gets diabetes has one or all of these risk factors," Cobin says.

The good news is that even if you are at risk, diabetes doesn't have to be your destiny. A recent large-scale study called the Diabetes Prevention Program (DPP) found that by making moderate changes in diet and exercise, pre-diabetics can reduce their risk of developing the disease by 58 percent. "You're not doomed to a lifetime of diabetes if you're diagnosed with pre-diabetic glucose levels," says David Nathan, M.D., a professor of medicine at Harvard Medical School and one of the leaders of the DPP study.

For Maria DePasquale, this meant losing 8 pounds, in part by taking up salsa dancing and working out several times a week. After two years, her glucose levels dropped back into the normal range. "I'm at the point of my life where I would like to have a child one day, and I knew that diabetes would make it much harder," she says. "Knowing that I can do something to prevent the disease has pushed me to take action."

sexual side effects Diabetes can also take a toll in the bedroom: A study in *Diabetes Care* found that 27 percent of women with the disease reported sexual dysfunction, compared with 15 percent of nondiabetics.

Weigh Your Risks for Heart Disease

So your jeans are a bit tight around the middle—everyone gains a few pounds at times, right? Before you shrug off the snug fit, consider this: According to a recent study in the *New England Journal of Medicine*, being even moderately overweight can increase your risk of heart failure by over a third. For people who are obese, the danger doubles. To determine your chances, figure your body-mass index (BMI) with our chart at Health.com (click on "Fitness" and look under "Charts & Guides" for "Are You Overweight?"). Use your height and weight to find your corresponding BMI. (A 5-foot-5-inch woman weighing 162 pounds, for instance, has a BMI of 27 and is considered overweight. If she reaches 180 pounds, her BMI increases to 30, pushing her into the obese category.)

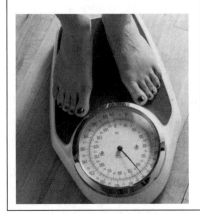

New Drug Can Help You Lower "Bad" Cholesterol

If you're taking statin drugs to lower your cholesterol, ask your doctor about Zetia, a new prescription medicine approved by the Food and Drug Administration that researchers are touting as the next pharmacy blockbuster. Studies have shown that people who take Zetia in combination with statins have significant reductions in LDL (bad) cholesterol.

Pucker Up for Health

You nurse them when they're chapped, nibble them when you're nervous—heck, the president's dad once challenged an entire nation to read his. Yet for all the lip service, rarely do people appreciate what's right under their noses. Why you really should love 'em now: They can help you stay warm. A serious smooching session can raise your body temperature, says James G. Pfaus, Ph.D., associate professor at the Center for Studies in Behavioral Neurobiology at Concordia University in Montreal. You can also think of puckering up as disease protection. Frequent kissers may be more resistant to stress, making their immune systems better able to handle bacterial and viral infections, Pfaus says.

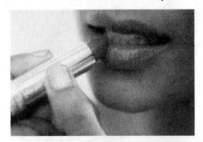

What *Really* Aggravates Asthma

A new study in the *British Medical Journal* shows that while many people blame pet dander and pollen for bothering their asthma symptoms, the likelier culprit is mold. Researchers say that the tiny spores, which multiply in the fall, easily enter and tickle people's airways.

During the winter, when your house is closed up tightly, the problem can become even worse. So fight the fungus: If you use a humidifier, empty out the reservoir daily, because mold loves moisture. And crack open the windows—you could use a breath of fresh air.

Quit Smoking—for Your Cat's Sake

Here's yet another reason to quit smoking: your cat's health. Exposure to secondhand smoke more than doubles the risk of feline lymphoma, a cancer that kills, within a year, most of the cats diagnosed, according to a Tufts University study. And now it's even more important to look out for your kitty, since University of Buffalo researchers have discovered that curling up with four-legged friends relieves stress much better than hashing out problems with your human pals.

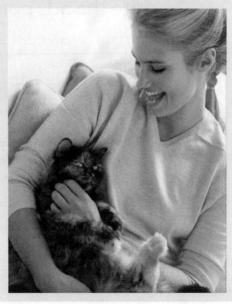

Q + A   FIGHT FUNGUS WITH FLIP-FLOPS

Can wearing flip-flops in the locker room and shower keep you from catching athlete's foot or toenail fungus?

The extra protection is worth the few bucks you'll shell out for a pair of flip-flops.

For showers to be completely fungus-free, they'd have to be wiped down with a fungicide after every use, and even the cleanest gyms can't do that. Antifungal sprays and powders are ineffective under running water, so wearing some kind of shoe while you rinse off and drying your feet well afterward are really your only defenses. Of course, going barefoot doesn't necessarily doom you to infections; some people are more susceptible to them than others.

What They <u>Don't</u> Tell You in *TV Drug Commercials*

Are the ads popping up on television screens as realistic as they should be?

BY STEPHANIE JO KLEIN

When I first saw ads for my antianxiety medication on TV, I was delighted. More than that, I felt a sense of pride. "Check that out!" I marveled. "My pills are on TV during *Friends!*" Maybe, I thought, the commercials' prime-time placement signaled progress in combating stereo-types about mental illness. "Stephanie," my friends might now say, "you're manic-depressive. How totally normal. You're not insane like we always thought people with chemical imbalances were."

After I viewed the Paxil promos a few more times, however, my euphoria over their one-minute explanation of a mood-stabilizing drug's intricate workings began to fade. Given the quick-hit nature of TV commercials, the company sells its product with catchphrases: "I'm back to being me," proclaims the newest pitch; prior ads advised, "Your life is waiting." Evidently, it doesn't have to wait long. In one spot, distressed family members quiz

> **Chronic anxiety and depression aren't always as easy to spot in the real world as they are in a Woody Allen movie.**

chemically imbalanced loved ones about why they don't sleep and why they worry so much. In another, symptoms of anxiety disorders flash across the faces of glum-looking people. In the end, the result is always the same: The previously morose, anxious insomniacs suddenly frolic with their families and friends, having found an instant pharma-ceutical solution to their problems.

In real life, it ain't so easy. My life wasn't waiting for me to discover it immediately after I washed down a handful of pills with a Diet Coke. Once I finally admitted something was wrong, it took most of my senior year of college, therapy sessions with three doctors, and two different diagnoses before we uncovered a family history of manic depression. From there, a combination of medica-tions and therapy got me through the worst. With the support of my family, friends, and doctor, I held it together and stood proudly in my cap and gown in the University of Michigan's stadium. When I returned home to New York City, things continued to improve. There were no more frenzied 3 a.m. closet reorganizations, no more locking myself in my room and weeping while listening to Sarah McLachlan on repeat. A few months after graduation, I got my first job at a magazine. The meds were the springboard—my life was something I had to work for.

I don't mean to say that publicity has no place in raising awareness about diseases, just that drug manufacturers owe it to the public to make pills seem less like fast-acting magic beans. Chronic anxiety and depression aren't always as easy to spot in the real world as they are in a Woody Allen movie, and chemicals aren't the exclusive solution. The commercials don't acknowledge that. Instead, they just list symptoms implying that every cranky, overworked person should get a prescription. Chronic anxiety for everyone! Of course, the ads end with a quick voice-over stating that prescription Paxil is not for everyday anxiety. If it's not, then why not explain what it *is* for? Remind people that therapy can help. Talk about the importance of family support. Get rid of the stigma.

Can all this really be done in less than a minute? Probably not. But it wouldn't hurt if the drug companies at least tried to inject some realism into their soft-focus minidramas. Although commercials might be the quickest way to introduce new products and ideas to the public, they may not be the best venue for explaining major medical problems. That's what watching documentaries—or heck, even *ER*—is for.

Stephanie Jo Klein is a freelance writer who lives in New York City.

Why Redheads Need More Pain Relief

It's often said that flame-haired women tend to have fiery personalities. That could explain some new research: A study at the University of Louisville in Kentucky found that women with naturally red hair need 20 percent more anesthesia than brunettes to achieve the same level of sedation. Researchers believe this phenomenon stems from the gene mutation that causes hair to be red or orange. "The finding is the first to link a visible genetic trait to a person's anesthetic requirements, so it may help us learn how anesthesia works—something that's not entirely clear," says Edwin Liem, M.D., assistant professor of anesthesiology at the University of Louisville and the study's principal investigator. So what should you do if you're a redhead preparing to go under the knife? Don't panic. You may want to mention this study to your doctor, but anesthetic procedures are now so advanced that doctors can tailor drug levels to each patient's needs, no matter what color her hair.

vital *stats*

64
Percentage of women who would rather receive high-tech ELECTRONIC GADGETS than diamonds as gifts

509,000
Number of American homes with TiVo, a device that AUTOMATICALLY RECORDS your favorite TV shows

671,000
Number of American households with OUTHOUSES

26
Percentage of traffic FATALITIES attributed to accidents caused by driver distractions

1
Rank of COFFEE among foods most likely to DISTRACT a driver

2
Rank of SOUP

14
Annual number of MEALS per capita eaten while driving

100
Percentage by which the risk of a FOOD-RELATED ACCIDENT can increase if someone is driving a STICK SHIFT

385
Number of NATIONAL PARKS in America

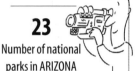

23
Number of national parks in ARIZONA

3
Number of the 10 most DANGEROUS national parks that are in Arizona

44
Percentage of Americans who take TWO or fewer SICK DAYS a year

16
Percentage who take NINE or more

68
Percentage of EMPLOYEE NO-SHOWS that aren't actually due to illness

63
Percentage of moms who keep all their MOTHER'S DAY CARDS

136 MILLION
Number of MOTHER'S DAY cards sent annually in America

84 MILLION
Number of FATHER'S DAY cards sent

54
Percentage of MEN under age 45 who are very pleased with their FACIAL APPEARANCE

47
Percentage of WOMEN who are

37
Percentage of WHITES who are very confident in their looks

62
Percentage of NONWHITES who are

41
Percentage of people in the WEST who are

35
Percentage of people in the MIDWEST who are

40
Percentage of people in the EAST who are

47
Percentage of people in the SOUTH who are

37
Percentage of Americans who get a "great deal" of their HEALTH INFORMATION from DOCTORS

23
Percentage who get a "great deal" of it from TV

61
Percentage who put a "great deal" of TRUST in the information they get from their DOCTORS

14
Percentage who put a "great deal" of TRUST in the information they get from TV

31.7
Percentage of Americans who get SUNBURNED each year

78
Percentage of WOMEN in one study who wore SUNSCREEN to the beach

73
Percentage of those who got SUNBURNED anyway

1
Rank of SKIN CANCER among most common cancers

Sources: Consumer Electronics Association, *Advertising Age*, Hallmark, Allergan, Hagerty Classic Insurance, *The New York Times*, *American Journal of Preventive Medicine*, American Academy of Dermatology, American Cancer Society, CCH Incorporated, Gallup Poll, National Park Foundation, National Park Service, U.S. Park Ranger Lodge of the Fraternal Order of Police —Reported by Laura Gilbert

female body

specific advice for
women-only issues

10 Issues You *Must* Discuss

with *Your Gynecologist*

Your time is limited—make the most of it.

BY MICHELLE DALLY

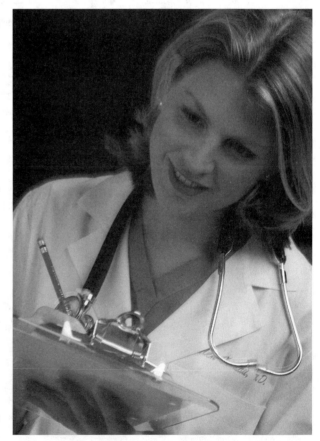

I t's a sad fact: Women often check their nerve at the door of the gynecologist's office. Sure, you'd rather be anywhere else when it comes time for that yearly exam, because of embarrassment, discomfort, or just plain boredom. But not asking questions at this appointment is asking for trouble.

Why? Because the doctor is busy. Really busy. The average OB-GYN sees 95 patients a week, and often she spends just 15 to 20 minutes with each patient. Now, that might be OK if most women also regularly saw a primary-care physician. But they don't. More than 50 percent use their OB-GYNs as their main doctors. So if you don't actively bring up your concerns and problems at the gynecologist's office, you might just miss out on new treatments—or even put your health at risk.

We've pinpointed 10 women's health issues that frequently get short shrift and revealed the surprising lowdown on why you simply can't ignore them. We've also assembled simple action plans so you'll know just how to use this information. Now it's your turn: During your next visit to the gynecologist, it's time to get vocal.

YOUR MEDICATIONS
MAY BE DANGEROUS.

Just being female puts you at 50-percent greater risk for adverse drug reactions, because your hormones, size, amount of body fat, and liver metabolism differ from a man's. Eight out of 10 medications pulled off the market by the U.S. Food and Drug Administration (FDA) between 1997 and 2001 caused more harm to women than to men. A woman is particularly vulnerable to problems when drugs are improperly combined—when she uses Claritin for allergies plus Nizoral for a foot fungus or a yeast infection, for instance. Although a number of relatively safe drugs can become toxic when taken together, studies suggest that some doctors unknowingly prescribe dangerous combinations and often don't know what other medicines patients are taking.

Drug interactions needn't be lethal to be life-changing, either. If you're on the Pill, you could get pregnant if you also take certain other medications: amoxicillin, tetracycline, or penicillin, for example. Other medicines, including some anticonvulsants,

Ask your doctor about the drugs you're taking. If you're on the Pill, you could still get pregnant if you also take certain other medications.

antifungals, and herbal remedies, such as St.-John's-wort, can also leave you unprotected.
Action plan: List your prescriptions and over-the-counter medications (including vitamins and herbal supplements) and remember to discuss everything you've noted at your next appointment. Or throw all the bottles into a zip-top bag and take them with you.

YOU'RE NEVER
TOO OLD TO CATCH AN STD.

Studies show that 4.5 million American women over age 40 (about 8 percent) engage in behaviors that put them at risk for sexually transmitted diseases (STDs). One consequence: People over 50 account for an increasing percentage of total AIDS cases. Yet only about half of OB-GYNs raise the ticklish topic with their patients.

Because women in their teens and 20s are more likely to contract most STDs, a doctor might assume you just don't fit the profile. Yet all it takes to make a married woman vulnerable to STDs are divorce or separation and unprotected sex with a new partner, says Diane Zablotsky, Ph.D., associate professor of sociology at the University of North Carolina at Charlotte and an expert on HIV and AIDS in middle-aged and older women. Even a "happily" married woman is at risk if her husband is fooling around.
Action plan: Tell your gynecologist about your sexual activity—all of it—especially if you're no longer in a long-term, one-partner relationship. Then ask for appropriate STD tests. Finally, use protection.

YEAST INFECTIONS
ARE NOT THAT COMMON.

If you think you've had recurrent infections, you may be misdiagnosing your problem. According to a 2002 study, 53 percent of women assumed that a vaginal itch was a yeast infection when it really wasn't, resulting in wasted purchases of over-the-counter products and potentially dangerous delays in getting a correct diagnosis. Why dangerous? Bacterial vaginosis (BV) also causes itching; left untreated, it can increase your risk of getting HIV from an infected partner. It may also increase the risk of premature birth if you're pregnant, and it makes complications more likely if you have certain surgical procedures (such as an abortion, a hysterectomy, or a cesarean section), says study author Daron Ferris, M.D., professor of obstetrics/gynecology and family medicine at the Medical College of Georgia. It's actually more common for a woman to have BV than a yeast infection. Fortunately, the former is easily treated with antibiotics.
Action plan: Don't just run to the pharmacy for creams and suppositories if you think you have a yeast infection. See your doctor for an accurate diagnosis.

THE **PILL** ISN'T YOUR ONLY OPTION.

Several new methods of preventing pregnancy have hit the market or are about to. One—a pill called Seasonale—gets rid of many of the hassles of birth control, along with the majority of your periods. It combines estrogen and progestin, just as in many of the familiar versions of the Pill. But you take the hormone-containing tablets for 84 days in a row, followed by a week of placebos. Result: the same contraceptive effect but only four periods per year. Side effects? About the same as those you would expect from the conventional Pill. The FDA approved Seasonale in September 2003.

With the contraceptive patch (Ortho Evra) and vaginal ring (NuvaRing), contraception doesn't have to be a daily thing. Both contain estrogen and progestin. According to studies by the company that makes the ring, both methods are likely to be more effective than the Pill, because they deliver the hormones more steadily and are less apt to be misused.

The patch is like a square Band-Aid that you apply to your stomach, buttocks, upper arm, or back. The ring, a flexible plastic device about 2½ inches in diameter, is inserted into the vagina. (Neither you nor your partner is likely to feel it during sex.) The patch must be applied weekly for three weeks, after which you take a week off. The ring should be kept in place for three weeks before you remove it for a week. Side effects are mild for both. The patch occasionally causes skin irritation, while the ring can produce vaginitis or headache. On the other hand, in a recent study, women formerly on the Pill reported having shorter and less painful periods while using the ring. Most were pleased with the method. The patch and the ring each cost about $400 a year.

Finally, don't forget about the IUD. Mirena, an improved version that has been on the market since 2001, contains progestin to make the mucus in your cervix thicker, so sperm aren't able to get through. It couldn't be any easier: The device prevents conception for up to five years, and if you want out, a single

doctor's visit is sufficient to remove it. Plus, the progestin tends to reduce period pain and bleeding. And since it costs about $550 for insertion—or about $110 per year of use—this birth control method can be more affordable than other forms of contraception over the long term.

Action plan: Many OB-GYNs talk about birth control with their patients, but they might not mention all the options if you're not assertive. Make sure to ask about new alternatives.

> In a recent study, women formerly on the Pill reported having shorter and less painful periods while using the vaginal ring. Most were pleased with the method.

HELP IS AVAILABLE IF YOU HAVE **UNPROTECTED SEX.**

There's a simple way to prevent an unwanted pregnancy should you, say, use a condom that breaks: emergency contraception. But your doctor probably hasn't discussed it with you. Emergency contraception (EC) is a set of pills that contain high dosages of the same hormones found in the regular oral contraceptives—estrogen and progestin (or just progestin by itself). When taken within 72 hours of unprotected sex, EC prevents pregnancy in the same way birth control pills do: It delays or inhibits ovulation, and it might also prevent a fertilized egg from implanting. Still, a substantial number of women surveyed in 2000 by the Kaiser Family Foundation didn't know that emergency contraception was available.

Though researchers have known for decades that birth control pills can be used as morning-after contraception, it wasn't until 1998 that the FDA approved a product specifically for this purpose. Now, the American College of Obstetricians and Gynecologists (ACOG) urges women to keep a prescription handy. That simple step could reduce unintended pregnancies in the United States by half. But remember: EC will *not* protect you from STDs.

Action plan: Ask your OB-GYN to prescribe you EC. If you do end up having unprotected sex, get your prescription filled right away, and take the pills.

THE JURY IS OUT ON
BREAST SELF-EXAMS.

For more than 50 years, women have heard how important it is to check their breasts each month. But a controversy about the effectiveness of breast self-examination (BSE) has been brewing for a decade. Recently, a major study out of China concluded that women who perform BSEs are no less likely to die of breast cancer than those who don't do them. So you can officially stop feeling guilty about forgetting to do an exam.

Susan Love, M.D., author of *Dr. Susan Love's Breast Book*, agrees that self-exams have little value. "I find that women get themselves scared to death and alienated from their bodies, feeling that they need to go on this monthly search-and-destroy mission," she says.

Action plan: Self-exams can't hurt you physically, but if they make you depressed or obsessed with breast cancer, take a pass. Whatever you decide, make sure you get a hands-on exam by your doctor at every annual visit. Changes in a breast that persist through a period should be checked right away.

Ask your gynecologist whether you should have a thyroid test. If you're over age 40, you've got a 1-in-10 chance of having an undiagnosed disorder.

YOU MAY NEED
A THYROID TEST.

If you're over age 40, you've got a 1-in-10 chance of having an undiagnosed thyroid disorder. Because the thyroid, a gland in your neck, produces hormones that help the cells in your body get the energy they need, a malfunction has far-reaching consequences. You may suffer exhaustion, weight gain or loss, poor concentration, depression, and changes in your period. If the disorder goes untreated, it can cause serious long-term complications, such as high cholesterol, heart disease, infertility, muscle weakness, and osteoporosis.

Women are five to eight times more likely than men to have a thyroid problem. So it's no wonder the American Thyroid Association urges women over age 35 to request a simple blood test of their thyroid-stimulating hormone, or TSH. The group suggests repeating the test every five years, more frequently if you have symptoms of a thyroid disorder.

Action plan: If you've never had a thyroid test, ask your doctor whether you should—especially if you notice such symptoms as off-the-charts exhaustion. They could signal trouble.

YOUR BONES NEED SOME TLC.

Beware: Youth doesn't guarantee strong bones. New research suggests that roughly one in four white women between ages 21 and 50 has osteopenia, or a dangerous thinning of the bones. That's a precursor to osteoporosis. Does that mean you should be tested for low bone mass? The U.S. Preventive Services Task Force recommends that women age 65 and older, as well as women age 60 or older who have at least one risk factor for osteoporosis, get a DXA scan, a painless, low-dose X ray of the spine and hips.

Ordinarily, most healthy premenopausal women don't need this test, but osteoporosis experts say some younger women should be tested in certain circumstances. If you have irregular periods (or no periods) because you have an eating disorder or because you're extremely athletic, estrogen deficiency puts you at risk for early osteoporosis. A bone-density test can help determine if you should go on the Pill, for instance, to help protect your bones. Testing might also make sense if you regularly take certain medications, such as steroids to treat asthma or thyroid hormone in larger-than-usual doses.

ACOG says that testing might also be useful for a relatively young woman if she smokes or has had endometriosis, lymphoma, multiple sclerosis, or rheumatoid arthritis, all of which increase osteoporosis risk.

Action plan: If one of the factors we've mentioned applies to you—or if you're simply concerned that you might be at risk—ask your doctor about having a DXA scan. It's the best way to measure your bone density.

9 IT'S TIME TO GO BEYOND THE PAP SMEAR.

About 2 million women each year have Pap tests that show atypical cells or some other abnormality, and many spend several months worrying, understandably, while they wait until they can have a follow-up test. But a human papillomavirus (HPV) test can give them an immediate answer. The test looks for certain strains of HPV that researchers have identified as the primary cause of cervical cancer. If your HPV results are negative, your abnormal Pap smear almost certainly does not indicate a problem.

Do you need to have an HPV test when your Pap smear results are normal? Experts say no. In the vast majority of cases in which the Pap is negative and the HPV test is positive, the immune system will get rid of the virus. That's important to remember, considering that HPV is the most common sexually transmitted disease in the United States.

Action plan: The U.S. Preventive Services Task Force recommends that women have a Pap smear at least once every three years. But because lab technicians sometimes miss signs of cancer when they examine cell samples, it's safest to have the test done every year. And if your Pap comes back with an abnormal result, don't panic: Ask your doctor to give you an HPV test.

10 HYSTERECTOMY IS RARELY THE RIGHT DECISION.

Roughly 600,000 hysterectomies are performed every year in the United States, as many as half of them to remedy ailments associated with fibroids,

> Insist that your doctor discuss alternatives to a hysterectomy. Studies show that 98% of women really do not need one.

which are noncancerous tumors. Roughly four-fifths of women who are told that they need a hysterectomy agree to have it done, and in the past decade, there has been little change in how often the procedure is performed.

Yet researchers who have studied the issue say far too many women needlessly subject themselves to this life-changing surgery. After being told that they needed hysterectomies, fully 98 percent of women referred to board-certified gynecologists by Hysterectomy Education Resources and Services, a nonprofit organization, discovered that they, in fact, did not need the procedure.

That's especially unnerving when you consider that hysterectomies can have extremely serious side effects: diminished sexual sensation, bone and muscle pain, depression, fatigue, heart disease, incontinence, and many others.

Fortunately, there are alternatives. One that women should think about is myomectomy, an operation to remove only the fibroids that are causing problems. It even allows a young woman to retain her ability to get pregnant—although the procedure can weaken the uterine wall, possibly making a C-section necessary.

A newer approach, uterine-fibroid embolization, involves cutting off the blood supply to the growths by injecting tiny plastic spheres into blood vessels. The procedure is not as invasive as myomectomy. But it is still fairly new, so the long-term side effects and success rate are unclear.

Action plan: If hysterectomy is suggested to you, insist that your doctor discuss the full list of alternatives. Then get a second opinion. You owe that to yourself. ■

Michelle Dally also writes for U.S. News and World Report.

Solving Period Puzzles

Discover the culprit behind five common menstrual irregularities.

BY JENNIFER PIRTLE

Even the healthiest women experience occasional blips in their menstrual cycles, but how do you know whether to chalk them up to lunar shifts or to something more serious? "Time-zone travel and medications, such as steroids or antibiotics, can all temporarily affect a woman's period," says Orli Etingin, M.D., director of the Iris Cantor Women's Health Center at New York Weill Cornell Medical Center. "Changes should be checked by a doctor if they occur for two or more cycles in a row."

Out-of-kilter periods can signal underlying health problems. Erratic menstruation may indicate metabolic abnormalities that raise disease risk.

Below are five of the most common period permutations and what to ask your OB-GYN to check for.

1. BLEEDING BETWEEN PERIODS
A dip in estrogen around ovulation can cause midcycle spotting. "Repeated spotting over two or more cycles could also be a sign of an ovarian cyst, endometriosis, or a uterine polyp," Etingin says. If you're taking oral contraceptives, off-cycle bleeding may mean that your pill's estrogen content is too low (this is fairly common with some of the newer low-dose tablets). Ask your doctor to prescribe a different brand.

2. MISSING A MONTH
As with other menstrual disturbances, skipping is often induced by stress: A major life change or sudden weight gain or loss can disrupt your schedule.

Missed periods can also signal premature ovarian failure (POF), a mysterious condition that causes ovaries to stop producing eggs and reproductive hormones, sometimes decades before menopause. POF increases a woman's risk of osteoporosis, so early diagnosis is a must.

3. SHORTENING/LENGTHENING OF CYCLE
Shorter periods often occur when a woman isn't ovulating and the uterus doesn't shed all its lining. One explanation: natural hormone shifts that happen when a woman enters her 40s. Lengthening cycles become an issue when a woman is trying to get pregnant. "It may be difficult to determine when she ovulates," Etingin says. "She may have to have hormonal testing in order to determine the exact date."

4. BARELY BLEEDING
An extralight flow usually means the uterine lining hasn't built up much and can simply signify that you haven't ovulated. If light periods become the norm, they could point to fertility problems; in some cases, an overactive thyroid could be to blame.

5. CRIPPLING CRAMPS
Intensely painful periods that get worse each month could be a sign of endometriosis, a disease that affects between 10 and 20 percent of American women of childbearing age. For unknown reasons, the tissue lining the uterus migrates to places in the body it shouldn't.

Massage Away Menstrual Cramps

Some health practitioners say an ancient technique may be your ticket to painless periods.

BY MICHELLE DALLY

Since she was a teenager, Elizabeth Hauptman had suffered from menstrual cramps so intense that she sometimes vomited or passed out. At 29, she was diagnosed with endometriosis (a painful condition in which uterine lining grows outside the womb) and underwent a four-hour surgery to remove the excess tissue. But the pain persisted. Six months of synthetic-hormone injections to temporarily prevent her from having periods also proved useless. Frustrated, Hauptman looked for new answers beyond her gynecologist's office. Enter Shelley Torgove, the owner of an herbal apothecary in Denver, Hauptman's hometown. Torgove told Hauptman that Mayan uterine massage (MUM) would change her life.

MUM isn't your typical spa treatment: It supposedly coaxes the uterus into prime position for trouble-free periods. Derived from an ancient Central American practice that Chicago alternative healer Rosita Arvigo learned while in Belize, the technique has been gaining popularity in the United States. Across the country, MUM devotees swear by the touch of the approximately 100 Arvigo-trained and -certified practitioners like Torgove, though many mainstream doctors reject the idea that you can massage away menstrual cramps.

The $85 treatment is a relaxing way to spend an hour, Hauptman says. A typical session involves a series of deep, scooping strokes from the pubic bone up to the belly button, then diagonally from each hipbone to the navel. The exact method depends on the position of an individual woman's uterus and is designed to nudge it into its proper place. "Torgove worked on me twice and taught me how to do it on myself," Hauptman says. "My next period was normal. I couldn't believe it was so easy."

Neither can some mainstream doctors. Reproductive endocrinologist Veronica Ravnikar, M.D., chairwoman of obstetrics and gynecology at St. Barnabas Medical Center in Livingston, New Jersey, questions whether the position of the uterus is the actual cause of pain and cautions that

Mayan uterine massage involves a series of deep, scooping strokes from the pubic bone up to the belly button, then diagonally from each hipbone to the navel.

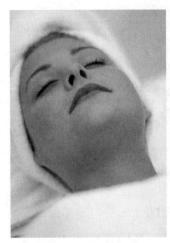

> **You can't hurt a woman by giving her a Mayan massage, and you may do her some good.**
> —Raphael S. Good, M.D.

women who use the treatment might be overlooking more serious problems that could affect fertility. "At times, the uterus is scarred and tipped because of endometriosis, pelvic adhesions, or pelvic inflammatory disease," she says. "If you get rid of the endometriosis and scar tissue, the typical patient does better." And even if repositioning can alleviate pain, says Suzanne Trupin, M.D., clinical professor of obstetrics and gynecology at the University of Illinois College of Medicine, actually being able to move the uterus and keep it in place through massage sounds—and is—too good to be true.

Other experts, however, are more open to the idea. Raphael S. Good, M.D., clinical professor of psychiatry and obstetrics and gynecology at the University of Miami School of Medicine, says many OB-GYNs have long suspected that a so-called misplaced uterus can cause painful periods. "A tipped uterus may require more intense contractions to discharge the menstrual flow," says Good, who notes that a number of his patients with the condition have complained of bad cramps. He says he wouldn't be surprised if external manipulation could ease the pain: "You can't hurt a woman by giving her a Mayan massage, and you may do her some good."

Nearly five years after Hauptman's first MUM session, she still massages herself several times a week—and she's free of menstrual pain. In fact, Hauptman has traveled to Belize to receive Arvigo's training firsthand. "I always tell women it's just not normal to suffer through cramps," Hauptman says. ■

Denver-based freelance writer Michelle Dally regularly contributes to U.S. News & World Report.

The Healing Touch

To locate a certified practitioner near you, go to www.arvigomassage.com/practitioners.html. Always see your OB-GYN to rule out problems before you seek alternative treatments.

Prevent Menstrual Migraines with This New Drug

There's good news for the approximately 5 million women a month who suffer from migraines during their periods: The new prescription drug Frova (frovatriptan) could prevent recurring pain. In a three-month study of 545 women who deal with these killer headaches, half of those treated with twice-daily doses of Frova—beginning two days before their periods were expected to start and continuing for a total of six days during their cycles—reported no headaches. (Only 26 percent of women who took placebos got the same results.) Because it stays in the bloodstream longer than other medications in its class (selective serotonin agonists called triptans), researchers think that Frova may work better for hormonally triggered migraines, which tend to last longer than typical ones.

Medicine That
STICKS

See why more and more women are throwing away their pill bottles and relying on the latest pharmaceutical trend—the patch.

BY EVA MARER • PHOTOGRAPHY BY KATE POWERS

It may be stuck firmly in place, but the latest pharmaceutical trend—the patch—is a huge leap forward. Pressing one onto your arm, back, or stomach makes taking your medicine easy. In many cases, it's also safer and more effective than popping a pill.

Patches deliver drugs in a steady stream, so your body doesn't have to handle a sudden flood of medication or a drought before the next dose. Plus, medicine that the skin absorbs goes directly into the bloodstream, bypassing the liver and stomach. That means a patch often works faster than its oral counterpart, says Alexander Bodkin, M.D., of the Clinical Psychopharmacology Research Program at Harvard University's McLean Hospital. Patch users report fewer side effects, too, because they avoid digesting drugs that can irritate the stomach or cause nausea, vomiting, and other problems.

Patches aren't for everyone, Bodkin says. If you have sensitive skin, they might cause redness,

> A patch often works faster than a pill because the medicine can go directly into the bloodstream, bypassing the liver and stomach.

itching, or rashes. Still, they're becoming more popular. In the past year or so, the U.S. Food and Drug Administration (FDA) has approved several, and more should be in drugstores soon. We think the following patches are among the most promising.

OVERACTIVE BLADDER

Patch: Oxytrol

What it does: Releases the drug oxybutynin, which relaxes the muscle that causes the urge to urinate.

The good news: Clinical trials have shown that the patch, which can be worn for up to four days, causes neither dry mouth nor constipation. Both complaints plague many women who take Ditropan (oxybutynin in tablet form) or Detrol (tolterodine), which works similarly.

Precautions: Whether in pill or patch form, oxybutynin can relax not only bladder muscles but also those of the stomach and intestines. That can cause discomfort and bloating in people whose stomachs cannot empty completely, since the relaxation sometimes intensifies this condition, which is technically known as gastric retention. **How to get it:** Approved by the FDA in February 2003, Oxytrol is now available by prescription.

BIRTH CONTROL

Patch: Ortho Evra Contraceptive Skin Patch

What it does: Delivers estrogen and progestin, the same hormones in most oral contraceptives.

The good news: You're less likely to miss a dose. One study in *The Journal of the American Medical Association (JAMA)* found that women were more apt to change out the patch once a week than take the Pill once a day.

Precautions: The JAMA study reported more breast tenderness in women who used transdermal birth control than in Pill takers. And if you weigh more than 198 pounds, the patch's hormone dose may not be high enough.

How to get it: Ortho Evra debuted in 2002; talk to your gynecologist about trying it.

DEPRESSION

Patch: EmSam

What it does: Transfers selegiline, a monoamine oxidase inhibitor (MAOI) that promotes the buildup of mood-elevating brain chemicals.

The good news: Doctors say the drug works quickly because it goes directly into the bloodstream. A recent study in *The American Journal of Psychiatry* showed that many patients using this patch felt better in one week, compared with the two to four weeks an oral antidepressant usually takes to kick in. EmSam also prevents a potentially dangerous (and sometimes fatal) side effect: Taken by mouth, MAOIs shut down an enzyme needed to digest the amino acid tyramine, which is found in wine and certain cheeses. The combination of tyramine and MAOIs can cause your blood pressure to skyrocket into stroke range. Because it bypasses the digestive system, selegiline delivered through the skin averts this problem.

Precautions: In the same study, 36 percent of patch users experienced redness and itching at the application site. Even so, most reported that the benefits outweighed the discomfort.

How to get it: Currently awaiting FDA approval, EmSam could be on the market in 2004.

CHRONIC PAIN

Patch: Duragesic

What it does: Provides around-the-clock relief with fentanyl, an opiate that attaches to and blocks pain receptors in the brain.

The good news: A single patch works continuously for three days—a boon to people suffering from such conditions as osteoarthritis, cancer, or persistent lower-back pain.

Precautions: Fentanyl is addictive; use it only when less potent painkillers don't work. Pregnant or nursing women should never use it.

How to get it: The FDA approved Duragesic more than a decade ago. Ask your doctor about it. ■

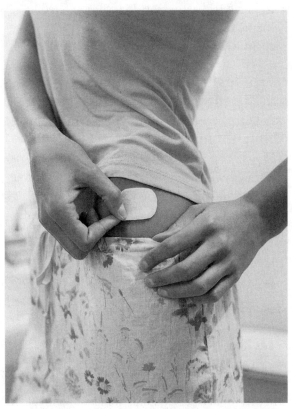

All-Natural Birth Control
The Latest in Contraception

Discover why a growing number of women are tossing aside pills and paraphernalia for no-tech birth control.

BY LYNDA LIU

When 30-year-old Kristin Murphy started taking birth control pills, she experienced Jekyll-and-Hyde mood swings. One minute, she'd be snuggling with her husband; the next, she couldn't stand to be in the same room with him. Her healthy sex drive also suffered. Nonetheless, she stuck with the Pill because she thought it was more reliable and easier to use than

> **Once the domain of Catholic women, natural birth control has been attracting a broader range of users who want to give their bodies a break from hormones.**

other methods of contraception. Murphy took four different kinds of pills in as many years, hoping to find the right match for her body. By the time she quit, she was so frustrated that even an unintended pregnancy would've seemed a better choice than the emotional roller coaster she had been on.

Then Murphy stumbled upon the fertility-awareness method (FAM), an all-natural birth control option, on a women's Internet message board. Today, she is one of a growing number of women who, for reasons more practical than religious, are going low-tech with contraception. Once the domain of Catholic women, natural birth

control has been attracting a broader range of users, like Murphy, who want to give their bodies a break from hormones, explains Joseph Stanford, M.D., associate professor of family and preventive medicine at the University of Utah and former president of the American Academy of Natural Family Planning. He estimates that 40 percent of women who follow natural contraceptive methods are actually non-Catholics.

FAM was developed to meet the needs of women who want a secular form of drug-free birth control. It relies on the daily monitoring of cervical fluid; morning temperatures; and, optionally, position, texture, and openness of the cervix (which change as ovulation approaches). All these factors help a woman track her fertile times in order to avoid—or achieve—pregnancy.

"If a couple uses FAM for contraception correctly, they can expect to have a pregnancy rate somewhere between 1 and 5 percent," Stanford says. The pregnancy rates of women who choose to have sex during their fertile periods, however, will be only as good as the birth-control methods they use. Because FAM does not protect against sexually transmitted diseases, nonmonogamous women should rely on barrier contraception instead.

The difference between FAM and its Catholic counterpart, natural family planning (NFP), is philosophical. NFP requires its followers to abstain from sexual intercourse during the fertile period because Catholic doctrine forbids artificial contraception. FAM, on the other hand, lets individuals decide whether they will forgo sex or use another form of birth control on those days.

Women who use FAM have to check their fertility signs daily, because stress and illness can alter ovulation patterns. "This method is most effective in a motivated couple," says Margaret Polaneczky, M.D., an associate clinical professor of obstetrics and gynecology at Weill Medical College of Cornell University. Charting and learning to read fertility markers is "not as easy as popping a pill at first," Murphy says, but after a few months, FAM becomes second nature and requires very little time. Murphy also likes that it's something both she and her husband can be involved with. "We get up, I'll put the thermometer in, and we can snuggle for a few extra minutes," she says. Cervical-fluid checks have also become a part of her routine.

The vigilant monitoring required by FAM and NFP sets these techniques apart from the rhythm method, the notoriously ineffective system of natural contraception based on a woman's menstrual cycle. Fertility

Another Natural Option

A recent study reported in the journal *Contraception* found that the Standard Days Method, a new natural technique in which couples avoid unprotected sex during days 8 through 19 of the women's menstrual cycles, was more than 95-percent effective when used correctly. For the method to work, a woman must have menstrual cycles of 26 to 32 days, says Victoria Jennings, Ph.D., one of the study's authors and director of the Institute for Reproductive Health at Georgetown University. For more information, visit www.cyclebeads.com.

awareness is much more effective because it identifies a woman's potential to conceive on a day-to-day basis, says Toni Weschler, M.P.H., author of *Taking Charge of Your Fertility*, a book that is credited with introducing this method outside the Catholic Church.

Beyond birth control, FAM teaches women to better understand their reproductive systems. "It's worth looking into just to learn the basics about your body and what goes on through your monthly cycle," Murphy says. "I felt like this is what I should have learned when I was 16." ▪

Finally, a Birth Control Pill for Men ...
But can you trust them to take it?

If further tests go well, a birth control pill for men may be available in the near future. A recent study in the *Proceedings of the National Academy of Sciences* showed that a non-hormonal compound called NB-DNJ acts as a reversible male contraceptive in mice and has already been found to be safe in humans. But could you count on your mate to take the new Pill? More than 600 *Health* readers responded to our Web poll. The results:

No way: Almost one-third of survey participants wouldn't trust their men to bear the birth-control burden.

Yes, with conditions: Nearly half of the readers polled would trust their guys, but only if the women picked up the prescription, reminded their men to take it, or used a backup method.

Go for it: About 22 percent totally trusted their honeys. Would you?

Keys to CONCEPTION

Real women and fertility experts sound off on what it takes to make a baby at any age.

BY DONNA FREYDKIN • PHOTOGRAPHY BY ANN ELLIOT CUTTING

For years, 20-something women were more concerned with careers and dating than strollers and nursing bras. They felt reassured by the doctor-supported belief that prime baby-making time lasted until their mid-30s. A recent study, however, has found that fertility actually begins to decline much earlier than that: at age 27. That's made some women rethink their priorities.

But don't ditch your birth control and jump into the sack just yet. We asked fertility experts to take a look at what the findings really mean. Yes, according to the study published in *Human Reproduction*, women ages 27 to 34 were 10 percent less likely to conceive during any one menstrual cycle than their 19- to 26-year-old counterparts. Women ages 35 and older, meanwhile, were half as likely to get pregnant during one month as women under age 27. Still, says study author David Dunson, Ph.D., the findings don't mean you've missed your chance at motherhood if you're not changing diapers by your late 20s. "Every woman is different, and there are no absolutes. You should just expect it to take a little more time to get pregnant after age 27," explains Dunson, a researcher at the National Institute of Environmental Health Sciences.

Sure, pop star Brandy might have made the biologically correct choice to have a daughter at 23, but early motherhood doesn't work for many women. Here are sound bites from women at various life stages, plus fertility experts' takes on their situations. The consensus: Making babies is as much an art as an exact science.

THE AGE OF DISCOVERY (26 AND YOUNGER)

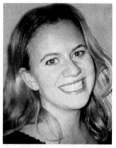

"I got a big promotion at work and am living in a dream apartment," says Lauren Weedon (left), 25, an editor from Jacksonville, Florida. "The last thing on my mind is having a baby. I can't even remember to water my plants, much less begin thinking of raising a child."

Baby Rx: "Your fertility is at its peak now, but women in their 20s should be using condoms, not worrying about popping out babies. The sexually transmitted disease chlamydia is one of the main reasons that women don't get pregnant," says Stephanie Teal, an OB-GYN at New York City's Columbia-Presbyterian Medical Center. "I also tell women to get regular gynecological checkups, quit smoking, lighten up on their alcohol consumption, get lots of sleep, and maintain a healthy weight."

THE TRANSITION YEARS (27–34)

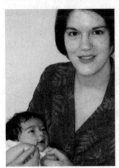

"My husband and I decided to try to get pregnant when I hit my early 30s," says stay-at-home mom Kristin Lemmerman (left), 33, of Atlanta. "I just assumed it would happen right away. But it wasn't so easy. I was in great shape, totally healthy, didn't smoke or drink—and it took us about six months to conceive. I started to worry that something might be the matter, although I had gotten a clean bill of health from my doctor."

Baby Rx: "Does fertility go down a bit here? Sure," says David Adamson, M.D., director of Fertility Physicians of Northern California, a clinical practice in Palo Alto and San Jose. "But does it go down so much that people should worry? I don't think so. At this stage of the game, women should decide whether and when they want to have kids, and get regular Pap smears and checkups. If they're healthy and don't conceive within a year, they should see a doctor."

THE SETTLED DECADE (35–39)

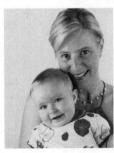

"I needed to have my financial independence, as well as the right partner, to embrace the idea of having children. When I finally met my soul mate, conceiving became a full-time job," says former Manhattan stockbroker Jill Lloyd (left), 39. She tried to get pregnant for 19 months before turning to artificial insemination and scoring on the first try. "We knew it was serious business when watching the calendar, using ovulation kits, taking my temperature, and shagging even when we were both exhausted didn't work at all."

Baby Rx: "Yes, being healthy is a good thing, but as you age, your lifestyle becomes less relevant—a good workout can't compete with the effects of aging. You just start to run out of healthy eggs," Teal says. "Women ages 35 and older can use ovulation predictors to make sure they're having sex at the optimum time, have their partner get a sperm count, and make sure they don't have blocked fallopian tubes. If they can't get pregnant spontaneously, they should get an evaluation within six months."

THE TAKE-CHARGE TIME (40 AND OLDER)

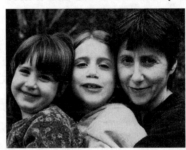

"I waited this long to have children because I simply was not ready," says Julia Indichova (left), now 53, a fertility counselor and mother of two from Woodstock, New York. "I naturally conceived my first daughter at age 41 in just one month and my second daughter four years later, after being told that I would never be able to have any more children because of an untreatable hormonal imbalance. So, I gave myself a total physical, emotional, and spiritual overhaul, and I conceived naturally eight months later."

Baby Rx: "Yes, women can conceive naturally, but they should be aware that the fertility loss here is dramatic. At age 40, fertility is half of what it was when it was optimal. By age 42, it's down to half of that," Adamson says. "By age 43 or 44, it's almost gone. But people do have options. Couples can choose to undergo standard hormone treatment, try in vitro fertilization, use egg donors, or adopt." ▪

Writer Donna Freydkin also contributes to USA Today *and* Marie Claire.

The Downside of Fertility Treatment:
Too Many Babies

Ana and her husband struggled for years to get pregnant. They never expected the anguish success would bring.

BY ANA MYERS*
*NAMES IN THIS STORY HAVE BEEN CHANGED.

Lying on the examination table, I can't help but worry that something has gone wrong. Nurse Lucy is taking an awfully long time on the ultrasound images of my uterus, and my stomach is in knots. I am pregnant with twins; my husband and I are nervously tracking their development.

Lucy moves her pointer around the computer screen and prints out images of the tiny fetuses. Finally, she stops, looks at me, and says, "There's a third fetus." I can tell by her face that this is not good news.

I've been through a lot with Lucy at this fertility practice. After three years of trying naturally, I had come here and become pregnant, only to lose the baby at 10½ weeks. The loss devastated me and my husband, Peter; in vitro fertilization (IVF) had been an emotional, physical, and financial ordeal. Now, two years and six IVFs later, we're pregnant again.

At first, just one fetus was detected and dubbed "Baby A." My visit a week later revealed "Baby B,"

and suddenly we were the parents-to-be of twins. We knew what that meant: a difficult pregnancy, the danger that the babies would be born too early, and an increased likelihood of surgical delivery. Then would come all the challenges of raising two children of the same age at the same time. Still, we thought, it was probably for the best. We had spent six years trying to conceive, and we might never have the opportunity to try again. Reeling, we nervously celebrated the news.

But now, eight weeks into the pregnancy, we have to adjust again. "Triplets? *Three* babies?" I ask, incredulous. Lucy nods, although she notes that Number Three looks very small. Our doctor comes in and confirms the news. "It might not make it," he says. "It doesn't seem to be as well-developed." He also repeats what we've read about triplets: While some are born healthy, they are far more likely than twins to arrive prematurely and can suffer serious lifelong health problems or learning disabilities.

If "Baby C" survives, he suggests that we consider a fetal reduction—that is, eliminating one fetus so that the other two have a better chance.

It's the first we've heard of this procedure. It seems unthinkable. By a miracle of science, we've managed to get pregnant. And now we have to decide whether to terminate what we tried so hard to create? We find ourselves hoping that one fetus just disappears so we won't be faced with two impossible decisions: whether to eliminate one, and if so, *which one*.

In the back of our minds, we've known the risk. We've consistently implanted more than one fertilized egg at a time to increase my pregnancy chances; this is standard at fertility clinics, though we've been warned that it also increases the odds of multiple births. As time and money began to run out for us, our doctor agreed that we should implant more embryos. On our fifth IVF, we implanted five, hoping one might take. On our sixth roll of the dice, we implanted six. And now we find we have succeeded all too well.

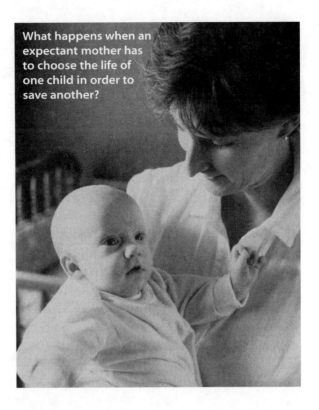

What happens when an expectant mother has to choose the life of one child in order to save another?

WEEK 9: Baby C shows no signs of disappearing on its own. Our physician recommends that we visit a fetal-reduction specialist. Six patients in our doctor's practice have chosen to go forward with their triplet pregnancies; half of the women ended up miscarrying all three babies. Tormented by the idea of losing ours or watching them suffer lasting hardship because of birth defects, we decide to consult the specialist.

He explains the procedure: Guided by ultrasound, the doctor inserts a long needle into my abdomen and injects potassium chloride into one of the fetuses to stop its heart. The fetus will then be absorbed into my body, as sometimes happens, apparently, when a woman miscarries naturally. He tells us more about the risks of carrying triplets, which experience "extreme preterm birth" (delivery between 20 and 27 weeks) at twice the rate of twins and 12 times the rate of single pregnancies. Among the defects more likely for triplets, he says, are cerebral palsy and problems with eyesight, breathing, hearing, and learning. Dazed, we return home.

WEEK 10: We reluctantly decide on a reduction. Our doctor advises us to keep the two embryos that appear largest and healthiest, because they seem to have the best prospects for survival. From this point on, nurses will no longer show us ultrasound images of Baby C. Instead, we're to focus on the shadowy figures of the larger babies and on giving them every possible chance to make it through the pregnancy.

WEEK 11: The reduction is days away. We return to the specialist for another ultrasound. Stunningly, he finds that Baby C is too low in the womb for the abdominal approach. If we insist on Baby C, he says, the needle will have to be inserted vaginally, a more difficult procedure. Our doctor says he'd rather continue with the lower-risk approach. He advises us to choose the fetus that is easiest to reach—one of the two he had recommended that we keep.

Besides, he says, the new ultrasounds show that Baby C has nearly caught up in size and seems as viable as the other two. For weeks, I've abhorred the very notion of a reduction, coming to accept it only as a way to save the stronger fetuses. And now my world is upended again as Peter and I learn that we will lose one of the babies we thought we were saving.

WEEK 11½: We've just spoken to another specialist. He concurs with the first: The procedure will be less dangerous if it targets the easiest-to-reach fetus. Numbly, we agree to the safer option, wondering when—if—this emotional roller coaster will end.

WEEK 12: I've lain on a gurney in the waiting room for nearly an hour, next to a crying woman I can only assume is in the same unimaginable position. At last, I'm wheeled into the operating room. Peter is allowed to stay; I press his hands over my face while they insert the needle into my abdomen. It's over in minutes. We wait an hour for a recheck to be sure the procedure was successful, then leave, driving home in exhausted silence.

WEEK 13: The emotional pain is compounded by my fear that the procedure will cause me to miscarry. I lose some fluid in the days after the reduction, but the twins survive and start clearly doing well. We begin to enjoy watching them grow.

WEEK 32: The twins are here! After endless bed rest and a scare three months ago when I had contractions, my water breaks. We rush to the hospital for a C-section. The babies, both boys, weigh in at 4.6 pounds and 5.1 pounds. That's a little below average for a twin (5.5 pounds in the United States), but way ahead of the 3.5-pound average for triplets.

THEIR FIRST DAYS: Our two sons are in the neonatal intensive care unit, in incubators with dozens of wires crisscrossing their tiny bodies. Getting them to the point where they can eat and breathe on their own is maddeningly slow. Peter and I find it hard to leave them each night and even harder not to be allowed to snuggle our newborns. We hold them only for brief intervals so they can rest and get stronger.

THE REST OF THE STORY: After a month in intensive care, Austin and Harry were able to come home. They cried almost constantly for six months, since their underdeveloped digestive systems made eating painful. But after their rough start, they thrived and have grown into energetic 6-year-olds. Peter and I have decided we won't try to have more children, but instead to take pleasure in our wonderful family. We're deeply grateful for the miracles of IVF, but having dealt with a multiple pregnancy, we could not bring ourselves to take another risk.

> We have no regrets about seeking fertility treatments. But knowing what we do now, we would no longer choose to implant so many embryos at once.

Some would argue that eliminating one fetus to help the other two is playing God. Others say we'd already taken on that role by conceiving artificially. We have no regrets about seeking fertility treatments. But knowing what we do now, we would no longer choose to implant so many embryos at once. It was a heartbreaking experience. When I look at the bright, expressive face of the firstborn of our twins, I am still haunted by a painful memory. He was Baby C—the fetus who originally was to have been eliminated. Had it not been for his position in the womb, he would not be here now.

As agonizing as the experience was, I'm writing this to spread awareness of the problems sometimes associated with fertility treatments. Perhaps one day, specialists will be better able to help infertile couples, while preventing multiple pregnancies. Expectant parents might then be spared the emotional toll of a reduction, anguish that dims a little through the years but never entirely disappears. ■

Find the Best Fertility Clinic

Trying to get pregnant can be stressful enough without having to worry about whether your fertility clinic makes the grade. You don't want to waste time and money at a center with a low success rate, or end up at one known for producing multiple births.

But you *can* find the help you need. The Centers for Disease Control and Prevention (CDC) puts out a biannual report (at www.cdc.gov/nccdphp/drh/ART0 0/index.htm) that lists information about clinics nationwide. It's not foolproof—critics say some of the info is inaccurate. Still, David Hoffman, M.D., former president of the Society for Assisted Reproductive Technology, which collects data for the CDC, says the report can be useful. "It gives you an idea of how many cases the clinic handles, whether the lab's certified, and what the success rate is for different age groups," he says. "It's not perfect, but it's good."

Start with the report to narrow your options. Before making a final choice, Pamela Madsen, executive director of the American Infertility Association, suggests that you ask the following four questions during your initial consultation with a physician.

1. Is a health-care provider accessible by phone, 24 hours a day, seven days a week? Clinics control egg development, so most retrievals can be scheduled during the week; nevertheless, you want someone on hand to answer your questions any time of day or night.

2. Does the center treat people my age? It looks successful because it deals primarily with younger couples, Madsen cautions. "What do they do for their over-40 population?"

3. Will the lab be able to handle the specific procedures I need? Suppose you've been told that you need sperm injection or testing for genetic diseases. Not all clinics provide these services, Madsen says. If yours doesn't, ask about off-site procedures.

4. What kind of emotional support does the clinic offer? You may be receiving treatment for some time, and the stress can take its toll. Some clinics employ therapists; others work with low- or no-cost support groups.

Eggs: A Limited Resource

Blame the fertility fallout on the dramatic drop-off of your eggs. At puberty, most women have a treasure trove of 300,000 to 400,000 healthy eggs raring to get fertilized, but only 300 to 500 of them will develop to maturity. Compare that to the reproductive capacity of guys, who continuously produce fresh sperm every 90 days. The older women get, the fewer quality eggs their ovaries release. By their late 30s, most women have about 25,000 good ones remaining. When women reach age 45, only several thousand eggs are left, and many of those aren't viable because of genetic flaws.

More than 90 percent of new prescription drugs approved since 1980 have not been adequately screened to ensure they don't cause birth defects, according to a recent report in the journal *Obstetrics & Gynecology*. Talk to your doc before popping any pills while pregnant.

The Fatty Acid for Moms-to-Be

What moms-to-be eat now may mean a well-rested little one later. A University of Connecticut study found that babies born to women who had consumed several servings of docosahexaenoic acid (DHA) a week during their last trimester slept more soundly than newborns whose moms skimped on the fatty acid. A safe source of DHA is cold-water fish, such as salmon and sole; eggs enriched with DHA are now available in some grocery stores.

Mixing Medication with Pregnancy

Until recently, if a pregnant woman got sick, she had to choose between her health and her baby's. If only more doctors knew things have changed.

BY CHRISTIE ASCHWANDEN

Lisa Radel was only 17 weeks pregnant when she found a lump in one breast. The diagnosis—cancer—forced questions with ugly answers: Should she immediately attack the disease, perhaps endangering her baby? Or should she wait five months, protecting the baby at the risk of her own survival? "I was worried about what treatment would do to my unborn child," says Radel, a registered dietitian from Buffalo, New York, "but also whether I'd be around to watch my children grow up." On the face of it, delay seemed the inevitable choice. After all, if there's one thing doctors and women learned from the 1960s thalidomide disasters that left thousands of children with missing or deformed limbs, medications and pregnancy are a dangerous combination.

The fact is, this old wisdom doesn't always hold true. By piecing together reports from women who conceive unintentionally while on medications, researchers are learning that pregnant women can safely take drugs for many common conditions, from asthma and allergies to heartburn and pain. They're also finding that abruptly stopping treatment for a chronic illness is often the riskier option for both mother and child.

By piecing together reports from women who conceive unintentionally while on medications, researchers are learning that pregnant women can safely take drugs for many common conditions.

Now more than ever, women and their doctors need to be armed with the latest information. But that's no easy task. Because cancer is uncommon during pregnancy, for example, most physicians lack firsthand experience with it. And many oncologists hesitate to treat pregnant patients altogether.

When faced with her dilemma eight years ago, Radel was lucky enough to find a specialist familiar with the latest research on chemotherapy and pregnancy. To her immense relief, he said she didn't have

112

to choose between her life and her baby's. Although chemotherapy drugs target rapidly dividing cancer cells, which behave much like the cells in a growing fetus, Radel's doctor assured her that the medications he was recommending were safe.

"My husband and I did a lot of research, and we just had to believe that this was true," Radel says. So they decided to go ahead with the therapy. And except for the chemo and the emotional toll of a life-threatening disease, her pregnancy continued just like her first one, with son Matthew, did two years earlier. Eventually, she delivered another healthy baby boy. Today, Radel is 42 and cancer-free, and second son Connor is a normal 8-year-old who has never met a video game he didn't like.

Others aren't so fortunate. Radel says that women referred to Pregnant With Cancer, a support group she helped found, still come to her with stories of doctors who refused to give them chemotherapy if they planned to carry their babies to term. Many practitioners either don't know where to turn for information or they're unaware that it exists in the first place, says Gideon Koren, M.D., a clinical pharmacologist at Toronto's Hospital for Sick Children.

WOMEN WHO ARE DIAGNOSED with cancer during pregnancy need to know there are other women who have gone through this and are OK," says Elyce Cardonick, M.D., a doctor at Thomas Jefferson University in Philadelphia. Cardonick has conducted two studies showing that pregnant women who undergo chemotherapy after the first trimester later deliver normal babies.

Yet drug companies rarely update their product labels to reflect studies like Cardonick's. The reason? "They're not required to," says Sandra Kweder, M.D., co-chair of the U.S. Food and Drug Administration's Pregnancy Labeling Task Force. And because of liability concerns, she adds, "most are happier not saying anything."

The federal government first stepped into the information vacuum in the late 1970s, rating drugs' risk during pregnancy with one of five letters: A, B, C, D, or X. A is the safest, Kweder says, while X means the medicine's potential risks outweigh its benefits. But most products end up as Cs, which usually means there wasn't enough evidence to assess the risk. And that affords little guidance in determining safety.

Choosing older drugs over newer ones is smart when you can do it. The longer a drug has been around, the more time researchers have had to document any troublesome side effects it may cause.

Kweder says she hopes a new labeling system that requires more complete information will address the dilemmas that pregnant women face in real life (her task force expects to finish work on that system later this year). "What's the risk of not treating a condition with the drug versus the risk of keeping the mother healthy with the drug?" she says. "Right now, the labels don't speak to that."

Every pregnant woman wants to err on the side of caution. That may mean continuing to take medicine. Many women with asthma, for instance, assume they must go drug-free if they get pregnant, says Nancy Sander, president of the Allergy & Asthma Network and Mothers of Asthmatics in Fairfax, Virginia. "But remember that you're breathing for two," she says. "If you're having asthma symptoms, your baby's oxygen supply is lower than it could be."

And if you die, your baby won't get any air at all: One expectant mother died of an asthma attack after forgoing her medication, says Michael Schatz, M.D., an allergist at Kaiser Permanente Medical Center in San Diego. "There's increasing recognition that the risk of asthma is greater than the risk of most asthma drugs," he says.

QUITTING ANTIDEPRESSANT DRUGS while pregnant could prove harmful—even deadly—to both mother and baby. When Cari Gagan's doctor took her off Prozac during her 1996 pregnancy, her depression flooded back. "Nothing mattered to me," the 33-year-old Sault Ste. Marie, Ontario, mother recalls. "I stayed in bed all day and cried. I really just wanted to die." Her doctor was unsympathetic: "He said it was just something I would get over."

113

Some women have an even harder time than Gagan. "We have had very sad cases of women committing suicide after stopping antidepressants cold turkey," says Koren. In the *Journal of Psychiatry & Neuroscience*, he reported cases of 36 pregnant women who abruptly quit antidepressants and went on to suffer physical or psychological problems. Many of those drugs are considered safe for expectant mothers, Koren says, stressing that women should not stop taking them without getting the facts beforehand.

When Gagan got pregnant again in 1998, she dreaded another nine months of hell so much that she sought out a different doctor. Her new obstetrician consulted Motherisk—one of the world's largest clearinghouses for information on drugs and pregnancy—and learned that the published risks of early delivery and low birth weight were not so great that Gagan needed to stop taking Prozac. "I was really worried about side effects for the baby," Gagan says. "But my doctor said it was worse for the child's mental and physical health to have a depressed mother." She weathered the pregnancy with no downward spiral. Her son James, now 4 years old, is healthy and active.

None of this means a pregnant woman can blithely pop pills. Even when a condition can be safely treated, prudence often requires switching drugs. For example, research has shown that a class of blood pressure medicines called ACE inhibitors causes birth defects, while many other hypertension drugs appear safe. Patti Taylor, 35, a human resources manager in Baltimore, was diagnosed with high blood pressure just before she conceived her

Which Drugs Are Safe?

Most don't come with clear answers, but these do.

OK to Take

Tylenol (acetaminophen): "Tylenol is probably the safest drug you can take during pregnancy," says pharmacist Donald Sullivan, Ph.D. This is the remedy of choice for pain and fever.

Sudafed (pseudoephedrine): Although you should avoid it during the first trimester, this is the best medicine for a bad cold during the second and third trimesters.

Tums (calcium carbonate) and Zantac (ranitidine): Both safely treat heartburn, one of the most frequent complaints among pregnant women.

Asthma medications: Expectant mothers with asthma should consult their doctors to develop a treatment plan. But most asthma drugs, especially inhaled ones, are OK during pregnancy, says Michael Schatz, M.D., an allergist at Kaiser Permanente Medical Center in San Diego.

Nasalcrom (cromolyn sodium): This is the nasal spray to use for allergies during pregnancy.

Not OK

Accutane (isotretinoin): Used to clear severe acne, this drug causes serious birth defects. Women should stop taking it at least a month before they try to become pregnant.

Lipitor (atorvastatin) and Mevacor (lovastatin): These cholesterol-lowering drugs have been linked to birth defects and may also increase the risk of miscarriage.

Aspirin: Unless your doctor prescribes a low dose for a specific condition, such as high blood pressure, abstain. Because Pepto-Bismol contains a similar drug, you should avoid it during the last trimester as well, Sullivan says.

Valium (diazepam) and Xanax (alprazolam): These antianxiety drugs can cause floppy-infant syndrome, characterized by fatigue and difficulty sucking. High doses can induce withdrawal symptoms in the baby after birth.

Tetracycline antibiotics: Taken in the last few weeks of pregnancy, these can discolor or deform a baby's permanent teeth, which form at this time.

third child. It was high enough to increase her risk of complications, so her doctor prescribed a drug known to be safe for mothers and babies. Taylor had also been taking Nexium for heartburn, but her doctor switched her to Zantac, an older—and more studied—alternative.

CHOOSING OLDER DRUGS over new ones, in fact, is smart when you can do it, advises Donald Sullivan, Ph.D., author of *The Expectant Mother's Guide to Prescription and Nonprescription Drugs, Vitamins, Home Remedies, and Herbal Products.* The longer a drug has been around, the more time researchers have had to document any troublesome side effects, he says.

With so many factors to consider, making any decision might seem overwhelming at first. But several credible resources are available, including Motherisk, the clearinghouse that Koren runs at the Hospital for Sick Children in Toronto. "More than 50 percent of pregnancies are not planned, and millions of women thus take medications into pregnancy," he says. Motherisk tracks cases all over the world and handles queries from hundreds of women and their doctors every day. Over the last decade, Motherisk researchers have published more than 300 peer-reviewed papers about drug safety during pregnancy.

Other resources include an online database of drugs and their risk ratings at Perinatology.com, affiliated with the San Gabriel Valley Perinatal Medical Group of California. OTIS, a North American network of services offering up-to-date information on the ways drugs and chemicals affect human embryos, can provide referrals to local databases. There are also registries for specific drugs, such as the migraine remedy Imitrex and the antidepressant Wellbutrin, that track the health of babies exposed to them in the womb.

The essential point is still this: Discontinuing any drugs before pregnancy should be your first choice—if you can do it without harming your health. A fetus is most vulnerable to medicines during the first 4 to 12 weeks and the last month of gestation (most damage, if there is any, would prevent a pregnancy from continuing beyond the first few days). "The first trimester is when all the organs form, and the last month is crucial because that's when the finishing touches are put on the lungs and heart," Sullivan says. "The second trimester is probably the safest time to take medications."

But if you or someone you love is taking a medication when a pregnancy is confirmed, don't panic. Call your doctor straightaway to get some answers before doing anything else.

And then take a deep breath. For now, at least, every medication decision involves some unknowns, despite your physician's level of expertise and the reliability of research. This is why Lisa Radel had to throw the dice when she chose chemotherapy—and why a part of her remained fearful.

"I was afraid to look at the sonogram because I was so scared I would lose the baby," she recalls. Her choices required faith in her doctors and a willingness to accept some risk. In that respect, Sullivan says, Radel was no different from any other pregnant woman. "In a sense, every pregnancy is uncertain," he says. But Radel says that when she sees her sons—both of them—zipping by her on their inline skates, she knows that she, at least, made the right choice. ◼

Contributing editor Christie Aschwanden is a former genetics researcher who helped map the human genome.

Info Sources
Allergy & Asthma Network, call 800-878-4403 or log on to www.breatherville.org to order the free pamphlet "Breathing for Two."
Motherisk, 416-813-6780 or www.motherisk.org
OTIS, the Organization of Teratology Information Services, 866-626-6847 or www.otispregnancy.org
Perinatology.com, www.perinatology.com/exposures/druglist.htm
Pregnant With Cancer Support Group, www.pregnantwithcancer.org
Registry of Pregnancies Exposed to Chemotherapeutic Agents, Children's Hospital of Oklahoma, Oklahoma City, 405-271-8685

Sayonara, Stretch Marks

New research shows that you can make them fade.

Stretch marks are an inevitable part of life for most women. But a new procedure looks promising: The U.S. Food and Drug Administration has approved the Xtrac excimer laser to treat these annoying scars. "Currently used for psoriasis and other skin conditions, this laser stimulates cells in the area to produce more pigment, which makes stretch marks less visible," says David J. Goldberg, M.D., director of laser research in the department of dermatology at Mount Sinai School of Medicine in New York City. The effect is like a tan, making the blemishes blend into surrounding skin (they don't disappear completely, though). Stretch marks are remarkably common: About 90 percent of pregnant women develop them, but they can also result from weight gain, growth spurts, genetics, or long-term use of certain prescriptions, such as cortisone creams. The marks start as raised red lines, then flatten and fade to white streaks in about a year. In the past, doctors were able to remedy stretch marks at the earliest stages, but once they turned white, nothing seemed to work—that's where the laser comes in. Results last up to six months, but they come at a cost: Most women need at least 10 weekly sessions at about $250 to $750 each (depending on the size of the area being treated and where you live).

Workout Wear Goes Maternal

Most expectant moms know regular exercise is a good idea, but who wants to hit the gym wearing a big pastel smock or a pair of plus-size sweats? Fortunately, big-name companies, such as Adidas, Nike, Reebok, and Title 9 Sports, have begun to offer fitness wear for mothers-to-be with all the style, support, and wicking power found in the companies' regular lines, plus a little extra room for your growing belly. We have only one complaint: Sure, black (and the occasional navy) is slimming and chic, but c'mon—even pregnant women like to wear a little color.

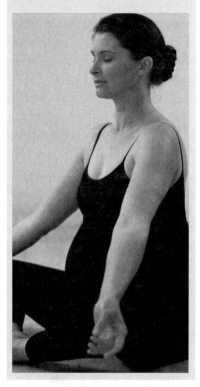

Mothers Know Best When It Comes to Baby Talk

A new study supports what moms have always suspected: Women seem to be better at baby talk than men. Researchers at Lehigh University in Bethlehem, Pennsylvania, asked a small group of parents to make approving or disapproving noises as they either encouraged their babies to play or warned them away from dangerous objects. The recorded sessions were fed into a computer program designed to peg parental speech as supportive or critical. In the end, the software correctly ID'd 12 percent more cues given by moms than dads. The program was accurate only 70 percent of the time, and the scientists admit men may communicate effectively in ways technology can't grasp. But babies respond to the emotional content of voices—and it's possible that Mom's coochy-coos are easier for them to understand.

Coming Soon: Blood Tests That Can Detect Breast Cancer

A study led jointly by Duke University, the M.D. Anderson Cancer Center in Houston, the U.S. Food and Drug Administration (FDA), and the National Institutes of Health found that a simple blood-protein test may be nearly as effective as mammograms in spotting breast cancer. The exam is still one-and-a-half to three years away from FDA approval, but it may someday replace routine screening for healthy women and be used alongside mammograms for those at high risk.

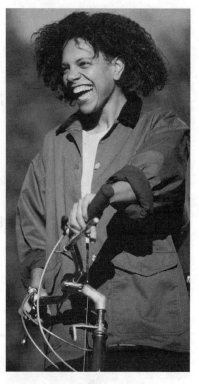

Discovery Gives New Hope for Fighting Breast Tumors

Until now, doctors have been frustrated by the 20 percent of breast cancers that recur and spread even after aggressive treatment. But a new study may ultimately lead to more effective, less invasive treatments for the 180 thousand women who are diagnosed with the disease each year.

Doctors have long believed that all types of breast-cancer

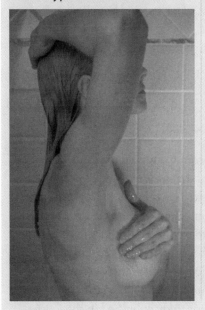

cells were malignant and capable of spreading. But researchers at the University of Michigan have, for the first time, isolated stem cells in breast tumors. They suspect that these cells—capable of maturing into any kind of tissue, whether brain, bone, or breast—are responsible for spreading the disease. In the new study, injecting mice with as few as 100 stem cells from breast cancers caused tumors in every case. But mice injected with as many as 10,000 nonstem cancer cells developed no tumors. "The goal of current therapies has been to shrink tumors across the board; our research suggests we may need to target the stem cells with very precise treatments," says Max S. Wicha, M.D., director of the University of Michigan's Comprehensive Cancer Center. Within the next five years, the discovery could lead to new drug regimens, he says.

Motivation to Exercise—It May Prevent Breast Cancer

Recently published research from the University at Buffalo found that premenopausal women who had exercised strenuously for three-and-a-half hours a week at age 16 cut their chances of getting breast cancer by 40 percent, compared with women who were inactive as teens. The risk was 20-percent lower in postmenopausal women. But even if you were an adolescent couch potato, it's still not too late: Fitting in physical exercise at any age can help ward off cancer, the researchers say.

do-it-yourself BIRTHING

A growing number of couples are boycotting hospitals, doctors—even midwives—and delivering their babies without professional help. Meanwhile, a debate heats up over the safety risks.

BY CHRISTINA FRANK

When Lesley Cross went into labor with her second child, she got into an inflatable kiddie pool set up in her home and, a few hours later, reached down and delivered her daughter. The only other people present were her husband and their 5-year-old son. "It was the most amazing thing," says Cross, 30, who runs a scrapbook-making business in Boyertown, Pennsylvania. "It felt like the perfect, normal, natural way to give birth." The delivery of her first child, Logan, was just the opposite, she says. It took place in a hospital, where Cross thinks the doctoring was excessive. "I told my obstetrician that I wanted a natural birth," Cross says. Despite her request, when she got to the hospital, she says her doctor gave her medications to speed up delivery. After her son was born, she recalls, the staff didn't let her hold or breast-feed him for 45 minutes. "I decided that my next child

> **Just because one woman delivers five normal babies herself doesn't mean the lady next door won't have a disaster.**
> ——**Laura Riley, M.D.**

would be born at home, and that I'd be the one to deliver her," she says.

Cross isn't the only one who believes that birthing solo is the way to go. She's part of what could be called an underground movement to fight the perceived pregnancy-as-disease mentality of some doctors and midwives.

In the past decade or so, medical interventions have increased: The number of labor inductions has more than doubled (from 9 to 19 percent), and the cesarean section rate, after a slight dip, has crept back up (from 20.8 percent in 1995 to 24.4 percent in 2002). Also on the rise is the number of Web sites, books, and videos devoted to unassisted delivery.

Natural childbearing is fine when a professional is on hand, say doctors and midwives, but turning your bedroom into a delivery room is both radical and risky. A recent study published in the journal

Obstetrics & Gynecology proves it: Home births double the risk of newborn death and increase the likelihood of problems in the mother.

Scary stats hardly faze do-it-yourselfers. As they see it, having a baby is a completely natural process—like breathing or digestion—that will "just happen" if you let it. Even doctor-supervised prenatal care is dismissed as superfluous. Midwives are vetoed because they resort to many of the same procedures as doctors. "When a midwife comes to your home, she has a list of things she's required by law to do, such as check dilation and time contractions, which interferes with the natural process," says Laura Shanley, who delivered her five children by herself and wrote the book *Unassisted Childbirth*. "Giving birth is like having sex. It's an intimate act that requires privacy, and it shouldn't include an outsider unless the couple wants someone there."

However, privacy might not be so great if things go awry. "When bad things happen and you're not in an environment that can handle them, they can snowball into something worse," says Laura Riley, M.D., chairwoman of the obstetric-practice committee of the American College of Obstetricians and Gynecologists. "Just because one woman delivers five normal babies herself doesn't mean the lady next door won't have a disaster." She cites emergencies such as the baby's head getting stuck in the birth canal; leakage of amniotic fluid into the mother's bloodstream, which causes maternal death in 80 percent of cases; postbirth bleeding, which can also be fatal; and life-threatening bacterial infections in newborns. Though uncommon, these problems should not be discounted if you're thinking about home delivery. "Catastrophic events are rare, but when they do happen, it's preferable to have a professional present who can handle the situation," Riley says.

Riley and other physicians do concede that some interventions take control away from the mother-to-be. For example, fetal monitors, machines that are strapped to a woman's belly to measure the baby's heart rate, have become standard in many hospitals and limit the mother's mobility. Having an epidural can stall labor, sometimes leading to a C-section. "There's no question that intervention in low-risk pregnancies has increased," Riley says. "Are these procedures often unnecessary? Yes." She suggests that women who are unlikely to have complications stay at home until they're in active labor to avoid these treatments in the early stages.

Some experts say you can stay home during delivery as long as you have medical help. "Light candles or deliver in a lawn chair," says Marion McCartney, director of professional services for the American College of Nurse-Midwives. "Just have a professional there. If something goes wrong, she'll know what to do. It's a safer way to have a natural birth experience."

Alternatives to Going It Alone

You've decided to use an obstetrician or midwife, but you're determined to have as natural a birth as possible. Here's how to exercise your options.

Nurturing: Midwives are often considered more attentive to women's emotional needs than OB-GYNs. If you'd rather use a doctor, ask around to find one who's known for a caring attitude. Another option is a doula, someone trained to provide emotional support during labor and act as an advocate on your behalf. Your practitioner should be present along with your doula at home or in the hospital.

Control: Write a plan that includes your wishes, such as forgoing anesthesia or an episiotomy, and give it to your physician several weeks before your due date. Bring a copy with you to the hospital when you go into labor and give it to the nurse. Your goal is to eliminate conflicts or misunderstandings.

Drug-free pain relief: Acupuncture, hypnosis, massage, and aromatherapy all have been shown to relieve labor pain in some cases. Find out what your hospital's policy is on allowing such practices in the delivery room and talk to your doctor about these alternatives.

DANGER
in the delivery room

Some call Cytotec a boon to doctors and patients. Others say it's a killer, putting women and babies at risk needlessly.

BY JUDITH NEWMAN

Arlene Matejka was certainly no stranger to childbirth. She and her husband, David, already had five daughters tearing around their cozy, countrified home in Fort Myers, Florida. Matejka, 35, knew her body, knew what was normal and what wasn't. "Which is why it was so awful that no one would listen to me when I said something was wrong," she says today.

On November 12, 1998, Matejka, then 39 weeks pregnant with her sixth daughter, Emily, says she was informed by her midwife that her blood pressure was elevated and the baby was larger than average, so the child would have to be delivered immediately. (The actual medical necessity of this decision has been disputed in subsequent depositions.)

Two of Matejka's previous labors had been induced with Pitocin, a synthetic hormone that replicates the uterine-contracting effect of a chemical produced naturally in a woman's pituitary gland. About 20 percent of all labors are induced, most with Pitocin, according to the American College of Obstetricians and Gynecologists (ACOG). "I was told I'd be given a drug that was another form of Pitocin," Matejka says. In fact, the midwife had consulted with Matejka's obstetrician, who ordered misoprostol, aka Cytotec, a pharmaceutical originally created to treat gastric ulcers. The drug, which also happens to be a powerful agent for softening the cervix and inducing uterine contractions, is not approved by the U.S. Food and Drug Administration (FDA) for this use.

While she was at the hospital, Matejka received one 50-microgram dose vaginally around 2:30 in the afternoon and another early the following morning.

Women get Cytotec and are not being told that the drug they've been given was neither manufactured nor tested for use during labor and delivery.

Her contractions were about three minutes apart. After two more doses that same day, Matejka's water broke around 5 p.m. Then she heard a popping sound. "I told them, 'Something's not right,'" she remembers. "I'm very capable of tolerating pain, but this wasn't going away, and it was excruciating." Alarmed, she asked the nurses to check her baby's heartbeat. A normal one is between 125 and 175; Emily's was 40.

Even though her cervix was dilated only 5 centimeters instead of the 10 that signals imminent birth, Matejka says a nurse got on top of her and began to push on her abdomen. When baby Emily came out, she wasn't breathing. The nurses stuck a tube down her throat and revived her. Meanwhile, Matejka herself was gasping for breath. Her blood pressure was dangerously low—40 over 20—and dropping. The nurses kept insisting that something was wrong with the blood-pressure machine. This is the last part of Emily's birth that her mother remembers.

Matejka was slipping in and out of consciousness, blood pooling beneath her. The nurses were now in a panic, but they still hadn't paged her obstetrician. Matejka recalls that her husband grabbed a nurse and said, "Look, I know you're afraid to call a doctor, but if you lose your job, I'll pay your wages for the rest of your life." The nurse found an OB-GYN in the elevator. After a quick assessment, the physician demanded, "Why didn't you call someone earlier? Get her to the OR now—she's dying." By the time Matejka's doctor showed up, she was on the operating table, fighting for her life.

The average human body holds 8 to 10 pints of blood; Matejka received 37 pints before the obstetrician got her hemorrhaging under control. The pop she had heard was the sound of her uterus splitting like a watermelon from her sternum to her cervix. If the tear had been horizontal, as is often the case with uterine rupture, Emily would have been born into her mother's abdominal cavity, and she would have suffocated. Fortunately, because of the vertical split, Matejka was able to deliver her daughter vaginally, thus saving her life.

Matejka spent the next two days on life support; Emily stayed in the neonatal intensive care unit for 10 days. The Matejkas, who had wanted at least two more children, were forced to abandon their dreams because of the emergency hysterectomy Arlene underwent after the rupture was discovered. Emily, now 4, weighs only 27 pounds (most little girls her age weigh about 45 pounds) and has breathing and speech problems. She can't tolerate strong smells, so her diet is limited to such bland foods as macaroni and cheese, and she is so averse to certain sensations that she can hardly stand to wear shoes and socks. "I never had a problem separating from my other children," Matejka says. "But I'm so afraid of being without Emily, I'm homeschooling her. I can't let her out of my sight. I have this fear I'm going to lose her."

Matejka is grateful that her daughter is alive, but when she sees Emily struggling with little things most mothers take for granted, she is angry. "The baby's heart rate dropping, the severe pain not going away—every sign was pointing toward a ruptured uterus. They knew the effects of this drug," she says.

"THIS DRUG" IS CYTOTEC, the labor inducer currently being used in at least 5 percent, or 201,000, of all births annually, according to ACOG. Depending on whom you ask, it's a safe and inexpensive pill that gives doctors and patients precise control over the delivery process—or it's a potential killer that needlessly risks women's and babies' lives to achieve conveniently timed births, for the sake of families and medical staffs alike.

Most labors induced using Cytotec result in healthy births. "My gut feeling is that Cytotec is only slightly more risky, and more efficacious, than other labor inducers," says Charles Lockwood, M.D., chairman of obstetrics and gynecology at Yale University and former head of ACOG's obstetric-practices committee, which examined the Cytotec issue.

Then there are also the disasters, recalled in Internet support groups and at Web sites like UterineRupture.com: These are the women who lost their fertility, their babies, and in some cases, their lives. At last count, the FDA received 49 reports of uterine rupture and 10 reports of infant death during labors in which Cytotec was used between 1988 and 2000. (Susan Cruzman, an FDA spokeswoman, says, "Uterine rupture is associated with several risk factors, so we can't know if the drug was responsible or not.")

Cytotec is one of the most controversial women's reproductive treatments in many years. But because litigation has ended with hospital settlements and gag orders against plaintiffs, few women have heard of the drug's potential problems—and many of the OB-GYNs who use it aren't telling their patients that the drug they've been given was neither manufactured nor tested for use in labor and delivery.

The sliver of Cytotec is either swallowed or inserted into the vagina. After this, there's no turning back, and the effects can take hours to wear off.

Legally, mothers who are giving birth don't have to be informed that inducing with Cytotec is off-label (that is, a use unapproved by the FDA) or that the package insert clearly states the risk of uterine rupture in pregnant women who take the drug. Of course, the FDA allows doctors to prescribe many other medications for off-label uses. Botox, for example, was only OK'd for smoothing out wrinkles in 2003; for the last 10 years or so, the muscle-paralyzing agent was approved solely to treat severe muscle spasms.

"OBSTETRICIANS RATIONALIZE IT like this," explains Carolyn Rafferty, R.N., a labor and delivery nurse in Maryland and executive director of the Association of Nurse Advocates for Childbirth Solutions. "They say, 'Well, we administer plenty of drugs off-label. We don't tell patients we're using magnesium sulfate, an anticonvulsant, or terbutaline, an anti-asthma drug, to stop their preterm labor—we just stop their labor.' That's true, but when things go bad with Cytotec, even though it's rare, they go horribly wrong." Unquestionably, all medicines carry dangers, but many practitioners question whether this particular drug's benefits really outweigh its possible side effects.

"If you know there are already induction agents that work well, are relatively safe, and have been studied sufficiently," Rafferty asks, "why would you want to risk the potential problems of Cytotec?"

THE MEDICATION'S WIDESPREAD USE "is not what you call science," says Marsden Wagner, M.D., a neonatologist, reproductive scientist, and retired director of the women and children's health division of the World Health Organization. "It's what you call experimenting on women without telling them."

In 1988, the G.D. Searle Corporation (which has since merged with Pharmacia) started marketing Cytotec, a synthetic prostaglandin that reduces acid production in people who need to take stomach-irritating anti-inflammatory drugs like aspirin.

Prostaglandins naturally produced by a woman's body cause uterine contractions, and it didn't take long for physicians to figure out that this lab-created version had the same effect and could be useful in the delivery room. But unlike Pitocin (an analog of the pituitary hormone oxytocin, which also causes contractions), Cytotec softens a woman's cervix as well.

"Induction of labor is one of those aggravating things," says Donald Shuwarger, M.D., an obstetrician in private practice in Lynchburg, Virginia; as editorial adviser for Obgyn.net, he helped write an online protocol for prescribing Cytotec. "If you start off with a cervix that isn't ripe, your chances of having a C-section with induction are very high—50 percent or more." Pitocin causes powerful contractions but doesn't change the elasticity of the cervix, and if this part of the uterus is not ready to permit the passage of a child, "it's like knocking on a closed door," Shuwarger says. "Cytotec opens the door. It does the job better than anything else we have."

Cytotec is often not enough on its own, however. It may ripen the cervix without actually causing contractions, so about 70 percent of the time, according to ACOG, it is used in conjunction with

Pitocin. But for some women who are sensitive to prostaglandins, Cytotec alone causes powerful contractions, sometimes too powerful. And predicting a woman's response is difficult because of the way the drug is manufactured and administered.

Even though ACOG has established guidelines for Cytotec's use, there is still disagreement regarding the correct dosage; the spacing of those doses; or even the most appropriate route of administration, oral or vaginal. "Cytotec is this tiny 100-microgram pill that has to be cut up manually into four pieces, and each piece is supposed to be a 25-microgram dose," says a veteran labor and delivery nurse at Highland Hospital in Oakland, California. Dosage preferences vary: Some obstetricians give 25 micrograms every four to six hours; others give 50 micrograms or more at shorter intervals." These imprecise standards can give Cytotec an unpredictable quality.

THE CRITICAL DIFFERENCE between combining a cervix softener like Cervidil with the contraction-eliciting Pitocin on one hand and using Cytotec on the other is one of control. Cervidil, also a synthetic prostaglandin, is administered in a tamponlike insert that can be removed from a woman's vagina if anything goes wrong; similarly, Pitocin is given intravenously, so the needle can be taken out if contractions become too intense. But the sliver of Cytotec is either swallowed or inserted into the vagina; after this, there's no turning back, and the effects can take hours to wear off.

When physicians began experimenting with the drug off-label in the early 1990s, the manufacturer already included an explicit warning that Cytotec could cause the uterus to rupture if used during pregnancy. "Uterine rupture," the label said, "may result in severe bleeding, hospitalization, surgery, infertility, or death."

Barring a tear, there is also the risk of an amniotic fluid embolism. Violent contractions can cause microscopic debris to leak from the uterus into the

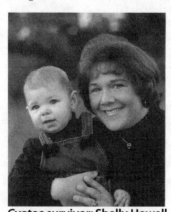
Cyotec survivor: Shelly Howell with Megan, now 2½

bloodstream; if a major vessel becomes blocked, heart failure or stroke can result. This is exactly what happened on December 27, 2001, to Tatia Malika French, 32, a Berkeley, California, psychologist. After she received the drug—unaware that Cytotec wasn't FDA-approved for inducing labor—her blood pressure and her baby's heart rate plummeted, she had a massive seizure, and both mother and child died.

A lawsuit against the hospital is still pending, and French's husband, J.B. French, cannot yet bring himself to talk about the event. But in an E-mail to *Health*, the high school teacher wrote: "The reverberations of my wife and child's horrible passing shake me with deep agony and anguish."

Embolisms like Tatia Malika French's are rare, but instances of uterine hyperstimulation are not. A baby gets blood through the placenta by means of the umbilical cord. When the uterus contracts, it temporarily stops blood flow to the baby. Of course, contractions are necessary to expel the fetus from the uterus, and babies in effect hold their breath during the normal course of labor. But if contractions are too strong and too close together over an extended time, the baby becomes deprived of oxygen and goes into a state of distress. The outcome of hyperstimulation can be brain damage—either subtle, as with Emily Matejka, or severe.

Such was the case for Megan Howell. Her mother, Shelly Howell of Topeka, Kansas, had already miscarried five times before giving birth to her in August 2000. After 20 hours of labor and eight failed doses of Cytotec, Howell, 29, was forced to have an emergency C-section. Her blood pressure skyrocketed, and her daughter went into fetal distress. The OB-GYN struggled for 10 minutes to remove the baby, who was trapped in the birth canal. Prolonged oxygen deprivation caused Megan to suffer a stroke at birth, followed by severe seizures.

At 9 months, she was on five different types of anticonvulsant medications and was still having hundreds of seizures a day. Four months later, to minimize further brain damage, surgeons removed most of the left side of Megan's brain, where the convulsions were originating. Now 2½, she is seizure-free but visually impaired and partially paralyzed. Howell says she believes that her daughter's brain injury resulted from the administration of Cytotec and the doctor's slow response when it became horrifyingly clear that the drug wasn't working.

WHILE DEBATE STILL EXISTS about the drug's appropriate uses, physicians now agree universally that it should not be used in cases of vaginal birth after a prior cesarean (VBAC). Most cases of uterine rupture have happened along the "fault line" of the prior surgical scar. "You would eliminate all cases of uterine rupture associated with Cytotec if you follow the guidelines we've set out: Use no more than 25 micrograms every four to six hours and do not use on VBACs, women with multiple births, or women who've had more than five children," Lockwood says. "And the one thing I always emphasize: Don't do an induction unless it's medically indicated. Don't do it because the patient is whining or because you're tired."

Lockwood, who has used the drug in his own practice, argues that uterine rupture occurs with other ripening agents as well, in about 2.5 percent of cases, and that the risk with Cytotec is only marginally higher. But according to Wagner, who has gathered statistics from the Centers for Disease Control and Prevention and ACOG, the risk with Cytotec is much higher. According to his figures, uterine rupture without induction in a normal, unscarred uterus occurs in 1 in 33,000 births. The risk in a VBAC, also without drugs, is 1 in 200. The risk in a VBAC using Cytotec is 1 in 20 births (despite ACOG's recommendations, some OB-GYNs continue to use Cytotec in VBAC births, according to anecdotal reports), and the chance of a baby dying or suffering brain damage after a rupture is 30 percent. Given the increased risk, Wagner argues—and given

doctors' uncertainty about the magnitude of that risk—why use Cytotec to induce labor at all?

For one thing, there's the cost: pennies per dose compared to approximately $175 for a dose of Cervidil and $85 for Pitocin. But far more critical to Cytotec's popularity is its ability to ensure quicker, somewhat more predictable deliveries. Since 1989, the number of births induced has doubled, according to the National Center for Health Statistics. And the number of vaginal births that take place Monday through Friday has increased significantly over the past decade. "For many working women, there's pressure to deliver near the due date so they can plan maternity leave. And many women are worried about complications, or they just get tired of being pregnant and want it over with," says William F. Rayburn, M.D., chair of obstetrics and gynecology at the University of New Mexico Health Sciences Center in Albuquerque and an expert on the rise of medically unnecessary inductions. "From the doctor's perspective, there are three main reasons to induce. Many OB-GYNs want to be present at delivery. Plus, there's the unspoken reason of financial reward; they want to collect the fees. And then there's liability—they're afraid of problems arising if they wait."

Wagner and other critics do not claim that Cytotec is uniformly dangerous. On the contrary, numerous studies have borne out its safety and efficacy in two phases of pregnancy. If a woman is bleeding profusely after giving birth, administering Cytotec will cause uterine contractions that stop the bleeding. In addition, Cytotec is routinely used in conjunction with mifepristone (RU-486) as part of the protocol for early abortion. Mifepristone is an artificial steroid that blocks the action of progesterone, the hormone that maintains the uterine lining in early pregnancy. Cytotec plus RU-486 causes contractions that allow the uterus to expel the lining and its contents effectively. (In fact, a physician in Dayton, Ohio, is serving prison time for secretly spiking his former fiancée's drinks with Cytotec after she became pregnant and refused his demands that she get an abortion. She eventually miscarried.)

In order for Pharmacia to market Cytotec as a labor-inducing drug, "they would have to go through our approval process," says FDA spokeswoman Cruzman. Securing this approval is costly and time-consuming. More importantly, it would make Pharmacia a target for litigation—likely the last thing the manufacturer wants. Spokesman Mark Wolfe has only this to say: "Cytotec was developed for prevention of gastric ulcers. We have not studied it for any purpose but its approved indication."

Until April 2002, Pharmacia warned pregnant women against taking Cytotec. The label now acknowledges for the first time that the drug is used to trigger labor, albeit off-label. Several reports indicate that pressure from OB-GYNs brought about the change.

Women who were left infertile, parents with damaged children, and bereaved relatives think it's time that labels and doctors alike inform people of the risks. "I cry myself to sleep every night," says J.B. French in his E-mail. "My wife was an intelligent, beautiful, and loving person whose bright future was snuffed out." ▪

Freelance writer Judith Newman's memoir on being an old new mother is due out on Mother's Day 2004.

Mammograms Can Detect Heart Disease, Too

If you have doubts about this breast-cancer test, here's yet another good reason to have it: According to researchers at the Mayo Clinic in Rochester, Minnesota, mammograms are able to spotlight calcified arteries, which can predict heart disease. The team studied 1,880 older women and found that those with calcium deposits around their breast arteries had a 20-percent higher risk of heart disease than those without. Ask your doctor about these findings at your next mammogram.

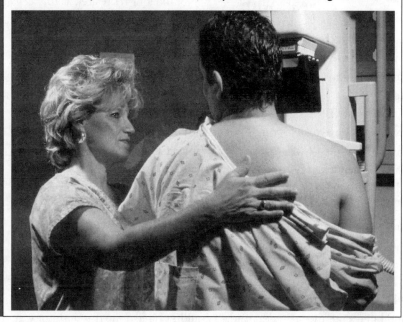

Women Win with Better Heart Meds

During the last 50 years, the rate of heart failure stayed the same for men but dropped by about 35 percent for women, says a recent study in the *New England Journal of Medicine*. Researchers credit the improved statistics to better medications for high blood pressure, a major component of heart failure in women (heart attack damage contributes more to cardiac failure in men).

Pap Tests Face Cutbacks

Most women over age 30 can safely skip their annual Pap smears and have one every two or three years instead, according to the American Cancer Society. If you've ever had an abnormal test, though, you should stick with the once-a-year plan.

When My OB-GYN Said Goodbye

BY BETH BERNSTEIN

Six months after I my 40th birthday, I received a letter saying that my OB-GYN, Marvin Zuckerman, M.D., was retiring. "I've enjoyed attending to your medical needs and your friendship," the note said.

That's it? A "Dear Patient" letter with secretarial initials typed under his name? I didn't expect a personal call; I just thought he would stick around to deliver my first-born. However long it might take.

My 30s were punctuated by losses: my mother to an aneurysm; my father to cancer; Muffin, my dog of 18 years, to old age. Losing Dr. Zuckerman to retirement did not just mean saying good-bye to an old friend. It was saying good-bye to the hope that I'd one day have a child.

"Who's going to deliver my babies?" I asked when I called to say that I'd miss him and to discuss who would be my new doctor.

"To tell you the truth, Beth, the thought of you calling me with every symptom for nine months was never terribly appealing."

This is why I spent 25 years with Dr. Zuckerman: He knew me. He made me laugh. He believed that "even at my age," I'd get married and have a family.

> This is why I spent 25 years with Dr. Z: He knew me. He made me laugh. He took my calls in the middle of the night.

Besides, I am what therapists call "change-averse." (I prefer to think of it as an appreciation for continuity.) Merida has been my hair colorist for 10 years; Larisa at Elizabeth Arden has been doing my bikini wax for eight years. On the table I inherited from my great-grandmother rests a wedding photo of my parents, even though they divorced when I was 12.

Not too long thereafter, at 15, I began seeing Dr. Z in my hometown of Fort Lee, New Jersey. My mom told me that she and his wife, Jeannie, had grown up in the same apartment building in Brooklyn. For some reason, this tidbit of information put me slightly more at ease the first time I put on the paper gown, lifted my feet into the stirrups, and had my first encounter with the huge metal salad clamps.

Over the years, Dr. Zuckerman's other patients became like close relatives, freely sharing gossip and Entenmann's cookies. There were home remedies traded as well, such as yogurt for a yeast infection and Mallomars for a broken heart. The walls were lined with framed collages of bald, scrunched-faced babies and accompanying notes from their mothers that said, "I couldn't have done this without you,

Dr. Z." Delivery after delivery, he had met his patients at the hospital, rubbed their backs, and coached them through labor. I ended up counting on him for much more than that.

During most of my late teens, I asked Dr. Z for pregnancy tests. Lots of them. I had an inexplicable hormonal imbalance and would go for months at a time without menstruating. Even though I was using birth control, I would worry each time I missed my period. Both my mom and Dr. Zuckerman thought I was overly anxious. Yet whenever I showed up at his office, Dr. Z would dutifully draw my blood and later call with the happy news that the test was negative.

Until the one time it wasn't.

I had defied the laws of nature, getting pregnant with a low probability of ovulation, a diaphragm firmly in place, and enough spermicidal jelly to kill an army of shifty little tadpoles on the make.

After the abortion, I woke up with Dr. Z holding one hand and my mother holding the other. "Don't try to sit up yet," he advised. He helped me drink from a straw, and he told me that he saw as many children in my future as I would ever want.

At 22, I moved to Manhattan and had my records transferred to Dr. Zuckerman's Park Avenue office. The friendly neighborhood chatter I had become accustomed to in New Jersey was replaced by the separate conversations of career women on cell phones. Sometimes, we'd put down our phones or our work and smile at each other. Now and then, I overheard talk of smooth or rocky deliveries, day care, and private schools.

After every examination, Dr. Z would call me into his office. Once, as I sat opposite him at his mahogany desk, he informed me that I had crabs. I learned about Quell, that condoms didn't cover enough territory for certain sexually transmitted diseases, and that my new boyfriend was sleeping around.

One night, when I was 23, my heart started racing so fast I thought I was going to die alone in my living room. I phoned Dr. Zuckerman's answering service. Within five minutes, he called me back and listened to my symptoms. It was a panic attack, he said, and he told me how to breathe into a paper bag. Then he waited until my pulse went back to normal.

When my mother died, I received a condolence card from Dr. Zuckerman and his wife that finally helped me put into words what I could never explain to my friends—the ones who extolled the "women understand women better" virtues of female OB-GYNs. Dr. Z had been there through most of my growing up. He took my calls in the middle of the night. He put up with my insecurities and flaws. He consoled me through every breakup and asked, "So when are you going to meet a nice emotionally available man to settle down with?" To which I could only reply, "When you find me one."

When I was 37, Dr. Z gave me the news that I had a fibroid tumor. "It's benign and extremely small," he said. "It's nothing to worry about."

Both my mother and my grandmother, though, had undergone hysterectomies when they were 40 because of fibroids. Dr. Zuckerman tried to reassure me. "Doctors performed hysterectomies more frequently back then," he said. Besides, my mother and grandmother had multiple fibroids that were five times larger than my pea-sized lump. "If it makes you feel better, you can come in every six months instead of annually," he said. "We can watch the size. But for now, just relax."

This was the one time that Dr. Zuckerman's words couldn't soothe me. Just the year before, my niece had been born. It was then that I discovered my biological clock. Now it began to go a little cuckoo, constantly repeating "too late, too late."

But so far, Dr. Zuckerman has been right. My fibroid has remained the same size for the past three years, and I feel fine. Now that he's retiring, I'll make an appointment with my new OB-GYN, the one Dr. Z said he'd handpicked to deliver my first-born. I'm still planning on a new family portrait to put on my great-grandmother's nightstand. After all, both Dr. Z and my mom said it would happen, all of it: love, marriage, and a child. If it does, I'll feel my mother holding my hand and hear Dr. Zuckerman saying, "Give the lovable pain-in-the-butt the epidural before it's too late." ■

Special Section

How to Handle the Curveballs of Menopause

From hormone therapy to alternative care, discover the best ways to stay in control during this time of your life.

BY ANNIE STUART

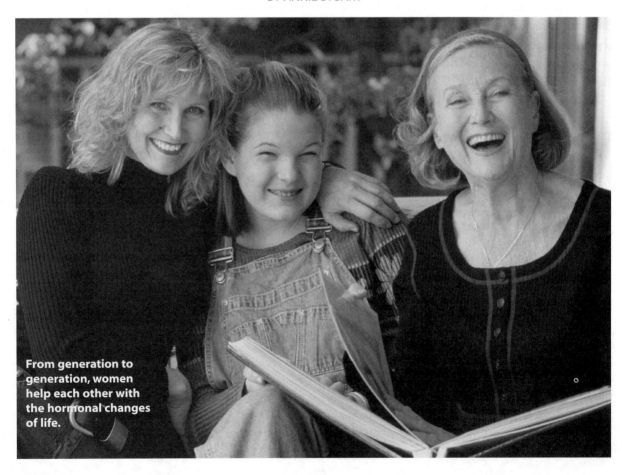

From generation to generation, women help each other with the hormonal changes of life.

You may view menopause as a journey lasting many years, but it's actually one day—the day that officially marks 12 months without menstruation. You could experience it as early as age 35 or as late as 55, the average being age 51.

Perimenopause, the sometimes tumultuous period before menopause, refers to the years during which you may start to experience menopausal symptoms, such as hot flashes and mood swings. This experience is different for each woman: You may be fortunate and breeze through it, while your best friend must cope with such symptoms as night sweats, anxiety, depression, insomnia, headaches, palpitations, and irregular or heavy periods.

These changes during perimenopause are triggered when your ovaries start to run out of eggs. Your hormone levels go through dramatic shifts: Estrogen

Menopause is a different experience for each woman: You may breeze through it while your best friend copes with night sweats, anxiety, depression, insomnia, headaches, palpitations, and irregular or heavy periods.

levels decrease, and your pituitary gland starts releasing more follicle-stimulating hormone (FSH) in order to try to get egg-releasing follicles to form. Menopause finally occurs after your estrogen and progesterone levels drastically drop, causing your periods to cease.

Menopausal Hormone Therapy in the News

Since July 2002, the media has been covering news from the Women's Health Initiative (WHI), which is sponsored by the National Heart, Lung, and Blood Institute. It is the largest research study ever conducted on the effects of menopausal hormone therapy (HT) on women. Here are key pieces of information you should know.

• Researchers halted part of the study when it became clear that women taking a particular form of hormone therapy, Prempro, faced a 26-percent increased risk of breast cancer, which was greater than the potential benefits of the treatment.

• Contrary to previous thought, the study found that HT does not prevent heart disease—in fact, it may increase the risk for heart attacks, as well as strokes.

• The study indicated that women taking HT have a 33-percent reduction in hip fractures and a 37-percent drop in colorectal cancers. However, these statistics weren't enough to offset the negative impacts.

• Part of the WHI study continues for women who have had hysterectomies and are taking only estrogen. The risk to them is reduced, since they are not taking progestin.

• HT taken for less than five years is not associated with significant risks, such as breast cancer.

• Since the WHI studied only Prempro, which is not considered natural to the human female body, further research is needed to see if bioidentical types of HT would prompt the same results.

Saying no to hormone therapy today doesn't mean you can't say yes later—and vice versa.

MY MENOPAUSAL SYMPTOMS

Share this form with your doctor. Check off the level of severity for any symptoms that you have.

Symptoms	Mild	Annoying	Unbearable
Hot flashes and night sweats	☐	☐	☐
Insomnia and fatigue	☐	☐	☐
Loss of libido	☐	☐	☐
Mood swings	☐	☐	☐
Thinning and less elastic skin	☐	☐	☐
Vaginal atrophy and urinary symptoms	☐	☐	☐
Worsened premenstrual syndrome (PMS)	☐	☐	☐

Check all that apply to help determine if menopausal hormone therapy (HT) is right for you.

Risk factors for osteoporosis, a condition that may improve with HT.

- ☐ I have a family history of osteoporosis.
- ☐ I went through menopause before age 45.
- ☐ I have a thin bone structure.
- ☐ I am a smoker.
- ☐ I take corticosteroids.
- ☐ I don't regularly do weight-bearing exercises, such as walking.

Cardiovascular-disease risks, which could increase if I take HT.

- ☐ I am a smoker.
- ☐ I have high cholesterol, high blood pressure, or diabetes.
- ☐ I am physically inactive.
- ☐ I am overweight or obese.

Breast-cancer risks, which could increase if I take HT.

- ☐ My mother or sister has had breast cancer.
- ☐ I have never had any children.
- ☐ I became pregnant for the first time after age 30.
- ☐ I started menstruating before age 12.
- ☐ I reached menopause after age 55.
- ☐ I have at least one alcoholic drink a day.
- ☐ I am overweight.

Other conditions that could impact my risks while taking HT.

- ☐ I have had a stroke, pulmonary embolus, heart attack, or other thromboembolic condition.
- ☐ I have had breast cancer, uterine cancer, or other estrogen-stimulated cancer.
- ☐ I have severe liver disease.
- ☐ I have had unexplained vaginal bleeding.
- ☐ I am pregnant, or there's a chance I could become pregnant.

10 Questions to Ask Your Doctor About HT

If you haven't done so already, there's no better time than menopause to develop a partnership with your doctor. Like many women, you may feel confused or uninformed about menopausal hormone therapy choices. In October 2002, the National Institutes of Health announced a name change from hormone replacement therapy (HRT) to menopausal hormone therapy (HT), since the previous name implied a full restoration of hormones, which does not occur. We'll use the new acronym: HT.

It's difficult to know what to ask your doctor to determine which hormonal regimen, if any, suits you best. It's easier to simply take your doctor's word, but you have a voice in this decision—it is *your* body, after all. Educate yourself so that you can work with your doctor to find the approach that works best for you. To help you get started, here are some questions to ask about HT.

1 What do you need to know about me before I decide whether or not to take HT?

Your doctor will help you weigh the risks and benefits of taking HT by discussing your menopausal symptoms, as well as your medical and family history. She may suggest certain tests, such as a cholesterol test or mammogram, to help evaluate your risks. In addition, she may order a follicle-stimulating hormone (FSH) test to confirm your estrogen loss, since a high level of FSH is an indicator of your body's attempt to boost estrogen levels. Fill out the questionnaire on page 130, take it with you to the doctor, and be prepared to discuss your situation.

2 Which method of HT should I use: pill, cream, ring, patch? It's all so confusing!

A lot depends on the symptoms you have. For example, if osteoporosis runs in your family, you may prefer to take pills, since they have been shown to increase bone mass, in addition to relieving symptoms. Is vaginal dryness your chief complaint? Then you may opt to use only a vaginal ring or cream. Worried about the impact of high dosages? Then you might consider a patch, which is absorbed directly into your bloodstream, achieving the same effect as with pills, but at a lower dose.

3 Does it make sense for me to take HT for reasons other than hot flashes and fatigue?

Doctors used to think HT would prevent or help treat heart disease, but the Women's Health Initiative (WHI) study found that after five years of treatment, HT slightly increased the incidence of heart disease problems and stroke. (You can read more about the WHI study on page 129.)

HT—specifically its estrogen component—is still thought to boost bone-mineral density, helping to prevent osteoporosis. The WHI study also showed that Prempro (a type of combination HT that

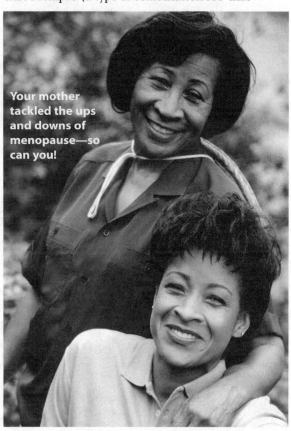

Your mother tackled the ups and downs of menopause—so can you!

131

contains estrogen plus a progestin) and Premarin (a type that contains conjugated equine estrogens) reduced the risk of hip fractures. Regardless of these benefits, doctors may no longer reach for hormone therapy as their first choice to help combat bone loss. Why? Because the benefits do not outweigh the risks of developing breast cancer, and osteoporosis can be treated with nonhormonal drugs that do not increase breast-cancer risk.

Some studies suggest HT protects women against such problems as cognitive function or Alzheimer's disease, age-related eye ailments like macular degeneration, colon cancer, wrinkles, and tooth loss. The jury is still out on several of these, though. Discuss your risk for these conditions with your doctor and keep alert to the latest research results.

4 *How will I know I'm getting the right amount of estrogen?* Even after menopause, your body continues to make some estrogen through your adrenal glands and fat cells. It

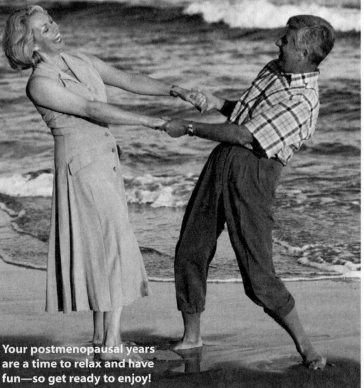

Your postmenopausal years are a time to relax and have fun—so get ready to enjoy!

produces three principle forms: estradiol, estrone, and estriol. Prior to menopause, estradiol is the main type of estrogen manufactured by the ovaries. After menopause, your body primarily produces estrone. Estriol is present at all times and is also produced by the placenta during pregnancy. How much—if any—supplemental estrogen you need depends on how much your body is already making. The only way to know that is by undergoing frequent saliva or blood tests to monitor your estrogen levels. Ask your doctor about monthly saliva tests that you can do at home, as well as how often you need blood tests. Some experts recommend monthly blood tests when you first start HT, then every three months to keep track of your changing needs.

5 *What is progesterone and do I need it?* If you still have your uterus, your doctor should prescribe HT that combines both estrogen and progesterone. Taking estrogen alone would allow the uterine tissue to continue to build up, with no hormonal cue to stop. Progesterone—or its synthetic form, progestin—tells your body to shed its uterine lining, which would cause you to start having periods again. But if you take the two together, you reduce the increased risk of endometrial cancer that you would otherwise have by taking only estrogen. Your HT treatment plan should include progestin for at least 10 to 13 days each month. Ask your doctor which regimen is preferable for you—and why. You can

> **Women need individualized hormone therapy. Be sure to discuss the risks and benefits with your doctor so you can find a plan that's right for you.**

take one estrogen and one progestin pill every day, as part of a 30-day cycle. Or you can take estrogen for the first 25 days, add a progestin tablet from Day 14 to 25, then no HT during the final five days of the 30-day cycle. In those five days, your uterus will shed its lining—in other words, you'll have a period.

Of course, if you've had a hysterectomy, you don't have a uterus so you no longer have the risk of developing uterine cancer. You can safely take estrogen without progesterone or progestin.

6 *Should I use conventional HT or bioidentical HT?* There are pros and cons associated with each. With conventional HT, such as that used in the WHI study, a large body of research has documented its benefits and risks. Other experts argue that bioidentical forms—those that more closely match the hormones your body once made in bigger supplies—are just as effective, yet carry less risk than conventional HT. Unfortunately, bioidentical types of HT have not been studied as much as conventional types.

7 *What else should I expect if I start HT?* When you take progesterone or progestin, you will still usually have a regular monthly period—minus ovulation, of course. Your healthcare provider may ask you to keep a record of any spotting or bleeding you experience to help your doctor fine-tune your regimen. In addition to saliva or blood tests, you will need to see your doctor several times a year to monitor the effects of treatment.

8 *Are there any danger signs I should watch for while taking HT?* As always, keep your regular appointments for breast, pelvic, and rectal exams. And whether or not you're taking HT, be sure to get a regular mammogram to check for any changes in your breasts. Call your health-care provider if you experience any of the following symptoms, which may be related to HT.

- Breast lump or breast tenderness that doesn't subside
- Severe headaches or aching muscles in your back or legs
- Unexpected, long-lasting, or heavy bleeding
- Unexpected vaginal discharge

9 *How do you decide which type of HT to prescribe for each woman?* Listen carefully for your doctor's response to this question. Does she have a one-size-fits-all approach? Or is there a concerted effort to evaluate your symptoms and risk factors in order to come up with a plan? Many women suffer from HT side effects—such as migraines, nausea, and breast tenderness—that are worse than the menopausal symptoms they were trying to alleviate in the first place. This may be because their doctors treat all women in the same manner. As a result, approximately 25 percent of the American women who try HT quit taking it within a month. And up to 80 percent quit within two years.

Women need individualized hormone therapy, best provided by bioidentical hormone therapy that more closely matches the makeup of the hormones your body produced before menopause. If you don't feel that your doctor is well-informed or open to this option, you may want to see a menopause provider, someone who specializes in menopausal symptoms and treatment options. (For more information, see page 136.)

10 *How long should I stay on HT?* Although certain health risks increase after you've been on HT for longer than five years, you may wish to continue in order to reap other potential benefits. HT may help prevent or treat osteoporosis and possibly ward off or delay Alzheimer's disease. Or you may choose to continue because of feel-good, look-younger perks you experience. In most cases, a physician will try to keep you on the lowest possible dose of estrogen and progestin.

Comparing Your HT Options

It's always good to be well-informed when you talk to your doctor about such significant decisions as menopausal hormone therapy (HT). Start by learning what's available to you. Estrogens and progestins come in both conventional and bioidentical forms. And, of course, there are advantages and disadvantages to each. Here are some of the basics.

Conventional estrogen comes from pregnant mares' urine or plant sources. This is the most commonly prescribed kind of estrogen. Research proves that conventional estrogens can relieve menopausal symptoms and improve bone mass. Potential side effects with long-term use include breast tenderness, fluid retention, heart disease, breast cancer, stroke, pulmonary embolisms, and worsening of liver or gallbladder problems. If you take a conventional estrogen without a progestin, you increase your risk of endometrial cancer, unless you've had a hysterectomy. Conventional estrogens include conjugated estrogens and esterified estrogens. They are made of the estrogens found naturally in the body—estradiol, estriol, and estrone—plus a type found in horses, called equilin.

Bioidentical estrogen comes from plant-based estrogens, such as from soybeans. These products are made of varying amounts of the estrogens found naturally in the body: estradiol, estriol, and estrone. Bioidentical estrogen is available commercially, or your doctor can use a compounding pharmacy to customize a hormone formulation to meet your individual needs. Unfortunately, not as much research exists for bioidentical estrogen, but its benefits and potential side effects are thought to be similar to conventional estrogen.

> **Talk to your doctor and learn what's available to you. Estrogens and progestins come in both conventional and bioidentical forms. And, of course, there are advantages and disadvantages to each.**

Conventional progestin is a synthetic form of the hormone progesterone, which your body produces naturally. Since it's not the same biochemical structure as your body's own progesterone, it may cause some side effects. You may experience PMS-like symptoms, such as mood swings, headaches, breast tenderness, and bloating. It could also lower your levels of HDL (the "good" cholesterol). And beware of the possible increased risk of breast cancer. Progestin may increase the chance of harmful blood clots, but estrogen is usually the culprit. If you already have asthma, epilepsy, migraines, heart failure, or kidney failure, note that this form of HT causes fluid retention, which can worsen your condition. Some women with a history of depression may experience depressive symptoms when using a progestin.

Bioidentical progestin comes from plant-based progesterone derived primarily from Mexican wild yams. It is biologically identical to human progesterone. The side effects tend to be fewer than that of conventional progestogen. For example, it does not seem to lower your HDL levels. However, this form may increase male hormone effects, such as acne. Watch your doses closely though—side effects increase if you take more than 400 milligrams a day.

You do not need any kind of progestin, conventional or bioidentical, if you have had your uterus surgically removed. But if you still have your uterus and you take estrogen, you must also take a progestin in order to protect your uterine lining from overgrowth, as well as from an increased risk for endometrial cancer.

COMPARING HORMONE TREATMENTS

The following chart lists several types of estrogens and progestins for both conventional and bioidentical menopausal hormone therapy. Unless noted otherwise, these hormone-therapy methods require prescriptions. This information will likely change over time, so do your best to stay well-informed. The Web site of the North American Menopause Society (www.menopause.org) is a good place to start.

Conventional Estrogen

Combination estrogens: include the hormones estrone, equilin (horse hormone), and estradiol
- Conjugated estrogens produced from pregnant mare's urine (Premarin)
- Conjugated estrogens synthesized from plant sources (Cenestin)
- Esterified estrogens synthesized from plant sources (Menest, Estratab; Estratab was discontinued in 2001, but may become available again.)
- Dienestrol vaginal cream (OrthoDienestrol)
- Conjugated estrogen vaginal cream (Premarin vaginal)

Bioidentical Estrogen   *All are synthesized from plant sources and don't contain horse hormones.*

Single-drug estrogens
- Estradiol (Estrace, various patches—Alora, Climara, Estraderm, Vivelle, and others)
- Ethinyl estradiol (Estinyl)
- Estropipate (Ogen, Ortho-Est)

These are available from compounding pharmacies.
- Tri-Est—estradiol, estrone, and estriol (usually in a 10%-10%-80% ratio)
- Bi-Est—estradiol and estriol (usually in a 20%-80% ratio)

Vaginal bioidentical estrogens
- Estradiol cream (Estrace vaginal, or compounded)
- Estradiol ring (Estring)
- Estradiol suppository tablets (Vagifem)
- Estriol cream can be compounded by a compounding pharmacy

Conventional Progestins

Synthetic form of the hormone progesterone
- Medroxyprogesterone (Cycrin, Provera)
- Norethindrone (available for menopause in combination products like Activella, Combipatch)
- Norgestimate (available in the combination product Ortho-Prefest)

Bioidentical Progestins

Derived primarily from Mexican wild yam
- Micronized progesterone (Prometrium) ***Note:*** *This product contains peanut oil, so some people may be allergic to it.*
- Progesterone cream (Crinone, or can be made by a compounding pharmacy)

COMPARING DISTRIBUTION METHODS

Estrogen Pill	• Is a pill that you swallow. • Requires a higher dose, since potency lessens as it moves through digestive system.
Estrogen Patch	• Resembles a small bandage and is placed on skin of abdomen, buttocks, or thigh; you change it twice a week. • Estrogen is absorbed through skin directly into bloodstream, so it does not impact the liver as much as pills. • Dispenses estrogen continuously, more closely resembling the body's own estrogen production. • Can achieve same effects as with pills, with lower doses. • Dosage not as flexible as with pills. • May irritate skin.
Estrogen Vaginal Cream or Ring	• Apply creams to vaginal or urethral area to prevent atrophy. • Inserted soft ring stays in vagina for 90 days to prevent atrophy. • Estrogen is absorbed through skin directly into bloodstream. • Eases vaginal dryness more quickly than other methods, but doesn't consistently ease other symptoms. • It is not known how much is absorbed beyond vagina or urethral area, making it difficult to assess benefits or risks to rest of body. • Ring may be expelled while straining during bowel movement.
Progestin Pill	• Is a pill that you swallow. • Is easily combined with estrogen to provide symptom-relief and uterine protection in one product. • Most pill regimens produce menstruation-like bleeding. • Requires higher dose for effectiveness than with other methods, since potency lessens as it moves through digestive system.
Progestin Creams and Gels	• Is typically applied vaginally. • Progestin is absorbed directly into bloodstream, bypassing liver where it could be destroyed. • Side effects are fewer than with pills. • Is helpful in management of menopausal symptoms, such as loss of libido. • Absorption varies from person to person—may not be adequate to offer endometrial protection.

Caution: Some companies falsely claim that their wild-yam creams contain progesterone or convert to progesterone in the body. Some over-the-counter creams may contain a small amount of progesterone, but it probably doesn't have much effect. Check labels and consult a physician.

MENOPAUSE PROVIDERS

If you feel you're not getting the individualized attention you need from your primary-care physician or gynecologist, it may be time to investigate what menopause providers have to offer. They specialize in menopausal symptoms and treatment options, and also provide emotional support during this life-changing period of your life. You may choose to see a menopause clinician who can prescribe medications. Or you may see a menopause educator, such as a nurse, who is licensed to provide health care.

Menopause providers are well-trained in the nuances of individualized hormone therapy. They take great care to listen to your specific complaints, test your serum hormone levels for both estrogen and progesterone, and tailor treatment to your specific needs.

For help in finding a menopause provider, check out the North American Menopause Society Web site at www.menopause.org.

ALTERNATIVES TO HT

What if HT isn't right for you? What if you feel the risks associated with HT are too high? Or you want to try a more natural approach? Should you just throw in the sweat-drenched towel and give up? Certainly not. The options may be confusing to sort through, but you have quite a few from which to choose to help you cope with the symptoms of menopause.

For starters, don't neglect good nutrition and exercise, especially weight-bearing exercises that help prevent osteoporosis. And, of course, it may be particularly helpful at this point in your life to get the emotional support that you need. You might also want to consider taking supplements. For example, by taking 400 to 800 International Units of vitamin E daily, you may minimize hot flashes and even reduce the risk of cardiovascular or Alzheimer's disease.

Beyond taking supplements, you also may want to try holistic herbal remedies. More than 20 percent of women ages 45 and older depend upon alternative methods to manage their menopausal symptoms. And 25 percent integrate these alternative approaches with conventional care in order to achieve relief.

Although much research still remains to be done, the following herbal remedies have shown some promise in easing women's menopausal symptoms, especially in undercutting the impact of hot flashes.

> Herbs may help relieve your symptoms, but they can be toxic if taken at certain dosages. Be sure you talk to an herbalist first.

• **Black cohosh** may mimic the brain chemical serotonin, which may reduce your menopausal symptoms.
• **Soy** contains isoflavones, which may mimic hormones, in particular estrogen. (Foods high in plant estrogens include soybeans, lima beans, nuts, and seeds.)
• **Red clover** is considered to be one of the richest sources of isoflavones, offering some of the same benefits as soy.
• **Dong quai** is a Chinese herb recommended for a wide variety of women's health problems, including menopausal symptoms. Dong quai contains phytoestrogens, or plant estrogens, which can help you with hot flashes.
• **Evening-primrose oil** may help by controlling inflammation.

Consult an herbalist to learn about safe dosages of each of these, since some herbs, in certain dosages, can be toxic. And always alert your primary-care doctor about any alternative supplements you're taking. Some interact adversely with certain medications.

KEEP AN OPEN MIND

You may have mixed feelings about HT—that's completely understandable. Even if you choose

It's easier to simply take your doctor's word
about which hormone therapy is right for you—but remember
that it is *your* body and you *do* have a voice.

not to use it in early perimenopause, you can still opt to try taking it later. And just because you decide to take it now doesn't mean you can't stop treatment later. What's important is that you make an informed choice.

The most current research shows that you're not likely to suffer any ill effects if you take HT for up to three years. Once menopause is a couple of years behind you, you can probably taper off HT without experiencing any recurring symptoms, since your body has adjusted to the hormonal changes of menopause. However, you may want to continue treatment because of other potential benefits. Whatever you choose, it's a decision you need to make with the input of your doctor.

Women still have many questions concerning HT, but scientists are working to answer them. For example, once the WHI study is complete (some time between 2006 and 2010), researchers will be able to reveal more information about the risks and benefits of HT. So stay tuned!

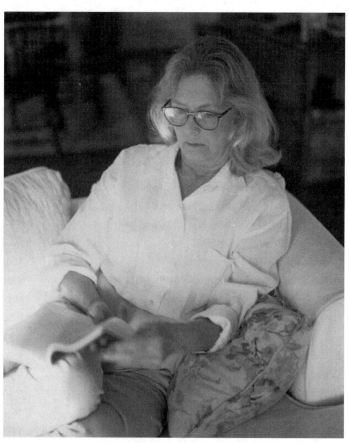

You may opt to try HT later or to take it now and stop it later. What's important is that you make an informed decision.

Warning: Depression Could Lead to Early Menopause

Women who suffer from depression are twice as likely to stop menstruating early as women without any mood disorders, according to a new study from Boston's Brigham and Women's Hospital. Researchers are still looking into theories to explain the connection. If you've been diagnosed with depression, ask your doctor for advice regarding extra precautions. Early menopause means you'll be living longer with less estrogen, and reduction of this hormone has been linked to heart disease and other serious illnesses.

Beyond a Single Solution

How one Oregan executive used multiple approaches in order to find relief from menopause

Olga Haley began noticing peri-menopausal symptoms at age 46. By the time she turned 51, she was feeling many of the distressing effects associated with this natural, but sometimes thorny, passage.

For Haley, insomnia was the worst symptom. Lying awake about three hours every night contributed to other maladies, including headaches, exhaustion, and lethargy bordering on depression. "Finally, I went to see my gynecologist, who prescribed menopausal hormone therapy (HT), telling me that the safeguards it provided for my heart outweighed the dangers of getting breast cancer." Haley admits, "I was dubious, but I took the prescription and got it filled anyway."

She also decided to resign from her position as a vice president at a public relations firm and begin working from home so that she could manage her life and menopause better. Although her workload was still fairly heavy, at least she could schedule rest breaks once or twice a day to make up for the insomnia.

About four years later, Haley felt a stinging in her left breast. She went for a mammogram, white with fear that she had breast cancer. Fortunately, the problem turned out to be cysts. Soon after, she heard a report that estrogen given as part of HT was linked to a 40-percent increase in breast cancer. "I was so frightened that I threw my prescription away and quit cold turkey," says Haley.

Abruptly stopping HT caused massive headaches for a few days, but they eventually subsided. Haley decided to quit seeing her male doctor and found a female gynecologist who encouraged the use of alternative treatments. Rather than advocating the one-size-fits-all approach that her other doctor took, Haley's new physician worked with her to design a program geared to her unique needs.

Haley began using herbal products, such as Pro-Gest, a natural progesterone, and valerian root, to help her sleep. She also took vitamin E, an antioxidant thought to have heart protective benefits, as well as vitamin D and calcium to stave off osteoporosis.

> Haley's new physician worked with her to design a program geared to her unique needs.

Vigorous exercise is now part of Haley's health regimen. She had been taking walks for years, but then she committed to a more regular routine and now pushes for longer distances. She started with small weights, doing 20 repetitions of six exercises every day, then she added sit-ups. And unless it's a Friday- or Saturday-night splurge—when she doesn't care if she's a little sleepless—Haley avoids alcohol and caffeine late in the day.

Listening to her body and charting her own course of wellness enabled Haley to return to work downtown. Today, at age 57, she owns a successful public-relations firm and is as active as she ever was. Yet she doesn't regret stepping out of the mainstream and taking time to evaluate her life.

"Menopause brought with it a real sense of loss," says Haley. "I would feel down in the dumps, even though I had everything I ever wanted: a great husband, wonderful home, good job. Then I realized that my life was far from over, despite all the foolishness women are fed by our society. I have a good third of my life ahead of me, so I started thinking about all that I could still contribute."

Foods
That Fight Fibroids

Could nuts, seeds, beans, and tofu heal these often debilitating tumors without surgery?

BY LINDA VILLAROSA

As Jacqueline Woodson shook off the after-effects of anesthesia, her doctor told her there was good news and bad news: Laparoscopic surgery to remove an ovarian cyst had been a success, but a lemon-sized fibroid was growing in Woodson's uterus. This noncancerous tumor, the doctor said, could be the reason that the New York City–based children's book writer was having trouble getting pregnant. The physician recommended that she take Lupron for six months to shrink the fibroid, then undergo surgery to remove it. Without the operation, her chances of getting pregnant were slim. But the medication would throw her body into temporary menopause. "I was 36, and I wanted to have a baby. I didn't want to spend six months on medication that would mess with my period, then have more surgery," says Woodson, now 40. "Plus, I really didn't want to get cut open."

So she researched and tried alternatives. She cut back on bread, fried foods, and dairy, and ate only organic products to avoid hormones and pesticides.

She signed up for weekly acupuncture treatments purported to help boost her fertility and massage sessions to ease her stress. Her acupuncturist also recommended *Vitex agnus castus*, an herb the woman said could help shrink the fibroid.

"Right away, my body started feeling different," Woodson says. "My periods were normal, and I didn't have to take medication for cramps. I just felt good overall. Most importantly, I got pregnant after being told that I probably couldn't conceive." Her daughter is now a year old, and Woodson no longer suffers from fibroid-related problems.

Although not thoroughly researched, many women swear by alternative approaches, such as changing their diets, to treat fibroids.

As many as 70 percent of women will develop fibroids at some time in their lives, and 25 percent of them will experience troublesome symptoms. Fibroids can interfere with fertility, cause debilitating pain, and bring about heavy periods. They are among the top three reasons women undergo hysterectomies, the most common treatment for the tumors. No one knows an exact number, but up to 100,000 women a year are unable to have children because of fibroids.

In the past decade, several new medical procedures have had measured success. Myomectomy, a surgical technique in which fibroids are removed while keeping the uterus intact, appeals to women who want to have children. In as many as 50 percent of cases, however, the growths come back. More recently, uterine-artery embolization (UAE) has gained popularity. In this minimally invasive procedure, small particles are injected into arteries that supply blood to fibroids, stunting the tumors' growth. But studies published in 2002 in the journal *Obstetrics & Gynecology* found that UAE may be less effective than previously believed and can cause complications in women who later become pregnant.

Alternative approaches are vying to offer solutions that conventional medicine has yet to provide women with fibroids. While most have not been researched thoroughly and are not recommended by traditional practitioners, many women swear by them. Allan Warshowsky, M.D., a board-certified OB-GYN who has been practicing for more than 20 years, wants to bridge the gap between mainstream and nonstandard medicine. The director of

the Women's Health Program at Beth Israel Hospital's Center for Health and Healing in New York City, Warshowsky began studying alternative strategies after realizing that nothing he learned in medical school, or later in his practice as a physician, could help a host of common female troubles.

"My patients come to me and say, 'Please save my uterus,'" says Warshowsky, who wrote the book

Women want ways to treat fibroids that don't involve surgery, which can impact fertility and cause complications during later pregnancy.

Healing Fibroids: A Doctor's Guide to a Natural Cure, which combines holistic and mainstream remedies. "Conventional medicine doesn't know what to do with fibroids beyond surgery. I take the position that the presence of a fibroid indicates other related, perhaps serious, health problems. You cannot heal a fibroid without addressing the underlying imbalances and dysfunction in your entire system."

When reproductive hormones, particularly estrogen, are thrown off-kilter, these benign tumors develop in and on the uterus. Outside of heredity, traditional doctors can't explain why some women get them and others don't. One hypothesis asserts that unhealthy foods, stress, and lack of exercise and sleep can alter your hormonal balance.

Q + A   HOW THE PILL AFFECTS FIBROIDS

If my mom had fibroids, should I avoid taking birth control pills?

Many OB-GYNs say that women with a family history of these tumors should avoid the Pill out of concern that hormones might "feed" them. But several large-scale studies have shown

that women who take oral contraceptives are less likely to develop fibroids than women who don't. Experts aren't sure why, but they suspect that the estrogen and progestin in birth control pills may protect against fibroids in the same way that pregnancy does. If you've had fibroids yourself,

though, check with your doctor about taking the Pill. You might want to use something else.

By the way, the fact that your mother had fibroids may have nothing to do with whether you get them or not. Scientists are beginning to question the long-held belief that the growths are hereditary.

Alternative healers posit other theories that conventional doctors aren't buying. Warshowsky and others believe that hormones in dairy products can feed fibroids. Proponents of natural therapies also worry that chemicals found in pesticides, insecticides, solvents, and plastics can enter the body and mimic estrogen. "When estrogen becomes dominant, fibroids occur," Warshowsky says.

Probably the most controversial and least studied theory—but one that many holistic specialists firmly stand by—is that fibroids result from emotions that are not completely expressed. "It is proven that stress and anger have physiological effects," explains Andrea Sullivan, Ph.D., a Washington, D.C.-based naturopath and author of A Path to Healing. "I see many fibroid patients holding their pain and emotions in the uterine area. Many have a history of molestation or incest, and there is a shutting down and hardening there. They have to deal with what has happened to them in order for their healing to begin."

The lack of science supporting such theories—and the remedies Warshowsky proposes—may make a typical healthcare provider balk at the idea of them. In fact, "there just isn't good data on the outcomes of any fibroid treatments, even the mainstream medical ones," says Evan Myers, M.D., associate professor of obstetrics and gynecology at Duke University Medical Center. But, he adds, "it's perfectly reasonable for women to experiment with alternatives. The only potentially life-threatening danger is if the bleeding is heavy and persistent and the woman becomes anemic." In addition to the dietary changes, acupuncture, and herbs that Woodson tried, experts advocate avoiding caffeine and sugar. Warshowsky also

Doctors aren't sure why some women get fibroids and others don't. One hypothesis asserts that unhealthy foods, stress, and lack of exercise and sleep can alter your hormonal balance.

recommends eating salmon, tuna, and halibut, as well as nuts, seeds, beans, and tofu. Other suggestions include quitting smoking, limiting alcohol, exercising at least three times a week, doing yoga to lower stress, and getting regular sleep.

Herbal supplements can be powerful—and dangerous—so talk to your doctor before using them. Common ones include black cohosh, evening-primrose oil, red raspberry, and Vitex agnus castus (chasteberry).

Nontraditional remedies may not work for every woman. "If the fibroid is causing severe anemia or just not responding to alternative medicine, surgery may be necessary," Sullivan says.

Linda Diane Seldt grudgingly turned to conventional medicine after trying to shrink her fibroids naturally. Diagnosed 11 years ago, she combined an organic vegetarian diet and herbs to avoid surgery. But in 1995, after both a miscarriage and the death of her mother, her hormones "went berserk," and the fibroid grew to the size of an 8-month-old fetus. "During my period, I wore a super pad and a super tampon at the same time, and I still bled down my legs sometimes," says Seldt, 44, a holistic practitioner and educator in Ann Arbor, Michigan. "I was severely anemic, and everybody was saying, 'Have surgery.'"

Three years ago, she chose to have UAE. Since the procedure, her fibroid has shrunk, and she is nearly symptom-free. "I managed to stave off surgery for nine years, but ultimately, I did the right thing." ▪

Linda Villarosa is a contributing health writer for The New York Times *and the author of* Body & Soul: The Black Women's Guide to Physical Health and Emotional Well-Being.

New Studies Discover a Hidden Cause of Bladder Pain

Does this sound familiar? Chronic, shooting pelvic pain; an unrelenting urge to pee (up to 60 times a day); and a doctor who doles out antibiotics faster than Prada sells out of shoes. More than likely, that doc thinks either you've got a bladder infection or you're a world-class whiner. But something else could be creating the havoc below. A handful of new studies hint that many cases of chronic pelvic pain could in fact be linked to interstitial cystitis (IC), a debilitating bladder inflammation that affects roughly 700,000 women in the United States.

The symptoms mimic those of bladder infections, but antibiotics won't alleviate the stabbing sensation or that got-to-go feeling. There's no cure, and the cause is just as elusive. Two likely theories: The organ's lining lacks protective molecules, or clusters of inflammatory cells settle into the bladder's wall.

Still, lifestyle changes and medication can ease the pain. Eliminating alcohol, caffeinated drinks, and acidic foods may lessen IC discomfort. Antidepressants, antihistamines, even aspirin and ibuprofen have helped some women, and in a recent study, a prescription drug called Elmiron relieved symptoms in 38 percent of sufferers. More extreme options include bathing the bladder in a medicated rinse, which reduces inflammation and blocks pain, or stretching it, which helps increase its capacity and cuts down on trips to the bathroom.

IC has fallen under the diagnostic radar mostly because there isn't a reliable test to detect it. As a result, the average patient—a woman, 9 times out of 10—suffers four years or more and consults five different physicians before she receives an accurate diagnosis. In the future, researchers hope to develop a urinary marker for IC, but for now, doctors detect it by ruling out other possibilities.

For more information, contact the Interstitial Cystitis Network (visit www.ic-network.com or call 707-538-9442).

Juice Arsenal Expands in UTI Fight

Any kind of unsweetened fruit juice, not just cranberry, may help ward off urinary-tract infections (UTIs), according to a new study published in *The American Journal of Clinical Nutrition*. Finnish researchers tracked women's diets for five years and found that the women who drank unsweetened juice daily remained UTI-free, compared with nondrinkers, who experienced frequent and acute symptoms. The scientists also found that women who ate fermented-milk products, such as yogurt with beneficial bacteria, reported fewer infections. If you're troubled by frequent UTIs, be sure to drink a glass or two of 100-percent juice every day or eat yogurt made with live cultures.

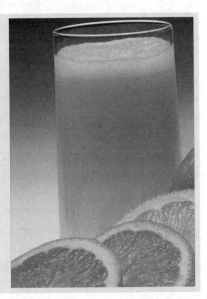

Costly Consequences Facing Women with
EATING DISORDERS

Many women struggle for years to admit that they need help, only to discover that their health-insurance companies won't pay for it.

BY KIMBERLY CONNIFF TABER • PHOTOGRAPHY BY JAYNE WEXLER

When Rebecca Walker started a Ph.D. program in economics in the fall of 1997, she faced the challenges of a typical student, juggling schoolwork with a new social scene. But unlike most of her classmates at Boston College, she was also fighting an illness that had controlled her life for the previous four years: anorexia. At age 22, Walker barely had enough energy to get out of bed in the morning, much less endure a day of intense studying and obsessive thoughts about ways to avoid eating or fit in her hour-long run. One October night, mentally and physically exhausted, she collapsed and was admitted to a local hospital.

Her parents rushed to Boston that same day and took her home to Hoosick Falls, New York, to get help. But despite Walker's obvious illness, her insurance company would only cover a stay at a psychiatric hospital without a specialized program for people with eating disorders. She would be placed in the same ward as women who were schizophrenic, manic-depressive, or actively suicidal. None of the outpatient therapists on her plan had any experience treating anorexia, and the company wouldn't cover anyone out-of-network. Walker knew she needed help—but her provider seemed unwilling to pay for it.

Thousands of other people with eating disorders are not getting the support they need for the same reason. According to experts who treat and study these diseases, behavioral managed-care companies (which are usually contracted by insurance firms to handle mental health claims) control what—and if—therapy is approved. In the traditional

A young woman with anorexia is 12 times more likely to die than other women her age.

medical hierarchy of what receives immediate attention, physical ailments generally supersede mental ones. Eating disorders, which fall into the latter category, are usually relegated to the bottom, below such illnesses as schizophrenia and bipolar disorder, which many HMOs consider more critical.

PART OF THE PROBLEM: Those who review cases for managed-care companies often lack the medical experience to offer an accurate assessment. "Many reviewers have never treated an eating-disorder patient in their lives," says Steve Wonderlich, Ph.D., co-director of the Eating Disorder Institute at the University of North Dakota School of Medicine and Health Sciences and former president of the Academy of Eating Disorders. "They're using general clinical knowledge and applying it to eating disorders. They may not have sufficient knowledge to offer a competent analysis."

The majority of eating-disorder patients end up staying in full-time care for short periods. A Cornell University study shows that the average stay dropped from 130 days in 1984 to 22 days in 1998. According to the Eating Disorders Coalition (EDC), sufferers need at least four to six weeks of around-the-clock care. Today, the average maximum stay many managed-care companies will approve is two or three weeks, according to EDC executive director Jeanine Cogan, Ph.D. As for outpatient counseling, the common 20-session cap can easily be exceeded by the typical client, who needs therapy two or three times a week.

Shortchanging care results in a cycle of recovery and relapse. "The current 'frequent flier' model of eating-disorder treatment is helping neither our economy nor our patients," says Katherine Halmi, M.D., author of the Cornell study and a professor of psychiatry at the university's Weill Medical College in New York City. In the end, only about 30 percent of anorexia and bulimia sufferers today get well completely, according to a number of studies. But with early intervention for both the psychological and physical aspects of these diseases, research shows that the statistic nearly doubles.

Federal legislators are now considering a law that might shift the odds in favor of recovery. Advocacy organizations, therapists, and treatment centers are pressing for passage of the Mental Health Equitable Treatment Act, which would require insurance companies to provide the same level of coverage for mental illnesses, including eating disorders, that they do for physical ones. A similar bill was passed by the House in 2001 but failed in the Senate. Thirty-four states have already passed mental health parity laws, yet most cover only large multistate employers or focus solely on five or six "serious" mental illnesses. This definition usually includes schizophrenia, schizoaffective disorder, bipolar disorder, major depressive disorder, obsessive-compulsive disorder, and panic disorder—but excludes anorexia and bulimia.

> Shortchanging care results in a cycle of recovery and relapse. Early intervention can double the number of those who get completely well.

Most managed-care companies oppose the latest federal bill. They argue that it will significantly increase health-care costs and will ultimately leave more Americans uninsured, since some employers won't be able to afford the expense of plans that include comprehensive mental-health coverage. However, the Congressional Budget Office notes that premiums would only increase by about 1 percent. The proposed legislation will likely come up for a vote in the near future.

Physicians and psychologists have made much progress in dispelling the misguided notion that overcoming an eating disorder is as easy as just saying yes to food. However, insurance companies (and employers who determine their workers' benefit packages) have not caught on. "The stigma and ignorance continue to result in denied care," says Ralph Ibson, vice president of government affairs for the National Mental Health Association.

Today, doctors recognize that if the psychological aspects of eating disorders are ignored, the physical complications can be grave, among them osteoporosis, infertility, gastrointestinal problems, heart problems, and, in the most serious cases, death. A young woman with anorexia is 12 times more likely to die than other women her age. "An eating disorder is addictive behavior, not just a change of habit," says Lorna Boyer Chase, Rebecca Walker's current therapist. "It takes time to create new behavior patterns. You can't expect to make those changes in a short period."

Rebecca Walker, who has been struggling to overcome anorexia for 10 years, is convinced—and her therapist agrees—that if she'd had access to targeted treatment early on, she would have had a much better chance of beating her disorder. Walker grew up in a small town where her father runs the family farm and her mother is a nurse at a nearby hospital. She was the picture-perfect adolescent: prom queen, three-sport athlete, class valedictorian. But in 1993, when she enrolled at St. Lawrence College in upstate New York, she realized she could no longer be the best at everything. Controlling her weight became a way to cope with her insecurities. Impromptu late-night pizza parties or even dinner with friends was out. A member of the school basketball team, she started running long-distance in the off-season to stay in shape. Soon, her behaviors developed into an unhealthy obsession; by the winter holidays, she had lost more than 30 percent of her normal body weight. She became so weak that she had to quit the team. "I was being buried by my own impossible expectations, and I always felt inferior to others and to the person I expected myself to be," she says now. "Being sick was a way to justify not being perfect."

During her sophomore year, her parents insisted that she start seeing a therapist. Although her insurance provider, Community Health Plans (CHP), wouldn't cover anyone near St. Lawrence since it was out of the company's network, she was able to see a counselor at school for a semester. (CHP went out of business in 1998, so we were unable to reach them for comment. David O'Grady, a spokesman for Kaiser Permanente, which assumed CHP's clients,

No Pictures, Please For Rebecca Walker, the decision to be photographed for this story was not an easy one. In the following E-mail excerpt, she talked about her hesitation.

"The problem with showing pictures where I look sick or anorexic is the same problem that I have with having my weight mentioned. When I got involved with this article, it was very important to me that it didn't turn into another sensationalized story about eating disorders. These stories focus on weight and the dramatic parts that inevitably become part of living with an eating disorder. But they don't help the general public to understand the disease. They don't show that this can happen to anyone and that it doesn't have to be dramatic to ruin a life. It's the everyday silent struggle that is really crippling. More importantly, when an eating-disordered person reads an article like this, they look for two things: weights and pictures. If the person in the article is thinner, then they feel like they are not 'good enough' at their disorder. If the person is heavier, then they get this distorted sense of pride that they are doing OK—almost some sort of validation. Neither effect is beneficial."

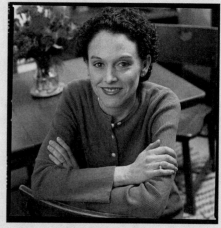

says it is common practice not to cover outpatient care outside a plan's service area.) But by the following summer, her weight was tumbling again, and her parents were pushing her to check in to the hospital. The only place her insurance would cover was Brattleboro Retreat Healthcare, a psychiatric center in Vermont that offered no specific program for people with eating disorders. Walker says that, far from helping, some aspects of the treatment exacerbated her problem. She recalls having to undress with other women before showering, for example, and reveal her weight in her first therapy group—both frightening propositions for someone who has severe body-image problems. In her first individual therapy session, she says a frustrated social worker asked her, "So why are you here? Are you just trying to piss Mommy and Daddy off?"

When her parents came to visit her the next evening, they took her home. "I left with the determination never to put myself in the position where I'd have to go there again," Walker says. Chase says Walker was resistant to getting help later on because her first inpatient experience was so negative. (Citing patient confidentiality, Maria Basescu, a spokeswoman for Brattleboro Retreat Healthcare, declined to respond to specific questions regarding Walker's stay. But she says that in 1995, Brattleboro had "a specialized treatment team" and that its program was "designed to address the unique psychological, medical, social, and nutritional needs" of its patients.)

BEFORE SOMEONE WITH AN EATING DISORDER can even attempt to claim any benefits, she must first prove that her treatment is a "medical necessity"—a phrase that means different things depending on the managed-care company. Some say a patient must have lost more than 25 percent of her ideal body weight or have lost 15 percent of her body weight in one month. (A woman whose healthy body weight is 130 pounds would have to weigh 97½ pounds or have lost 19½ pounds within a month to get coverage.) Another criterion is the risk of "imminent, serious harm," such as a suicide attempt. Professionals who treat eating disorders say they often must also prove that their patients have such medical complications as abnormal blood work, low bone density, an irregular heartbeat, or unbalanced electrolyte levels to get care approved. (When Walker fractured her hip her junior year, necessitating surgery and three months on crutches, she had no trouble getting her insurance to pay—even though her injury was most likely a direct result of her eating disorder, since she had already been diagnosed with osteoporosis.) There's little consideration, these experts say, of the psychological factors that contribute to the disease.

"My health insurance doesn't even think I'm worth it, so I might as well die," says one eating-disorder patient.

This arduous evaluation process almost cost Beth Handler her life. The 28-year-old has suffered from bulimia since she was 17. Handler reached a crisis point in June 2002—not only was she bingeing and purging 12 times a day, but she was also actively suicidal. Cheryl Stayton, Handler's therapist, wrote to her client's insurer, Cigna Behavioral Health, explaining why she urgently needed specialized treatment, but her appeal was denied. Incredulous, Stayton, who now holds a Ph.D. in clinical psychology, called Cigna and was able to negotiate an emergency evaluation at the Renfrew Center in Philadelphia, the closest facility to Handler's home in central Pennsylvania. Renfrew agreed with Stayton, but the request was again denied since her patient was evaluated by a social worker and not a psychiatrist (Stayton says she was never informed of this stipulation). She arranged for another emergency evaluation, this time with a psychiatrist at a local hospital. Even though this physician also argued that Handler's situation was critical, Cigna once again ruled against her. "At this point, she was completely hopeless," Stayton says. "She had done everything they asked, and they were still rejecting her." Stayton finally had to have Handler hospitalized for her own safety after the psychiatrist's plea was turned down.

Cigna, the therapist says, argued that bulimia treatment was medically unnecessary, since it was Handler's depression, not her eating disorder, that was life-threatening. "The point at which it becomes medically necessary is often too late; patients' bodies have already become so damaged," Stayton says. "The real treatment needs to be around the psychological issues before they get to this point." Handler's struggle to receive coverage compounded her insecurities. "My mentality was, 'They don't even think I'm worth it, so I might as well die,' " she says. Thanks to fervent lobbying by the psychiatrist, Handler was eventually admitted to Renfrew. Her weight has stabilized, and she has since moved to Baltimore, where she is currently completing an outpatient program at a hospital covered by her insurance.

Cigna declined to answer questions about Handler's case. "Our job is to try and match what the patient needs with what her benefits allow," says Rhonda Robinson Beale, M.D., chief medical officer for Cigna Behavioral Health.

MANAGED-CARE COMPANIES insist that they offer the best treatment possible, but they have to work within the boundaries (including maximum allowable stays) of the plan that is chosen by the employer or individual. "We are not responsible for the design of the benefit plan that is available to a company's employees or a health plan's members," explains Erin Somers, a spokeswoman for Magellan Health Services, the nation's largest managed behavioral-health company.

Frustrated by her continued battle for treatment, Rebecca Walker has been forced to take the

The Cost of Illness *The pressure of paying for eating-disorder treatment can be a heavy burden. Sometimes, it's unbearable.*

Kathleen MacDonald

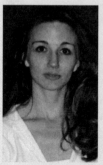

After 18 years of battling anorexia, MacDonald, 31, is still trying to dig herself out of debt. Following two inpatient hospital stays when she was 16 and 20, she was faced with paying the enormous sums that her parents' insurance didn't cover. In her 20s, MacDonald, who lives in Michigan, tried to scrape together enough money for outpatient care (about $100 a week for therapy and $80 for nutrition), but she was too sick to stay in college or hold a steady job. Now in recovery,

MacDonald has cashed in her mutual funds, depleted her IRA, and defaulted on her student loans—and she's still $60,000 in debt. "Every day, I look at my life and say, 'I don't think I can do this anymore,' " she says.

Anna Westin

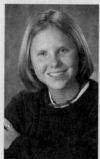

In 2000, Westin, a 21-year-old college student from Minnesota, learned that her parents' insurance company had refused to cover inpatient treatment for anorexia and that her mother

and father planned to pay $25,000 up front. No longer able to bear the pain of her disorder, she killed herself the next day with an overdose of pain medication. (Westin's parents eventually filed a lawsuit that forced BlueCross and BlueShield of Minnesota to reimburse the state $8.2 million for treating patients who had been denied coverage.) "I think that ultimately the passing of parity is going to be imperative," says Kitty Westin, Anna's mother, who now advocates for insurance coverage through a foundation in her daughter's name. "I don't think managed-care companies will necessarily jump on board just because it's the right thing to do."

responsibility for her recovery on herself. In 1999, with the help of a therapist, she decided to enter a full-time treatment program at the Renfrew Center. But her new insurance company, BlueCross BlueShield (BCBS) of Central New York, refused to guarantee coverage, even though Walker's physician and therapist attested to its necessity. Walker entered the program anyway, with her parents putting down an $8,000 deposit plus fees for the first three weeks of treatment. After three weeks, Renfrew's staff insisted that Walker was too sick to leave (she was still severely underweight). But BCBS still wouldn't guarantee any reimbursement—and determined that if they covered treatment at all, they would not cover more than 20 days. Her only other option was Brattleboro Retreat Healthcare—the same facility that had failed her previously. So, once again, Walker was forced to walk away untreated. BCBS of Central New York refused to comment on Walker's case, but spokeswoman Elizabeth Martin says that the organization "works closely with members and providers to maximize treatment whenever possible."

Today, Walker goes to weekly therapy sessions and lives with her sister for support. She works full-time,

but her lifestyle is not the one she imagined. "The eating disorder made me into a person I never wanted to be," she says. "I had different dreams. My goal had been to get a Ph.D. in economics; I now have a master's, and I am the manager of a fitness center."

"I know I need treatment, but it's such a process in order to get it when the insurance companies are saying 'you should be able to do this on your own'". —Rebecca Walker

Chase, Walker's therapist, says Walker has "been doing much better in terms of life functioning." But both know that Walker's physical and mental health are still compromised. "I get to these points where I know I need treatment, but it's such a process in order to get it," Walker says. "It's so hard to battle the eating-disordered mentality that you're OK, and it's hard to stick to treatment when insurance companies say, 'You should be able to do this on your own.'" ▪

Kimberly Conniff Taber is a freelance writer in Paris. Her work has also appeared in Brill's Content, The New York Times, *and* Philadelphia.

Q + A
LOW THYROID

I'm in my 30s and have always been active, but lately I feel like I'm in slow motion. Why am I so tired all the time?

It could be your thyroid. This gland produces a hormone that regulates your metabolism, sex drive, and energy levels, among other things. Feeling worn-out may mean that your thyroid is underactive, a condition known as hypothyroidism.

Other signs include weight gain, dry skin, sensitivity to cold, forgetfulness, and anxiety. You could also have such invisible symptoms as high cholesterol increasing your risks of stroke and heart disease.

Hypothyroidism is common in women your age; at least 13 million people suffer from it. In fact, the American Association of Clinical Endocrinologists recently changed its guidelines for normal thyroid-hormone levels, so the number of people who are deficient could be closer to 27 million.

Of course, extreme tiredness can also signal other illnesses, such as anemia or depression, so see your doctor to rule out those problems. The only way to know for sure if you have hypothyroidism is to take a blood test. If your thyroid-stimulating hormone (TSH) levels are low and no other problems are detected, your doctor may prescribe a synthetic equivalent. The downside: You'll have to take a pill every day for the rest of your life. The upside: You'll start to feel much better right away.

The Shocking Truth About Little Girls on Hormones

Many young girls turn to hormones to keep themselves at "ladylike" heights. But could this controversial method of stunting their growth also jeopardize their health?

BY MICHELLE DALLY

By the time she was 31, Laura Cooper had already suffered three miscarriages. She had undergone surgeries for blocked fallopian tubes and endometriosis. She'd also endured heavy, painful periods and ruptured ovarian cysts. At 40, when she miscarried a fourth time, she asked her gynecologist to tie her tubes. "I didn't ever want to go through that again," says Cooper, a 47-year-old bank teller in New Hampshire. She began searching the Internet for clues that might help explain her host of female troubles. She eventually discovered Tall Girls Inc., a group of Australian women who complained of similar problems. Like Cooper, they had all received high doses of estrogen as girls to stunt their growth.

Even today, with 6-foot-plus models sashaying down runways and the WNBA all the rage, doctors and parents are giving preadolescent girls estrogen to arrest bone growth and keep them at more "ladylike" heights. A national survey published in the *Journal of Pediatric and Adolescent Gynecology* found that one-third of pediatric endocrinologists still prescribe hormones to girls who are expected to grow taller than 6 feet. More than 100 girls are currently receiving the therapy, estimates Neal Barnard, M.D., who conducted the survey. The treatment requires as much as 10 to 15 times the amount of estrogen recommended for menopausal women, even though its long-term physical safety, not to mention its psychological impact, remains unknown. In spring 2002, Barnard, president of the Physician's Committee for Responsible Medicine, petitioned the U.S. Food and Drug Administration (FDA) to change the labeling on oral estrogens (such as the Pill and hormone-replacement medications, such as Premarin) to advise patients that these drugs have never been approved for reining in growth. So far, the FDA has not responded, and the major medical associations remain relatively silent.

Although estrogen has been linked to cancer, doctors and parents are still opting for the treatment in hopes of sparing girls the psychological trauma that can come with being tall, according to medical and anecdotal reports. "Being extremely tall is viewed by many girls and their parents as awkward," says Scott Rivkees, M.D., an associate professor of pediatrics at Yale University School of Medicine who is currently giving one girl high-dose estrogen therapy. He says the girls he has treated have "all felt the same—like it was the best decision of their lives."

But Barnard says that treating tallness as a medical condition just "compounds the body-image issue; it doesn't resolve it." And Elizabeth Berger, M.D., a child and adolescent psychiatrist and author of *Raising Children with Character*, says there's no evidence that above-average height makes girls depressed and suicidal. "In 25 years of practice, I can't recall a single patient whose psychological despair was related to being tall," she says.

For Laura Cooper, the physical traumas have outweighed any promised emotional benefits. During a routine exam when Cooper was 12, her pediatrician took one look at the 5-foot-6-inch preteen and recommended estrogen therapy to limit her growth. Cooper wasn't keen on the idea. "I liked being tall," she says. Now slightly less than 6 feet tall, Cooper recalls that her parents, both of whom hover around 6 feet 1 inch, told her, "We're saving you the pain your mother went through; you'll understand later." What they didn't know was whether or not the treatment would have any lasting health consequences.

Even today, no definitive long-term research on side effects exists. The longest study so far of high-dose estrogen and reproductive health involved 40 women in their early 20s who had taken hormones in their teens. Ten years later, the researchers found no distinct differences in fertility among treated and untreated women. Without studies that follow subjects into their 30s and 40s, however, even the study authors concede that it's hard to draw conclusions about the therapy's impact in the long run.

Nobody knows what high doses of estrogen can do in the long run, especially in young girls whose reproductive systems are still developing.

The fact that the medical community has yet to develop guidelines for hormonal growth suppression further confuses the issue. The American Medical Association (AMA) recently published a brief article on the subject in its newsletter, *AMNews*, citing the potential risks and the fact that "tallness in girls is not a disease." But the AMA stopped short of calling for a ban on treatment or supporting the relabeling petition, concluding that the practice will probably fall out of favor on its own. The American College of Obstetrics and Gynecology also has no formal position or written policy on using estrogen to control height. Neither does the Endocrine Society, although they did refer us to Alan Rogol, M.D., Ph.D., professor of pediatrics in the division of endocrinology at the University of Virginia. Compared with the amount of hormones women are naturally exposed to over their lifetimes, Rogol says, the additional dose isn't that significant. But he can't cite evidence to prove its safety. As for the cancer connection, Rogol is not concerned. "The absolute risk is still very low," he says.

Other doctors disagree. "I would tell my daughters not to touch this therapy," says pediatric endocrinologist Naomi Neufeld, M.D., clinical professor of pediatrics at David Geffen School of Medicine at University of California at Los Angeles. Nobody knows what high doses of estrogen can do in the long run, especially in young girls whose reproductive systems are still developing, Neufeld says.

Laura Cooper tried to dissuade one Texas family she met through Tall Girls Inc. from going ahead with treatment for their daughter. "But they just had this mind-set that they should never have brought this girl into the world because they were so tall," she says. "I couldn't convince them." ◾

Michelle Dally was part of the Denver Post *team that won a 2000 Pulitzer Prize for its coverage of the Columbine shootings.*

Who Has the Best Bones?

Osteoporosis isn't always linked to your birthdate or the amount of milk in your fridge. None of these five women thought she was at risk, but four of them were wrong.

BY LAMBETH HOCHWALD • PHOTOGRAPHY BY MATTHEW RODGERS AND BUFF STRICKLAND

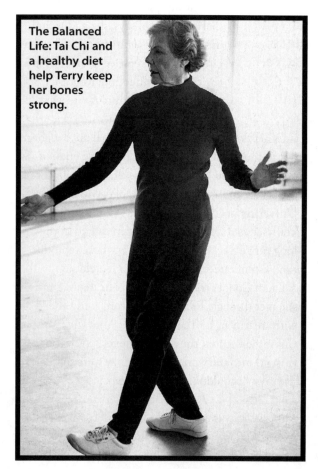

The Balanced Life: Tai Chi and a healthy diet help Terry keep her bones strong.

THE WINNER:
75-YEAR-OLD TERRY CHAYEFSKY
Grade: A+ • Home: New York City
Height: 5 feet 7 inches • Weight: 134 pounds

Surprised? You're not the only one. Most women think osteoporosis is something you don't have to worry about until you qualify for AARP membership. But the latest research says that isn't so. Osteopenia, a precursor to osteoporosis more commonly known as low bone density, affects an estimated 16 percent of Caucasian women between ages 20 and 29, and 25 percent of white women ages 21 to 50.

Of course, risk does increase with age: Bone regeneration starts to slow beginning in your 30s, and the drop in estrogen at menopause further accelerates loss. Nearly 40 percent of postmenopausal women have osteopenia, according to a 2001 report by the National Osteoporosis Foundation. Low calcium intake, as you probably already know, can also deplete your bones. But other factors—ones you may not have heard of—can set up a woman for osteoporosis as well. None of the women featured here, except maybe Terry Chayefsky, thought she was at risk. But

Chayefsky was the only one who wasn't. Each of the other four discovered that she already had bone problems for one of several reasons: family history, poor diet, low body weight, and years of taking epilepsy medication.

"You should be thinking about your bones even in your 20s," says Miriam E. Nelson, Ph.D., professor of nutrition at Tufts University and author of *Strong Women, Strong Bones*. "You're accruing the bulk of your skeletal mass throughout childhood, your teenage years, and your early 20s."

Thankfully, all five women found ways to reduce their odds of developing or halt the progression of a disease that currently afflicts 8 million Americans. Not all women are so lucky, though. For starters, you can't assume your provider will bring up the subject. In 2002, Howard University researchers discovered that osteoporosis counseling or treatment occurs in only about 10 percent of the 267 million doctor visits that women over age 40 make every year. Making matters worse, even women who are diagnosed with osteoporosis frequently avoid dealing with their disease. In a recent study conducted by the University at Buffalo, half of the 836 women who underwent screening for the first time were found to have osteoporosis. One year after being diagnosed, 50 percent hadn't even begun treatment, and 25 percent hadn't discussed the results of their screenings with their physicians.

These statistics are disturbing, because women who don't act fast when they're diagnosed increase their risk of bone fractures—which in turn can lead to pain, surgery, even death. Hip fracture in an elderly woman significantly increases her risk of death.

Fractures aren't the only risk, either. Bones are where your body stores lead, and in this industrial society, most people have absorbed at least some of the toxic mineral. As bones begin to thin, they may leak the lead they've accumulated over the years into the bloodstream—a situation that could contribute to high blood pressure, according to a study published in the March 2003 issue of *The Journal of the American Medical Association*.

To find out if your bones are at risk, take our quiz on page 156. If you answer yes to two or more questions, a growing number of experts say you may need to seek further testing, even though new federal guidelines recommend screening only for women ages 65 and older. Ask your physician to give you a DXA (dual-energy X-ray absorptiometry) scan, which most doctors consider the gold standard of bone-density tests. This 10-minute, noninvasive process, which costs about $200 and may be covered by insurance, images your spine, hips, and/or wrists to gauge how vulnerable your bones are. You can also request a CT (computerized tomography) scan or an ultrasound, which uses sonic waves to predict fracture risk by measuring bone-mineral density at the heel, shin, or kneecap. But neither is considered as accurate as DXA.

For added measure, take some hints—for what to do and what not to—from the women whose stories follow, and from Judith Andariese, R.N., director of the Osteoporosis Prevention Center at the Hospital for Special Surgery in New York City, whom we asked to comment on the progress of each.

"I'm one of the few among my friends who hasn't shrunk," says Chayefsky, an actress and grandmother of five. The only reason she got her bone density tested last year was that she felt she should know her number, just as she knows her cholesterol. She showed no signs of bone loss. One big factor: "I've been a big milk drinker since I was young," she says. "I remember being almost embarrassed to drink milk as a 30-year-old—I used to ask for it at PTA meetings—but now I'm glad I did." Chayefsky regularly performs exercises that may build bone, such as lifting weights and running in place. "I also do Tai Chi, which is great for balance," she says, "and I walk everywhere." In addition, she takes 630 milligrams of calcium citrate daily and eats such healthy foods as fish, shrimp, chicken, vegetables, and fruit.

Expert take: "Besides having good genes, drinking a lot of milk in her youth and doing a lot of walking have kept her bones in good shape," Andariese says.

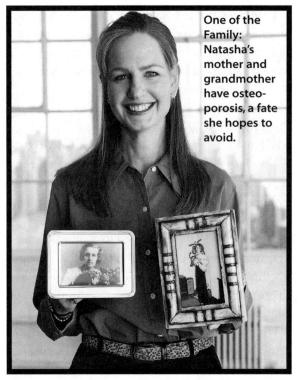

One of the Family: Natasha's mother and grandmother have osteoporosis, a fate she hopes to avoid.

NATASHA WEISCHENBERG

Grade: B • Age: 39 • Home: Bedminster, NJ
Height: 6 feet 2 inches • Weight: 161 pounds

A frequent horseback rider and runner, Natasha Wieschenberg had always felt healthy—until October 2001, when she got up from her couch, took a step, and fell to the floor. A hospital X-ray revealed a serious break in her foot, and she spent the next three months in a cast. This wasn't her first fracture, either—she'd previously cracked a vertebra and injured a hip after falling from a horse. Her history led her doctors to suspect osteopenia, a diagnosis confirmed by a DXA scan. "This was a real curveball," she says. "I wish I had supplemented with calcium more when I was younger, especially since both my mother and grandmother have osteoporosis." Now Wieschenberg takes 1,500 milligrams of calcium every day. She also works out on a stationary bike and elliptical machine. "Now that I know I have a problem, I want to take better care of my bones," she says.

Expert take: "Sixty to 70 percent of osteoporosis is hereditary," Andariese says. "While her active lifestyle is commendable, her multiple injuries may have played a part in her bone loss. She should keep taking calcium, plus vitamin D, every day."

DANIELLE ARCENEAUX

Grade: B- • Age: 28 • Home: New York City
Height: 5 feet 11 inches • Weight: 135 pounds

Danielle Arceneaux, a public-relations account supervisor, had experienced stabbing pain in her right hip off and on since she was in college. She found out in summer 2002 that the discomfort was due to torn cartilage, but her doctors also ordered a bone-density test to find out if anything else was wrong. The diagnosis: osteopenia in her back that may be related to her diet. Because she is lactose-intolerant, she'd avoided dairy foods and tended to eat on the run, often making a meal of a few olives or pieces of candy. Arceneaux was shocked at the

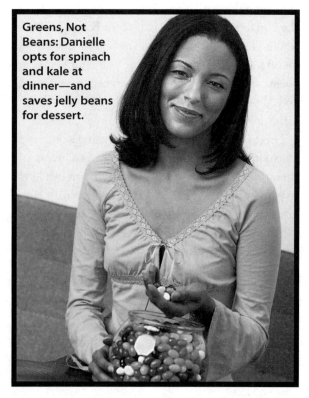

Greens, Not Beans: Danielle opts for spinach and kale at dinner—and saves jelly beans for dessert.

news. "I felt like I was too young to have this problem," she says. Since her diagnosis, Arceneaux has met with a nutritionist, started lifting weights and walking 30 minutes most days of the week, and begun taking 800 milligrams of calcium a day. She gets even more of the mineral from fortified orange juice, oatmeal, and such vegetables as spinach, broccoli, and kale.

Expert take: "Building bone density continues to age 24 or 25. The fact that she's 28 and has experienced some bone loss means that she was on her way to osteoporosis just because of her diet," Andariese says.

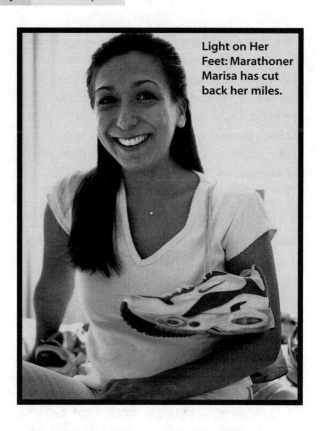

Light on Her Feet: Marathoner Marisa has cut back her miles.

MARISA DE MOURA

Grade: C • Age: 31 • Home: New York City
Height: 5 feet • Weight: 100 pounds

Marisa de Moura, a banking assistant and marathon runner, was preparing for a race in fall 2002 when her left leg started hurting so much that she consulted an orthopedic surgeon, who discovered a stress fracture. He advised her to take four months off to heal. She started running again as soon as she could, training five days a week despite growing pain in her other leg. After completing the marathon, she visited her orthopedist and found out that the bones in her hips and spine were dangerously thin. Her excessive running and low body weight were probably major contributors. "My doctor told me that if I didn't try to reverse it now, I could be 4 feet tall by the time I was 50. That definitely scared me." De Moura has cut back her running drastically, to about six miles a week; she also weight-trains to strengthen her legs. Plus, she's started taking 1,600 milligrams of calcium a day, drinking milk, and eating more calcium-enriched foods.

Expert take: "This is a big awakening for someone who is 31," Andariese says. "She definitely needs to strength-train, as she isn't bearing enough weight on her own to build bones."

RUTH BROWN

Grade: D • Age: 52 • Home: Philadelphia
Height: 5 feet 2 inches • Weight: 107 pounds

Ever since she was 13, Ruth Brown has taken antiseizure medication for her epilepsy. However, she never realized—and her doctors never told her—that the trade-off was increased risk for osteoporosis. She discovered she had it in 2002 when she underwent a routine bone-density test recommended by her gynecologist. "I was floored," Brown, an editor, says. "I drink two glasses of milk a day and eat a lot of cheese and yogurt, and I haven't even hit menopause." Brown, who takes 600 milligrams of calcium carbonate daily, has started exercising regularly. Several times a week, she rides her bike or goes to the gym, where she uses the weight machines and treadmill. She also takes Actonel, a once-a-week prescription drug, to help increase her bone mass.

Expert take: "Taking Actonel is an integral part of optimizing bone density, since it suppresses the rate of bone turnover and loss," Andariese says. "Medications for common conditions, such as asthma, arthritis, and thyroid disorders, can accelerate bone loss over time. This is going to be a lifelong challenge for her, but with bone health, it's never too late to start." ■

Diet and exercise are important factors in fighting osteoporosis. But you should still check with your doctor about medications that might affect your bones.

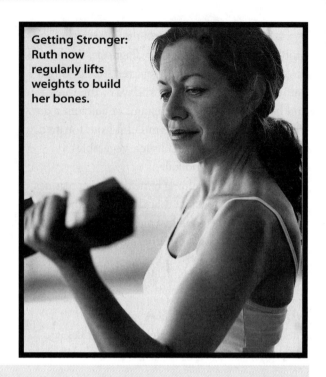

Getting Stronger: Ruth now regularly lifts weights to build her bones.

Are You at Risk?

If you answer yes to two or more of the following questions, see your physician or contact the National Osteoporosis Foundation (202-223-2226 or www.nof.org) for more information.

- Do you weigh less than 127 pounds?
- Are you Asian, Caucasian, or Hispanic?
- Have you ever stopped menstruating for a long period of time?
- Do you have a history of anorexia?
- Have you or a member of your immediate family ever broken a bone as an adult?
- Have you ever fractured a bone in the absence of a major trauma, such as a car accident?
- Do you have a family history of osteoporosis, and/or has your mother experienced an osteoporosis-related fracture?
- Are you postmenopausal?

- Have you undergone an early or surgically induced menopause?
- Do you take high doses of thyroid medication; high or regular doses of cortisone-like drugs for asthma, arthritis, or lupus; or antiseizure medications, such as Dilantin or Depakote?
- Do you have rheumatoid arthritis, inflammatory-bowel syndrome, or multiple sclerosis?
- Is your diet low in dairy products and other sources of calcium?
- Do you spend little or no time doing weight-bearing exercise?
- Do you smoke cigarettes or drink more than two alcoholic beverages per day?

What You Can Do

- Take 1,500 milligrams of calcium citrate or carbonate every day (or 1,200 milligrams a day if your diet is rich in calcium). To increase absorption, take half of your dose with breakfast, the other half with lunch.

- Ask your doctor whether any drugs you're taking could affect your bones.

- Perform some sort of weight-bearing exercise (such as walking or running) most days of the week and strength-train two times a week.

- Don't smoke.

- Keep your drinking in check.

Brittle Bones

Scientists in Iceland have pinpointed gene variations that significantly increase the chances of brittle bones. The team is working on a screening test that will identify the markers, enabling high-risk people to take preventive steps sooner.

New Osteoporosis Drug Boosts Bone Density

Teriparatide is a new medicine that, unlike other osteoporosis treatments on the market, builds bone and prevents loss. In a 19-month study of more than 1,600 postmenopausal women, those who received daily shots of teriparatide while also taking calcium and vitamin D showed significantly greater bone-mineral density in their spines and hips than women who took only supplements.

Build Bones with Vitamin K

More and more researchers now believe that vitamin K, the frumpy cousin of sexy antioxidants A and C, could be essential for strong bones.

Sarah L. Booth, Ph.D., of Tufts University, found in a recent study that low vitamin-K intake was associated with an increased risk of hip fracture among women in their 70s. Researchers theorize that a protein called osteocalcin, which promotes bone formation, requires vitamin K to function.

No one is suggesting that vitamin K is better than calcium, but some studies have shown that Americans fall short of the current recommendations of 90 to 120 micrograms a day. To get your daily dose, eat about $1/2$ cup dark leafy greens, such as broccoli or spinach.

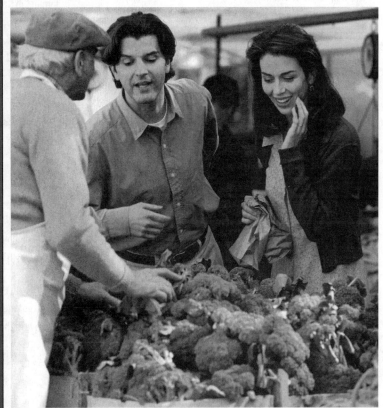

Be sure to add leafy greens to your grocery list. They are great sources of the vitamin K that your bones need.

vital *stats*

64
Percentage of FEMALE INSOMNIACS who cite irritation with their partners as the reason they can't sleep

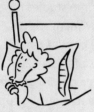

76
Percentage of these insomniacs who DAYDREAM of having an affair to bring on the z's

$1.50
State CIGARETTE TAX levied by New York and New Jersey (tied for highest)

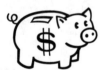

$.025
State cigarette tax in VIRGINIA (the lowest)

$16
Amount (in U.S. dollars) a smoker can be fined in downtown TOKYO for lighting up in public

2.5
Times more likely someone who works with PETS is to develop health problems (such as skin flushing, blurred vision, and asthma) if she uses chemical flea-control products

500
Times the safe level of PHOSMET (a pesticide used to treat fleas) a TODDLER WILL INGEST if she licks her fingers after petting a large dog on dipping day

0
Number of FLEA COLLARS the U.S. Environmental Protection Agency deems safe for kids under age 8 to be around

2
PINTS OF BEER you have to drink to make a person 25 percent more attractive to you

4
Number of GLASSES OF WINE required for the same effect

25
Percentage of American workers who have a mental disorder or SUBSTANCE-ABUSE problem

66
Estimated percentage of those workers who have NEVER BEEN DIAGNOSED

33
Percentage of marriages in which WOMEN EARN MORE MONEY than their husbands

80
Percentage of HOUSEHOLD spending controlled by women

80
Percentage of teenage GIRLS who expect to financially support themselves and their families in the future

87
Percentage of teenage BOYS who do

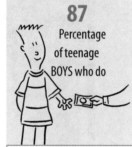

18.9
Percentage of the 9 million CHRONIC BRONCHITIS sufferers living in the Northeast

41.6
Percentage of those who live in the SOUTH

80
Percentage of Americans who clean out their REFRIGERATORS at least four times a year

55
Percentage who clean out their CLOSETS that often

42
Percentage who clean out their MEDICINE CABINETS at least once a season

63
Percentage who have OLD MEDS on their shelves

15
Number of minutes you should let an EGG SIT IN HOT WATER (after bringing to a boil) so that it's safe to eat

2
Number of hours an egg—even a hard-boiled one—can sit UNREFRIGERATED without risking SALMONELLA CONTAMINATION

Sources: American Association of Colleges of Nursing, Insurance Information Institute, *American Journal of Infection Control*, Durex Global Sex Survey, *International Journal of Eating Disorders*, SkyGuide, National Association of Nurse Practitioners in Women's Health, CDC National Prevention Information Network, National Marine Fisheries Service, American Meat Institute, Gallup Poll, *Divorce Magazine* —Reported by Laura Riccobono

nutrition

**fun foods and real
weight-loss solutions**

The Top 5 Diet Types ...
and Why They Don't Work

Wonder why you're not losing weight when your diet seems so healthy? We'll show you why these eating habits are flawed—and what you can do about it.

BY AMY YOUNG

Once upon a time, eating was simple. You plucked food from trees or hunted it in the wild. You ate when you were hungry and stopped when you were full. But then foods proliferated. They came in boxes and cans, with confusing labels and misleading names. Soon, book publishers unleashed hundreds of guides to help you make sense of it all; scientists and nonscientists alike churned out reports on what you should and shouldn't eat. What once was a completely natural endeavor became highly complicated.

Not surprisingly, the kinds of people who consider themselves healthy eaters have multiplied as well. There are vegetarians who abstain from animal protein but eat few vegetables, and snackers who nosh nonstop to keep their energy up. There are low-carb crusaders who steer clear of all breads, pastas, and fruits; fat-phobes who won't let a drop of oil touch their lips; and diet-food junkies who live off meal-replacement bars, shakes, and microwave entrées.

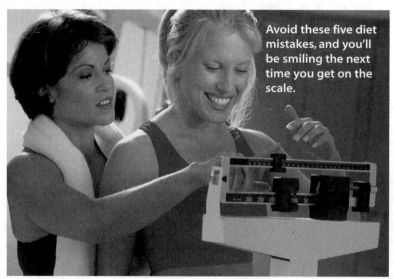

Avoid these five diet mistakes, and you'll be smiling the next time you get on the scale.

All popular eating plans have a sliver of truth to them. The problem is that many diet devotees become so fixated on extremes that they no longer appreciate—or enjoy—foods for the good things they provide (including flavor). This can lead to nutrient deficiencies, cravings, or bingeing.

With the help of several food and nutrition experts, we've identified five of the most common diet types—"healthy" eaters in dire need of makeovers—and offer some easy, practical suggestions to help them get the most out of their meals.

- Eat a big, colorful salad teeming with vegetables every day. Use bagged greens and precut veggies to speed things up.
- Replace processed cookies with fruit-juice pops or applesauce. But fruit you chew is even better, Heber says. Try some frozen banana slices or diced cantaloupe.
- Indulge in low-fat cookies if you must, but why not have a small square of rich dark chocolate instead? The fat and flavor satisfy a sweet craving, and you'll probably eat some later anyway.

THE FAUX-FOOD DIETER

She can't understand why she's still a size 14 when she's been dieting for 10 years. When it's not a frozen "lite" entrée, she's eating a sugar-packed cereal bar or protein bar for breakfast, then another "healthy" frozen meal for dinner. Nearly everything she eats comes in a package: diet margarine, nonfat yogurt, no-calorie sodas, and sugar-free ice cream. Fresh fruit never passes her lips—after all, it's full of sugar. The faux-food dieter does allow herself the occasional binge, though, because she feels she's earned a splurge after eating so much "diet food."

what the **faux-food dieter** eats
- sugar-free hot cocoa
- meal-replacement bars
- frozen vegetable lasagna
- diet soda
- sugar-free, low-fat cookies

what the **low-fat fanatic** eats
- applesauce
- baked corn chips
- pasta salad with fat-free Italian dressing
- boneless, skinless chicken breasts
- white bread

THE FLAWS
Diet-food junkies need the fiber and antioxidants in vegetables and fruits, says David Heber, M.D., Ph.D., director of the Center for Human Nutrition at the University of California, Los Angeles. Frozen entrées usually lack fiber, and they look disappointingly small (and unsatisfying).

THE MAKEOVER
- Instead of a microwave dinner, choose a frozen fish fillet, a ready-to-eat smoked chicken breast, or a speedy turkey burger.

THE LOW-FAT FANATIC

This diet type keeps better track of her fat grams than her 401(k). It's a life dictated by Nutrition Facts labels. She avoids good fats, such as in nuts and olive oil, filling up instead on nonfat snacks, such as bagels, fat-free pudding, and baked chips. *Bor-ing.* Because she never feels full, she's constantly eating—and consuming way more calories than she needs.

THE FLAWS
"This diet looks like it's from the low-fat '90s," Heber says. Then, the traditional food pyramid prevailed, with all carbs placed indiscriminately at the base (which implied you should eat them in abundance) and all fats at the tip (meaning you should eat them sparingly). So calorie-dense bagels and pastas were consumed with abandon, while beneficial foods, such as nuts and avocados, were avoided like the plague.

To revamp this diet, the low-fat fanatic needs to rethink a few long-held tenets: Some fats are good, and no matter what anyone says, calories from carbs *do* count. "The protein/high-fiber combination is the best solution to controlling hunger," points out Barbara Rolls, Ph.D., author of *The Volumetrics Weight-Control Plan*.

THE MAKEOVER

- Add more fat and protein early in the day to keep hunger pangs at bay: Instead of a bagel, substitute scrambled eggs with peppers, onions, and mushrooms.
- Increase the fiber intake: On whole-grain toast, spread reduced-fat cream cheese with vegetables or Nova lox in place of fat-free cream cheese.
- Use olive-oil vinaigrette or even pesto on a pasta salad instead of fat-free dressing, and toss in some chopped fresh tomatoes or other raw vegetables.

THE HOLD-THE-VEGETABLES VEGETARIAN

Diet irony: Some people aren't so much vegetarians as they are food-avoiders. There are two subtypes. One subsists on cheese pizza, pasta, and sweets, while the other uses vegetarianism to justify hardly eating at all. Either way, the only plant life you're likely to see on their plates is a pallid pile of iceberg lettuce.

THE FLAWS

We've got nothing against a meatless diet as long as it's approached properly. But some vegetarians simply don't eat enough vegetables, not to mention fruits and protein (the recommended dietary allowance for women is around 50 grams a day). Heber advises filling your plate with foods in a variety of hues to meet your daily quota for important vitamins, antioxidants, and fiber. Not a bad idea—especially from the author of *What Color Is Your Diet?*—considering you need 5 to 10 servings of fruits and vegetables daily for optimum health. To reach that goal, introduce them into every dish.

THE MAKEOVER

- Toss a handful of fresh blueberries into your next bowl of cereal.

- Order your pizza with plum tomatoes, spinach, and peppers rather than cheese alone.
- Instead of a brownie for a midafternoon refueling, try apple slices or grapes.
- Don't overdo cheese: Snack on 1-inch cubes of Parmesan, mozzarella, or feta to satisfy those cravings for salt and fat.
- Choose concentrated sources of plant protein, such as beans, soy (in its many permutations: edamame, tofu, patties, and sausages), and nuts.
- Good combos: soy-enhanced cereal (with fruit), a soy-chicken breast (with a salad), a small handful of almonds for a snack, and a six-egg-white-and-vegetable omelette for dinner.

THE SNACKER

This obsessive nibbler picks all day at nominally healthy foods, such as trail mix, raisins, pretzels, and reduced-fat cookies, most of which are at her fingertips (or in her desk). In the end, she's eating twice as much as she should. All those minimeals she consumes throughout the day add pounds without boosting her energy levels.

what the hold-the-vegetables vegetarian eats
- pizza
- pasta
- diet soda
- brownies

what the snacker eats
- M&M's
- snack mix
- peanut-butter crackers
- popcorn
- granola bars
- sourdough pretzels

THE FLAWS

"The philosophy behind snacking is that you eat several small meals throughout the day instead of three big ones," Heber says. "But I think most people have forgotten about the 'small' part." Frequent fueling is a great way to stave off fatigue. For many, however, it's also license to overeat. The more micromeals you indulge in, the smaller each portion should be, Heber says. If you're eating six of them a day, then none should stray much beyond 300 calories each.

THE MAKEOVER

- Stash all of your snack goodies in the cupboard or refrigerator where they belong, not beside your computer as a diversion from stress and boredom.

- Snack on proteins or complex carbs to maintain your energy over a longer period of time. Cookies and pretzels are digested quickly, leaving you hungry before an hour's up.
- Better snacks: turkey slices, some plain yogurt topped with fresh berries, a small handful of nuts, a hard-boiled egg, peanut butter spread on apple wedges.
- Better minimeals: a baked sweet potato with low-fat sour cream, tuna salad on flatbread crackers, a fruit-salad cup, a roasted salmon fillet.

her twice the protein she needs each day. Sticking to the low-carb mantra could be setting her up for some unhealthy consequences: at best, carb cravings (or binges); at worst, heart disease and kidney problems.

THE FLAWS

Atkins-diet adherents may not believe it, but not every carbohydrate is your enemy. It's the processed kind that you have to watch out for: white breads, white pastas, rice, and pastries. "They're high in calories and offer little nutritional payoff," Heber says. "And they don't sustain energy for very long." Even so, indulging once in a while to satisfy cravings is OK.

THE LOW-CARB LOSER

She fuels up on protein and fat but eats hardly any carbs at all, which also means no vegetables or fruit. T-bone steaks? Seconds, please! Cheese omelette too greasy? No problem! Her love of all things fatty leaves her with little desire (or room) for a fiber-rich salad—and sometimes gives

what the low-carb loser eats
- low-carb cereal
- low-carb protein shakes
- bag of cashews
- hamburger, Swiss cheese, bacon, no bun
- filet mignon with creamed spinach

THE MAKEOVER

- Instead of eating huge main courses of fatty meats, such as steak, think of proteins as side dishes to enjoy with small servings of brown rice or whole wheat pasta. This keeps your fat intake low without making you feel deprived.
- Eat more complex carbohydrates, such as whole grains, fruits, and vegetables. Because you process them more slowly than simple carbs, you feel fuller longer.
- Additionally, just like the no-veg vegetarian, the low-carb loser should help herself to more fruits by mixing diced peaches into cottage cheese, for instance, or adding lots of vegetables to a cheese omelette. ▪

The low-carb dieter should eat extra fruits and vegetables to ward off carb binges, heart disease, and kidney problems.

How You Can Avoid the Trans-Fat TRAP

If trans fats are so unhealthy, why aren't they on the label?

BY JOE MULLICH

You're watching your cholesterol as well as your waistline, so no one needs to tell you to eat less saturated fat. That's a given. So instead of decadent, dripping-with-butter microwave popcorn to accompany your Friday-night video, you opt for a lighter rendition. The choices? Jolly Time Butter-Licious (3 grams of saturated fat and 10 total grams of fat) looks to be better for you than Newman's Own Organics Pop's Corn With Natural Butter Flavor (4.5 grams of saturated fat and 9 grams in all). In reality, though, Butter-Licious is just as likely to gunk up your arteries as Newman's Own: It contains about 4 grams of undisclosed trans fatty acids.

Although you won't find trans fats listed on food labels (they're not required to be), it's in the majority of processed foods on supermarket shelves. And the obviously decadent treats—chocolate-chunk cookies, Krispy Kreme doughnuts, and neon-orange cheese curls—aren't the only offenders. Even seemingly healthful foods, such as granola bars, multigrain snack chips, low-fat cookies, and high-fiber breakfast cereals (we're not talking Lucky Charms), may harbor this hidden fat. Confusing things further, foods containing trans fats are allowed to make health claims such as "no cholesterol" or "low saturated fat," even though the other fat in the product may be just as bad for you as the saturated kind. Health experts aren't saying you have to banish all foods made with trans fats from your diet. But many top scientists and groups, such as the American Heart Association, are calling for labels to spell out the amounts—a move the U.S. Food and Drug Administration (FDA) is currently considering. Until that happens, though, how do you keep tabs on your trans-fat tally?

While negligible amounts of these fatty acids occur naturally in milk and dairy products, the majority of them are man-made, produced by a process called partial hydrogenation—adding hydrogen gas to corn, soybean, and other unsaturated oils to make them more solid. This arrangement keeps vegetable shortening and stick margarine from melting at room temperature; it also makes crackers crisp, cakes moist, and piecrusts flaky. In addition, trans fats prevent cooking oil from becoming rancid, so that it can be used repeatedly for deep frying.

At first, this chemically re-engineered fat seemed to be a healthier replacement for butter, palm and coconut oils, and lard. But increasing evidence suggests that it could be even worse for you than natural fats. What makes it a health hazard? Like their saturated relatives, trans fats raise bad LDL cholesterol. They also tend to reduce good HDL cholesterol, something saturated fats don't do. Along with this double-whammy, trans fats are believed to aggravate inflammation, clog arteries, and raise triglyceride and lipoprotein levels, all of which add up to an increased risk of heart attack.

It's been almost 10 years since a 1994 Harvard School of Public Health study surprised health experts and consumers alike, attributing 30,000 heart-attack deaths a year to trans fats. But it wasn't until recently that snack-food giant Frito-Lay removed trans fats from all of its products. (McDonald's, despite making a similar promise in late 2002, has yet to publicize any such change and did not return our phone calls seeking confirmation on the issue.)

In April 2003, Denmark became the first country to radically restrict companies from using trans fats in their products. The regulations ostensibly forbid all foods, both domestic and imported, that contain more than 2 percent trans fatty acids per 100 grams of fat. Denmark's decision might sway the FDA to start including trans fats on labels. U.S. food manufacturers are battling a proposal that labels also include a footnote, based on a National Academy of Sciences recommendation, directing consumers to keep their trans-fat intake as low as possible.

These fats are believed to make up as much as 2 to 4 percent of your daily calories, but other estimates are much higher, especially if someone eats a lot of fast food or bakery items made with shortening.

Until it's listed on the package, consumers are blind to the amount of trans fats in foods they think of as healthy. While it's no surprise that a glazed Dunkin' Donut has a whopping 4 grams of undisclosed fat (plus 2.5 grams of saturated fat), the substance also turns up in such snacks as "light" microwave popcorn, seemingly wholesome wheat crackers, and bran cereals.

"Some of the things that masquerade as healthy, like veggie burgers and high-fiber cereal, can be very high in trans fats," says Jana Klauer, M.D., a New York City physician who specializes in treating obesity. According to a recent study conducted by *Consumer Reports*, a quarter-cup of fiber-rich Cracklin' Oat Bran cereal contains 1.5 grams of trans fat (plus 2 grams of saturated fat)—as much as three Nabisco Chips Ahoy! Real Chocolate Chip Cookies. A handful of Wheat Thins has only 1 gram of saturated fat but an additional 2 grams of undocumented trans fat.

Trans fats are believed to aggravate inflammation, clog arteries, and raise triglyceride and lipoprotein levels, all of which add up to an increased risk of heart attack.

Still, some researchers caution against overemphasizing trans fats. Alice H. Lichtenstein, a nutrition professor at Tufts University, is among those who suggest that they be grouped with saturated fats on food labels and designated "bad fats," rather than being singled out. "If you start obsessing about one dietary component in isolation," Lichtenstein says, "the others can get knocked off-kilter." As a guide, she advises people to keep their grand total of saturated and trans fats below the current recommended guidelines for saturated, which is no more than 10 percent of calories. (If you're eating 2,000 calories per day, that's an allowance of 20 grams of saturated and trans fats combined.)

Even if the FDA implements the new labeling regulations, food companies may have up to six years to comply, so consumers need to be their own watchdogs.

- If you eat **lots of margarine**, switch to one with no hydrogenated fat, such as tub or liquid squeeze versions (or others labeled "trans-fat-free"). But you probably don't have to worry about small amounts of margarine (or butter, for that matter, which contains no trans fats but does contain saturated fats) that you spread on your toast.
- Limit the amount of **processed or fast foods** you eat, particularly those that are fried.
- Look for hydrogenated or partially **hydrogenated oil** on the ingredient lists of foods that you consume regularly. If you find it near the top of the list, then that means it's a primary ingredient.
- If you stick with foods that are **low in total fat**, they're likely to be low in trans fats as well.
- If you're really motivated (and have a calculator handy), **do the math**. Monounsaturated and polyunsaturated fats are sometimes listed along with saturated fats on the label (but because the government makes this inclusion optional, only

certain products note them to support their health claims). If these numbers add up to less than the total amount of fat, the difference equals the trans fats. Because fat content is rounded off to the nearest half-gram, the figures might not be precise, but at least you'll have a ballpark idea of what you're taking in.

- Don't try to reduce trans fats by selecting products with **higher saturated fats**. Klauer has noticed that some nutrition bars have eliminated trans fats by replacing partially hydrogenated oil with palm and coconut-kernel oils. "That's the most saturated fat there is," she notes. ∎

Freelance writer Joe Mullich has written for more than 100 publications. He is based in Sherman Oaks, California.

Update: *In July 2003 the FDA issued a regulation requiring manufacturers to list trans fats on the Nutrition Facts panel of foods and some dietary supplements. Food manufacturers have until January 1, 2006, to start providing this information.*

Q + A FDA PUTS TRANS FATS ON LABELS

I've heard that trans fats are bad for you, but I don't see them listed on many products. How do I know if they're in the foods I eat?

Tracking trans fats may soon get easier. In 2003, the U.S. Food and Drug Administration (FDA) is expected to make food companies start listing trans fats (created when vegetable oils are combined with

hydrogen to give foods longer shelf lives) on nutrition labels. That's big news, especially since these fats—as harmful to your heart as the saturated kind—are found in thousands of processed foods. Just a few grams add up fast: Six peanut-butter crackers can account for nearly a fifth of your total daily allotment of trans and saturated fats (20 grams combined).

As it stands now, most labels lump trans and unsaturated fats together under "total fat." Even if the FDA requirements go through, it may take several years for packaging to reflect them. Until then, check ingredient lists and go easy on foods with hydrogenated or partially hydrogenated oils. The higher these are on the list, the more trans fats the food contains.

5 Tips for Dropping 4 Dress Sizes

A pastry chef shares her strategies.

BY AMY YOUNG

The trouble with dieting is that there are so many tasty reasons *not* to. There is cheese, just begging to be savored on a fresh-baked baguette. There is wine, which couples divinely with the cheese. And there is dessert, which, of course, must be experienced with a steaming cappuccino.

Colleen Grapes, pastry chef at the Red Cat restaurant in New York City, knows all about these reasons. For her, dessert, in particular, is an occupational hazard. Yet, surprisingly, despite the high-calorie exposure, she's lost weight, dropping from a size 14 to a size 6 in a scant six months.

"I don't believe in cutting things out completely," says the 5-foot-5-inch brunette, who had lost and regained the same 20 pounds since graduating from culinary school nearly 12 years ago. One day she declared, "This has to stop!" and made a deal with herself to exercise more and eat better. The first part was easy: She signed up to take yoga classes four times a week and began walking 40 minutes to a distant subway station each day instead of using the one closest to her workplace.

Cutting calories and choosing healthier foods presented a challenge—especially when Grapes faced the daily task of chopping 3 pounds of chocolate malt balls for a mousse cake. Keeping sweets out of sight, out of mind—often the first diet defense—was impossible. Grapes knew she needed to manage what she ate rather than eliminate whole food groups altogether. So she whipped up the following five rules for enjoying food and cutting back.

1 COOKIES ARE MEANT TO BE SHARED.
Tasting freshly baked sweets is a job requirement as well as a weakness for Grapes, who used to eat eight cookies a day. But no longer: "I take one, immediately break it in half, and give the other half away."

2 CHIPS ARE OK IN SMALL PACKAGES.
Despite eating great restaurant meals every night, Grapes is a potato-chip junkie. But she prefers the gourmet chips cooked in olive oil rather than in hydrogenated fat. She buys a snack-sized bag when the craving hits and allows herself just 10 chips. Then she gives the rest away.

3 CHEESE TASTES BEST ON PIZZA.
One of Grapes' biggest fat traps was sampling cheese throughout the day. The only way to keep the calories from piling up was to quit nibbling. Now she enjoys this passion only at mealtime, on a hot slice of pizza.

4 A SANDWICH TASTES JUST AS GOOD ON HALF A BUN.
Grapes discards the thicker top bun and cuts the remaining bottom bun in two for a leaner sandwich (yes, it can get a little messy).

5 EAT ONLY THE BEST ICE CREAM.
"If it's not my own or Ben and Jerry's, I don't eat it." Grapes believes in *really* tasting your food. If you're not perfectly satisfied, why waste the calories?

Too Much of a Good Thing

When you get 100 percent of everything you need at breakfast, what's your tally at the end of the day? Discover how to avoid vitamin overload in a fortified world.

BY SHARON GOLDMAN EDRY

Sure, you eat right and exercise. Perhaps you also pop a multivitamin each day, have a bowl of fortified cereal with milk in the morning, and drink a glass of calcium-enhanced cranberry juice in the afternoon. Then there's the vitamin C and zinc tablets to ward off colds, the extra calcium pill (more osteoporosis prevention), and the energy bar you nosh on before heading to the gym.

You may have the best of intentions, but nutrition experts say some of these healthy eating efforts might be in vain—or even harmful. The negative effects of overdosing on certain supplements in pill form, such as iron and beta-carotene, have been well-publicized. Even if you're not gobbling handfuls of capsules, though, you might be getting way too many of some vitamins and minerals, thanks to the ever-increasing number of fortified foods on the market. The intricate web of nutrient interactions can range from confusing to mind-boggling, so you may be unaware of the ways your body can react to protein-packed nutrition bars, supercharged bottled waters and fruit juices, and cereals with 100 percent of everything.

> **Just because we know vitamins and minerals are key to all the body's processes doesn't mean more of them is better.**

To date, no hard data is available on the health consequences of megadosing on fortified foods, powders, and snacks. And there's no question that fortification has paid off in large part. In fact, since the U.S. government mandated in 1998 that cereals, breads, and other grain-based products be fortified with folic acid, the incidence of such common birth defects as spina bifida and anencephaly has dropped by at least 19 percent.

But a growing number of health experts think the potential for serious problems exists if you're eating enriched foods in addition to taking a multivitamin and certain other supplements. "It's a real concern as people buy more fortified products, particularly those that include nutrients we know have some toxicity associated with them, even at fairly low levels," explains Robert Russell, M.D., professor of medicine and nutrition at Tufts University School of Medicine. Case in point: A recent Swedish report in *The New England Journal of Medicine* confirmed several previous studies, including one from Harvard University, that linked high levels (more than 3,000 micrograms per day) of retinol-derived, or non-beta-carotene, vitamin A to decreased bone mass and hip fractures, both of which are symptoms of osteoporosis. Retinol-derived A is found in such fortified foods as cereal and skim milk, as well as meat, fish oils, and supplements. Along with the risk of bone loss, liver damage and birth defects are other potential dangers of over-consuming this form of the vitamin long-term. "I think health authorities should consider revising the current recommendations of retinol-derived vitamin A to lower levels," says Karl Michaëlsson, M.D., the lead author of the study.

As long as foods continue to be fortified, though, it pays to shop carefully. "You have to be careful with how you select foods," cautions Wahida Karmally, D.P.H., associate research scientist and director of nutrition at Columbia University's Irving Center

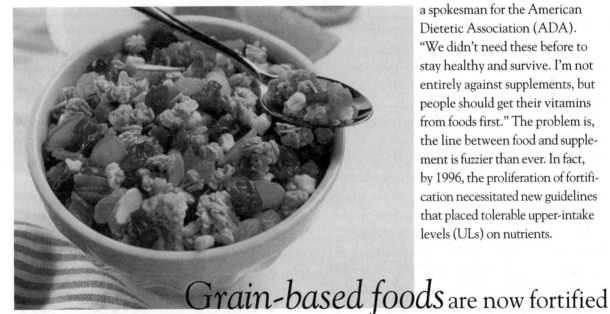

for Clinical Research. "Just because we know that vitamins and minerals are key to all the body's processes doesn't mean that more of them is better."

Aside from the side effects of overdosing on some vitamins, there may be repercussions for other nutrients—getting too much of one may lessen absorption of another, or one might depend on another to achieve the maximum benefit. For example, Russell says that high levels of vitamin E

can make vitamin K, which is essential for blood clotting, less effective. And calcium can interfere with iron absorption, so you shouldn't take a calcium supplement with a meal containing meat, which is high in iron. "The whole mind-set is more, more, more," says Ruth Kava, Ph.D., R.D., director of nutrition at the American Council on Science and Health in New York City. "Especially now that you might be getting 100 percent of your RDA (recommended dietary allowance) by the end of breakfast."

You didn't always have to worry about getting too much, though. In past decades, such nutrients as vitamin D, iron, and niacin were added to only a few staple foods, such as milk and bread, to combat rickets, pellagra, and other deficiency-related diseases. "Our bodies were designed presupplement and pre-protein powder," says Jeff Hampl, Ph.D., R.D., a spokesman for the American Dietetic Association (ADA). "We didn't need these before to stay healthy and survive. I'm not entirely against supplements, but people should get their vitamins from foods first." The problem is, the line between food and supplement is fuzzier than ever. In fact, by 1996, the proliferation of fortification necessitated new guidelines that placed tolerable upper-intake levels (ULs) on nutrients.

Grain-based foods are now fortified with folic acid, which is good, but most Americans are consuming double what they used to.

Even if you know what the limits are, though, it's hard to gauge just how much is too much. If you change brands or add and subtract new products, you probably have no clue what's in the stuff you're eating. Plus, food labels only list the amounts of certain nutrients, says Paula Trumbo, Ph.D., of the Food and Nutrition Board (a unit of the Institute of Medicine that created the new ULs). "It's been hard to get a handle on the actual amount that a person consumes," she explains.

For example, a report published in the January 2003 *American Journal of Clinical Nutrition* found that Americans are consuming more than twice as much folic acid as originally intended when mandatory fortification began five years ago. While synthetic folic acid isn't toxic, daily intake of more than 1,000 micrograms can reverse the anemia in a person with a vitamin B_{12} deficiency, interfering with diagnosis and delaying treatment—which can lead to permanent nerve damage.

How easy is it to cross the 1,000-microgram mark? A bowl of cereal, a multivitamin, two slices of bread, and a snack bar, and you're over the line. Vegans, who forgo such B_{12}-rich foods as meat, eggs, and cheese, are particularly vulnerable to deficiency and, thus, likely to experience problems if they overload on folic acid, says Lynn Bailey, Ph.D., professor of human nutrition at the University of Florida's Institute of Agricultural Sciences. "It's critical that a B_{12} deficiency is diagnosed early," she says. "So it's a problem if the accompanying anemia is covered up."

Going overboard on calcium? Chronically high intake (2,500 milligrams per day) can lead to kidney stones and block the absorption of such nutrients as iron and zinc. Double-dosing on vitamin D (50 micrograms is the UL for adults), which promotes bone formation by increasing blood levels of calcium and phosphorus, may cause calcium toxicity. Very high levels of niacin (more than 35 milligrams) can cause nausea and skin redness, while too much

The occasional energy bar is OK—but you shouldn't rely on it to replace a balanced meal of real food.

magnesium (350 milligrams from supplements and fortified foods) or iron (45 milligrams) can cause diarrhea.

Vitamin and mineral supplements or fortified foods can also affect the potency of prescription drugs, especially antibiotics. A recent study at the Bassett Clinical Pharmacology Research Center in Cooperstown, New York, found that taking the antibiotic Cipro with calcium-enriched orange juice reduced the medicine's absorption by up to 40 percent. Cipro is the frontline treatment for urinary-tract, bladder, and sinus infections, as well as anthrax. Patients are often encouraged to take such medications with food, but not with supplements; what most people don't realize, though, is that a given food may actually be a supplement. "We need to take into account how the fortified foods we eat can affect the drugs we take," says Guy Amsden, Pharm.D., who co-authored the study.

Such vitamins as A, D, and E are fat-soluble, meaning they are metabolized along with fat in the body and can be stored in large, potentially toxic, amounts. Other vitamins, on the other hand, may not be harmful in high doses, but you might be wasting your time and money if you consume more of them than you need. C and the B vitamins, for instance, are water-soluble, or stored in the body for only a short time before being excreted. So if you consume in excess of the RDA—say, by chugging vitamin water or chowing on a meal-replacement bar—there is no scientifically proven benefit, Karmally says. "You'll probably just have very nutritious urine," she explains.

That doesn't mean fortified cereals, drinks, and energy bars have no value. If you don't like milk or can't tolerate it, for example, you can get a bone boost from calcium-fortified orange juice. And if you miss lunch once in a while and need an energy bar to keep going, that's better than grabbing a candy bar or chips. Experts simply encourage women to not rely on these for their RDAs in lieu of a varied menu filled with lean protein, fruits, vegetables, and grains.

Crunching the Numbers

Are you overdoing your daily vitamins and minerals? You could be getting too many of them without even knowing it just by eating common fortified foods, such as cereal, milk, juice, energy bars, and nutritional drinks, in addition to multivitamins and other supplements. And if you exceed the limit on some important nutrients, including A, calcium, and folic acid, you might just pay a pill-popping price.

VITAMIN A	CALCIUM	FOLIC ACID
Too much vitamin A (retinol-derived) can cause bone loss, birth defects, and irreversible liver damage.	*Too much calcium can lead to kidney stones or can block the absorption of nutrients, such as iron and zinc.*	*Too much folic acid, the synthetic version of folate, can mask the anemia that accompanies a vitamin-B_{12} deficiency, leading to irreversible nerve damage if left untreated.*
RDA: 700mcg **Upper Limit:** 3,000mcg	**RDA:** 1,000 mg **Upper Limit:** 2.5g	**RDA:** 400mcg **Upper Limit:** 1,000mcg
One-A-Day multivitamin **900mcg**	One can Boost nutritional drink **330mg**	¾ cup Whole Grain Total cereal **400mcg**
1 cup low-fat milk **143mcg**	1¼ cups Harmony cereal **700mg**	Centrum multivitamin **400mcg**
28g (about ¾ cup) regular Quaker Instant Oatmeal **140mcg**	2 cups 1% low-fat milk **600mg**	Two slices Arnold Brick Oven white bread **45mcg**
Vitamin A fish-oil capsule **3,030mcg**	GeniSoy protein bar **250mg**	PowerBar Pria energy bar **240mcg**
	One carton Stonyfield Farms raspberry yogurt **250mg**	
	One-A-Day Women's Formula **450mg**	
	Viactiv Soft Calcium Chew **500mg**	
TOTAL: 4,213mcg	**TOTAL: 3.08g**	**TOTAL: 1,085mcg**

171

"You'll be missing out on a lot of other things that could benefit your body if you don't eat real food, especially fruits and vegetables," Russell says. The ADA's Hampl agrees: "We need a 'cocktail' of foods to get the full benefit of a nutrient. Taking a supplement or eating an energy bar might have some effect, but not close to the effect you get from whole foods."

Also, you shouldn't feel that you have to pop additional supplements to get all your nutrients from A to Z. For most women who eat healthy diets, a multivitamin or the equivalent fortified foods that contain no more than the RDA are sufficient to make up for any shortfalls. And if you're thinking about getting pregnant, consider consulting a physician or a dietitian about a healthy diet and supplement regimen.

Keeping track of the vitamins and minerals you take is the key to moderation. Before you whip out your calculator, though, remember that you would have to make a mighty effort over many months to go over the limit and suffer side effects. However, if you eat a lot of fortified products, a targeted assessment of your intake, especially of vitamin A and folic acid (the synthetic version of folate added to foods), is worthwhile, Russell says: "You have to read the labels and add everything up to make sure you're not going overboard on a regular basis."

You might also want to avoid taking a multivitamin on top of all those high-powered foods. "We want to feel like we're doing something good for ourselves," Kava says. "But in this case, trying to do everything right can potentially be harmful." ■

What's the Scoop on All That Soy?

Soy is everywhere, not just in tofu and veggie burgers. The high-protein additive is found in everything from energy bars, fruit drinks, and powders to a multitude of snacks, cereals, and even soups. Sales of soy have skyrocketed over the past few years, with claims of cholesterol reduction and heart-disease prevention. But can you get too much of it?

The jury is out about soy's hazards, but questions persist about isoflavones—plant hormones in soy that have estrogen-like effects on the body—especially as these chemicals pertain to breast cancer. A recent report from the United Kingdom's Committee on Toxicity of Chemicals in Foods, Consumer Products, and the Environment advises women with estrogen-dependent breast cancer against

consuming high amounts of foods containing phytoestrogens. "This is one of the most comprehensive reports I've ever seen on this topic," says Clare M. Hasler, Ph.D., founding director of the Functional Foods Program at the University of Illinois at Urbana-Champaign. "In terms of how much is too much, though, we still don't know what the recommendations should be."

A current claim approved by the U.S. Food and Drug Administration asserts that 25 grams of soy protein per day benefit heart health. But while concentrated soy supplements have caused the most concern among researchers for their estrogenic effects, some energy bars, drinks, cereals, and powders also tout high levels of

isoflavones, as much as 150 milligrams per serving. "We really don't know what the overall risk is in consuming isoflavones in a much more concentrated form," says Pat Murphy, Ph.D., professor of food science at Iowa State University. However, she believes fortified foods that contain soy protein and moderate amounts of isoflavones are relatively safe and well-understood.

While there may be some disagreement on how much soy is best, most experts concur that getting protein from foods with only small amounts of soy won't give you the most bang for your buck, Murphy says. "Traditional soy foods, such as soybeans, soy nuts, soy milk, and tofu, are a better and more economical way to get your protein and cholesterol-lowering benefits," she says.

172

Dieting Good Intentions *Do* Pay Off

You've probably heard that yo-yo dieting may be bad for your heart, not to mention your psyche. Well, new research from the Centers for Disease Control and Prevention suggests that trying to drop excess pounds, even if you fail, does offer health benefits after all. The study found that repeat dieters ended up living longer than those who kept packing away the cheesecake. Experts guess that good intentions lead to healthful changes, even if the love handles don't disappear.

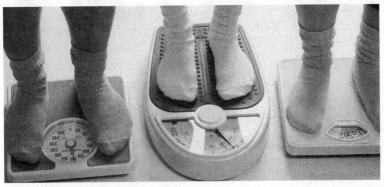

The Mindset That Drops Pounds

It always pays to think ahead—unless you're planning a diet. A recent study found that the mere thought of a future diet can

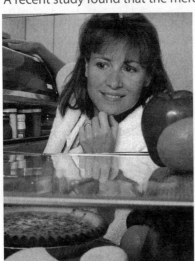

trigger overeating. "As soon as you put a prohibition on something, you leave yourself vulnerable to temptation," says study author C. Peter Herman, Ph.D., of the University of Toronto. If you're trying to shed a few extra pounds, don't focus on the food you're not going to have, says Joy Bauer, author of *The Complete Idiot's Guide to Total Nutrition.* "Think about what you are going to have: confidence and inner strength from knowing that you're in control."

According to a report released by the U.S. Federal Trade Commission, almost half of all weight-loss ads, whether in print, on television, or on the Internet, make false claims.

What the Japanese Know (That We Don't) About Healthy Eating

Eating healthfully is effortless in Japan, where small portions and beautifully prepared foods nourish the senses.

BY PEGGY ORENSTEIN

My husband and I like to play the castaway game. You know the one: If you were forced to spend the rest of your life on a desert island, which books, CDs, and videos would you bring? But instead of entertainment—since a contemporary Crusoe would simply take a laptop and download everything she needed from the Net—we play with food: If you could eat only one style of cuisine from here to eternity, which would it be?

He leans toward French for its sheer scope and excellent cheese. But for me, it's no contest: Japanese. With few exceptions, the whole of breakfast being one of them, I could eat Japanese food every day until the good Lord calls me home.

So when my editor asked me to eat like a local on a recent three-week jaunt to Japan, I felt like the last Survivor after the final vote. My editor's motives were, shall we say, more honorable: How, she wondered, did diet contribute to the legendary good

Only an American would think of all-you-can-eat sushi.

health of the Japanese, and could it have an impact on a Western body in such a short time?

According to the World Health Organization, the Japanese live longer than practically anyone on the planet (their life expectancy: 74.5 years; Americans': 70). They have far lower rates of obesity, heart disease, and breast cancer than we do. Good genes, you say? Maybe, except that one generation after immigrating to America, chronic-disease rates among people of Japanese descent shoot up.

But I wasn't concerned with all that. I don't have any health issues at the moment. If my blood pressure were any lower, I'd be dead. Ditto my cholesterol. Although I've come to terms with the fact that I kissed size 6 good-bye a decade ago, if I placed a personals ad describing myself as "slender," it would still qualify as truth in advertising. I was even a vegetarian for much of my adult life, includ-ing an ill-advised stint in college during which I

174

made my own tofu. I wasn't sure what a Japanese diet could do for me, but for the sake of research, I vowed to eat my favorite foods until I burst.

Within hours of arriving in Tokyo, it became obvious that the Japanese themselves don't necessarily eat like Japanese anymore. There was actually a Starbucks two blocks from my hotel (one of 165 in the city). The corner coffee shop sold bagels and lox in the morning. And McDonald's wildly outnumbered Mos Burgers, its Eastern rival, which serves a surprisingly tasty, White Castle-size rice burger. My Japanese friends begged to go out for Italian, which would be their desert-island pick. Meanwhile, Japan's annual tofu consumption has been plummeting while its consumption of beef has been steadily rising. Rates of childhood obesity have also climbed.

Yet beneath that layer of saturated Western fat still beats a vigorous cultural heart. As it turns out, with the exceptions of high sodium and low calcium, eating the traditional Japanese way basically means sticking to a healthy diet. And doing it effortlessly.

My first day in Tokyo, for instance, I met friends for *kaiseki*, the ne plus ultra of Japanese food, at Aoyama Asada restaurant. Centuries ago, rice was the centerpiece of a Japanese meal, accompanied by small side dishes of vegetables and fish. Over time, the side dishes took over. Now kaiseki consists of seven or more exquisitely presented courses, each about five bites, ending with a symbolic bowl of rice. Aoyama Asada's Kaga-style kaiseki (native to an area southwest of Tokyo, on the Sea of Japan) began with an earthenware bowl that held a dollop of spinach, lotus root, yam noodle, and shiitake-mushroom salad dressed in a smoky miso sauce. An accompanying lacquer box contained appetizers, including a smidgen of pâté in a tiny gold-rimmed cup, a single shrimp, and a fava bean suspended in aspic; a hollowed-out mandarin peel cradled a baby square of sesame tofu topped with a dab of orange-flavored miso. Next came a hexagonal bowl resembling a gazebo. Inside, a garden of miniature flowers surrounded a sashimi bridge made from precisely four bites of tuna and snapper. We paused to admire each dish's beauty and cunning,

which were essential to its pleasure. In Japan, eating is an aesthetic experience as well as a social one.

Which brings me to **Japanese Health Lesson Number One:** *It's not just what you eat, but how you eat it.* My trusty *Cambridge World History of Food* says that the Japanese have for centuries put a premium on presentation, particularly that which evokes the natural world. This means nix on the Styrofoam containers. The beauty, which incorporates a Zen-influenced appreciation of the empty space on a plate, encourages one to eat slowly, to savor each bite rather than shoveling it in. Even the more hearty home-style cuisine is meant to be enjoyed communally, over relaxed conversation: I shared sukiyaki, *shabu-shabu*, and *nabe*—a winter stew of vegetables, seafood, chicken, noodles, and tofu (and whatever else might be handy) that a friend cooked in a pot on her dining room table as we chatted. By contrast, we Americans seem to prefer high-fat fare that we can wolf down in our cars. *De gustibus*.

Every meal couldn't be a sensual feast—that would be cheating. Luckily, **Japanese Health Lesson Number Two is:** *Fast food can be good food.* I slurped buckwheat noodles in a tasty broth at a soba-noodle stand. I trolled the food halls found in every department store basement for premade sushi, grilled treats, or *bento* boxes stocked with fish and vegetables. One day, I tailed a group of young office workers and discovered the local 7-Elevens have surprisingly decent chow. I bought a bento box of grilled salmon; two seaweed-wrapped rice balls; *tamago* (sweet omelette); and a salad of spinach, grated carrots, and yam noodles with sesame sauce. The fish clocked in at about 155 calories, with 6.9 grams of fat and the heart-protective benefits of omega-3 fatty acids. That's a long way from a Big Mac, with its heart-stopping 590 calories, 34 grams of fat, and 1,090 milligrams of sodium. Don't even get me started comparing a side of fries with my spinach salad.

Speaking of "bigs," that's **Japanese Health Lesson Number Three:** *Like diet docs keep telling us, it's all about portion control.* Only Americans would think of all-you-can eat sushi. "By American standards, the courses Japanese eat are like the little things you pass around on a cocktail platter before dinner," says Marion Nestle, Ph.D., chairwoman of the department of nutrition and food studies at New York University. "True, we're larger people and need more food than they do, but not nearly as much as we eat. All the metabolic abnormalities—heart disease, obesity, diabetes, and high blood pressure—are associated with eating more calories than you burn."

Even fast food is good for you in Japan. Bento boxes of grilled salmon and rice balls are sold at 7-Elevens.

Perhaps because of that, I ate some things in Japan I never thought I would, though not the exotica you'd imagine. I'm talking about chicken skin. Beef. Cream puffs. Foods I usually consider taboo. I just didn't eat very much of them. The two bites of fried chicken in a bento-box lunch hit the spot but weren't enough to send me into a junk food shame spiral or amp up my LDL. Even the meals I grabbed on the train featured bite-size courses rather than a slab of an entrée. Maybe that's partly why Americans don't get the gestalt of tofu: We want to eat it like a steak, in a big soy-drenched hunk.

Originally, the Japanese didn't have a choice about their healthy habits. Their diet was foisted upon them by royal decree in the seventh century A.D., when a particularly devout Buddhist emperor banned the eating of cows, horses, chickens, monkeys, and dogs. Without a lot of cattle breeding, there wasn't much dairy, so butter, cheese, and cream were out, too. That pretty much left naturally low-fat fish and vegetables as the only menu choices for the next 1,200 years, when the country opened to the West. Luckily for their life expectancies, old habits die hard: Even now, the Japanese lead the world in seafood consumption. Meanwhile, since most types of wheat won't grow in Japan's climate, bread wasn't much of an option for millennia, either. Even rice was scarce, since there wasn't a lot of space for paddies. That's why, while Japanese eat a small bowl of rice at the end of a meal, they don't carbo-load the whole way through.

Aesthetics, royal edicts, portion control—it all fit, until I visited Hiroshima and sampled *okonomiyaki*, a local specialty that's the Japanese answer to a Philly cheese steak. A building downtown is dedicated to the stuff: four floors of identical vinyl stools all huddled around identical short-order grills. Okonomiyaki isn't complicated—a crepe piled high with cabbage, udon noodles, bean sprouts, green onions, bacon, and, if you want to get fancy, shrimp or squid. It's topped with a fried egg and doused with a glutinous, slightly sweet sauce that is supposedly the secret to its appeal. It's as heavy as lead, and twice as filling. Under normal circumstances, I wouldn't have gone near it. And yet—cabbage? Bean sprouts? Green onions? *Squid?* My arteries were hardly in mortal danger. Besides, in Japan, okonomiyaki is an indulgence, not a mainstay.

That's the genius of the Japanese way of eating, as well as **Japanese Health Lesson Number Four:** *It embraces the best of Western diet fads—without the deprivation.* It's low-fat enough for Dean Ornish, but it still leaves enough wiggle room for a little tempura or okonomiyaki. It's high-protein and carb-free enough for Atkins, yet you get a hunger-sating bowl of rice to finish a meal. And of course, there's that magical, miracle soy, but it's *tasty* soy. In Kyoto, I ate the most memorable food of my visit: *shojin ryori*, a tofu-based cuisine created for vegetarian Buddhist monks. I sampled chewy tofu, meaty tofu, plum-flavored tofu, green tea–infused tofu, and sticky tofu with a pickled-plum center wrapped, gift-like, in a taro leaf. Best of all, in the middle of the table, a pot of soy milk simmered. Periodically, a film called *yuba* formed on top. My companions and

I took turns lifting it with chopsticks, dunking it in a soy-based sauce, and letting it melt in our mouths. *Oishii desu!* (That's "delish" to you and me.)

As with any diet, I inevitably slipped. Breakfast remained a challenge. Most Japanese eat broiled fish, rice, miso soup, and pickles when they rise and shine. It drove me nuts. One morning, I couldn't face it and answered the siren song of a Starbucks maple scone. Strangely, it wasn't as delectable as I'd remembered. Actually, it was rather ... *large*. The next day, I went back to pickled seaweed.

After three weeks of happy gluttony, I was nervous about the moment of truth on my return. As I predicted, there was little change on the vital signs front. But to my surprise, I'd lost 5 pounds. But that may be due in part to **Japanese Health Lesson Number Five: *Get out of the car.*** Like everyone else, I walked or took public transport for most of my visit. If I lived there, I'd buy a bike; even

in Tokyo, you see folks well into their 80s zipping along on one-speed two-wheelers. That's what diet and exercise will do for you.

I fell back into my American-style health habits, sticking to low-fat frozen yogurt, light butter, sugar-free cola, platters of pasta, and those huge skinless chicken breasts that seem to be bred from the Barbie dolls of hens. In two weeks, I was my Western-size self again. And so we're left with **Japanese Health Lesson Number Six: *Stay in Japan.*** It turns out that next month, I'm going back. Odds are, I won't be stranded there. No, Japan is not a desert island, and it's hardly a backdrop for the sequel of *Castaway*. But maybe if we Americans ate and exercised a little more like they do, we could all be survivors. ▪

Peggy Orenstein, a former Japan Society Media Fellow, is the author of Flux: Women on Sex, Work, Love, Kids, & Life in a Half-Changed World.

Peanut-Allergy Help Is on the Way

A recent study led by the National Jewish Medical and Research Center in Denver found that the drug TNX-901 may help the 1.5 million Americans who are allergic to peanuts. That's big news, especially since even a whiff of them can cause serious reactions in certain people. Early trials offer some hope: A monthly injection of TNX-901 increased the number of peanuts people could tolerate from one-half to nine on average. More studies are still under way, so the shot may not be available for several more years.

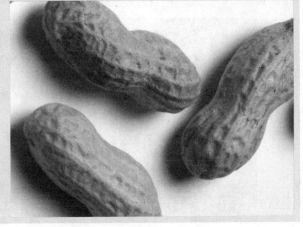

The Fat-Cancer Connection

You may have heard that packing on pounds increases your chances of breast, colon, and uterine cancers. A new American Cancer Society study has added cervical, ovarian, pancreatic, and liver cancers, among others, to the list. Researchers estimate that 20 percent of all cancer deaths in women are due to bulging waistlines. Fat cells produce hormonelike substances that encourage tumor growth. The antidote—diet and exercise—is within your reach.

The Cooking Wisdom of
YIN & YANG

These ancient Chinese principles teach balance in all things—including food—as the key to harmony and health.

BY GRACE YOUNG • PHOTOGRAPHY BY RITA MAAS AND CAREN ALPERT

When I first moved away from home, my mother would phone to ask what I'd had for dinner. If, in the dead of winter, I said I had eaten a big salad, her response would be pained silence. In Mama's mind, I was committing nutritional suicide, sustaining myself with chilled, raw "yin" foods during the coldest time of year. But she'd also caution me not to overload on "yang" dishes: "You must eat a combination of warming and cooling foods, with an emphasis on the warming ones."

In my Chinese family, food was central to a sense of well-being. My parents' cooking was based on the Taoist principles of yin and yang, opposites that, in balance, create harmony at the table and in the body. Mama would repeatedly remind us that without moderation in our eating habits, we were prone to illness. For

instance, rashes or fevers signaled too much heat, or yang; conversely, too much yin could make us feel weak and faint. Adding the appropriate foods to our diets would calm and cure our bodies.

The Chinese believe that all foods possess warming, cooling, or neutral natures. Meats, poultry, onions, and spices are said to be yang, tending to warm and invigorate; yin foods, such as cucumber, tofu, and watermelon, soothe and cool. Rice and fish are believed to be neutral. Cooking techniques are also

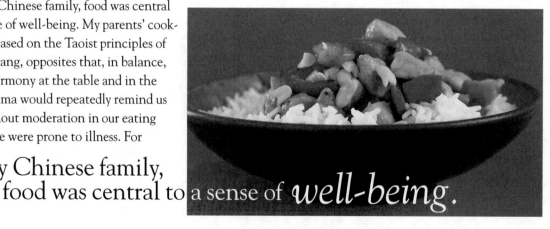

In my Chinese family,
food was central to a sense of *well-being.*

categorized as yin or yang: Stir-frying, deep-frying, and roasting impart a yang influence; gentler methods, such as steaming and poaching, are considered yin. To balance a meal, home-cooks like my mother typically serve a combination of stir-fried or roasted yang dishes, along with steamed or poached yin dishes and plenty of harmonizing rice.

The yin and yang of foods and cooking methods complement the seasons, which are also classified as yin or yang. During the yang seasons of spring and summer, my family would eat cooling foods, such as stir-fried bean sprouts with a little pork, tofu dishes, and plenty of fruit. (No one would ever make something as yang as a spicy lamb stew, for instance, in the summer.) In the milder yin months, my mother prepared hearty meat or chicken stews and stir-fries spiced with the warming flavors of ginger, garlic, and scallions. Essentially, we ate only what was in season, just as more people in the United States used to do before so many foods from around the world became available all year long.

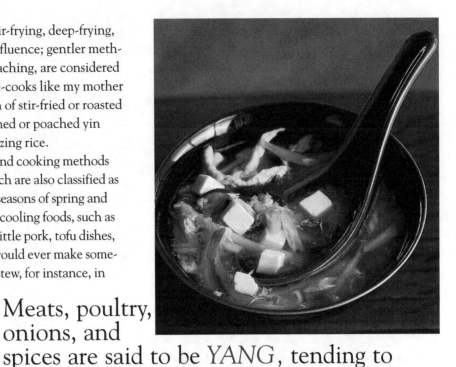

Meats, poultry, onions, and spices are said to be YANG, tending to warm and invigorate; YIN foods, such as cucumber, tofu, and watermelon, soothe and cool.

I was taught that eating in extremes was a recipe for digestive problems and other sicknesses. For example, the summer cookout not only includes such yang ingredients as chicken, spareribs, and hamburgers, but also it uses a yang cooking style in a like season. Beer and wine, two favorite summer beverages, are yang as well. Even though you might also be eating salads and watermelon, these are not cooling enough to offset the overabundance of yang elements. As my mother might say, no wonder we're out of balance.

Of course, there is little medical research in the Western world to support the theories of yin and yang, but they have been a way of life in China for centuries. Often when I explain this eating philosophy to friends, I am besieged with requests for lists of yin and yang foods. But eating in harmony is not as simple as a shopping list: It is much more, for example, than knowing that bok choy is yin and cheese is

Yin-Yang Cooking Tips

- For optimal balance, eat everything in moderation and cook seasonal vegetables.
- In the yin seasons of autumn and winter, eat more yang foods, such as chicken, lamb, beef, ginger, chili peppers, garlic, and spices. In the summer, you should increase your intake of such yin foods as cucumber, crab, watercress, clams, watermelon, tofu, and bananas.
- Throughout the year, serve a mixture of yang-style (stir-fried, deep-fat-fried, roasted, pan-fried, and barbecued) dishes and yin-style (steamed, poached, and boiled) dishes in a single meal, along with generous amounts of neutral steamed rice.
- When stir-frying such cooling vegetables as bok choy, Chinese broccoli, or watercress, cook them with warming ginger or garlic to make the dish more harmonious.

yang, and using both to create a balanced dish. Rather, it is about understanding the energetic properties of different foods and the effects they have on the body. Even most Chinese people cannot explain the yin or yang characteristics of most ingredients, as awareness of them comes so naturally. It would be akin to telling someone how to ride a bicycle.

Few books have been written about the subject in English, and those Chinese who are knowledgeable have learned from culinary traditions passed from one generation to the next. But this primer—and these recipes—can help get you started. Each is balanced and matched to chilly yin months, so you can take advantage of yang effects. If you want to learn more about the yin and yang of diet and good health, seek out a Chinese herbalist. They are plentiful in cities with Asian communities and usually are the best sources of guidance. Every individual's needs are different, and they vary with age and gender. But at its core, this seemingly mysterious concept is deceptively simple. I still believe the best advice I ever received came from an old woman I met on a visit to China: "Eat everything in moderation," she said, "and enjoy your food."

Grace Young is a writer in New York City and the author of The Wisdom of the Chinese Kitchen: Classic Family Recipes for Celebration and Healing.

Eating in Balance

The recipes that follow incorporate the Taoist principles of yin and yang, ensuring balance within the body as well as on the palate.

RECIPES BY GRACE YOUNG

CHINESE BROCCOLI WITH OYSTER SAUCE

prep: 15 minutes • **cook:** 5 minutes • **serves** 4

Chinese broccoli is a leafy green with florets, similar to broccoli raab.

1½ pounds Chinese or regular broccoli
1 teaspoon salt, divided
1 tablespoon canola oil
1 tablespoon peeled, minced fresh ginger
2 tablespoons oyster sauce
½ teaspoon granulated sugar
2 teaspoons toasted sesame oil

1. If using Chinese broccoli, trim ½ inch from bottoms of stalks; discard. (Stalks more than ½ inch in diameter should be halved lengthwise.) Slice stalks into 2½- x ¼-inch sticks. (With regular broccoli, just use the florets.)
2. Combine 6 cups water and ½ teaspoon salt in a large pot over high heat; bring to a boil. Add the broccoli stalks (or florets); blanch 2 minutes. Remove and drain in a colander. Add the leaves to the pot; blanch 1 minute. Drain broccoli in a colander.
3. Heat the canola oil in a large nonstick skillet over medium-high heat. Add the ginger; stir-fry 15 seconds. Add broccoli, remaining ½ teaspoon salt, oyster sauce, and sugar; stir-fry 1½ minutes, or until broccoli is crisp-tender. Remove from heat; drizzle with sesame oil.

PER SERVING (1¼ cups): Calories 107; Fat 6g (sat 1g, mono 3g, poly 2g); Protein 6g; Carbohydrate 10g; Fiber 6g; Cholesterol 0mg; Iron 1mg; Sodium 705mg; Calcium 70mg

SZECHUAN SPICY EGGPLANT

prep: 10 minutes • **cook:** 13 minutes • **serves** 4

Eggplant is yin. Cooking it with yang ingredients, such as chili-garlic paste, pork, and fresh ginger, balances the dish.

1 pound Japanese (or small) eggplant, halved and cut diagonally into ½-inch-thick slices
¼ cup low-sodium chicken broth
2 tablespoons brown sugar
2 tablespoons low-sodium soy sauce
1 tablespoon mirin (sweet rice wine)
1 tablespoon balsamic vinegar
2 teaspoons chili-garlic paste
1½ teaspoons vegetable oil
4 garlic cloves, minced
3 tablespoons finely chopped fresh ginger
¼ cup lean ground pork
¼ teaspoon salt

1. Arrange eggplant in a vegetable steamer. Steam, covered, 5 minutes, or until eggplant is tender; set aside.
2. Whisk broth and next 5 ingredients (through paste) in a bowl.
3. Heat oil in a large nonstick skillet or wok over medium-high heat. Add garlic and ginger; stir-fry 30 seconds. Add pork; stir-fry 2 minutes, or until pork loses its pink color. Add eggplant and salt; stir in the broth mixture. Cover; reduce heat, and simmer 5 minutes.

PER SERVING (³/₄ cup): Calories 155; Fat 6g (sat 2g, mono 2g, poly 1g); Protein 7g; Carbohydrate 18g; Fiber 3g; Cholesterol 19mg; Iron 1mg; Sodium 461mg; Calcium 21mg

SPICY STIR-FRIED CHICKEN AND PEANUTS

prep: 20 minutes • **cook:** 10 minutes • **serves** 4

1 pound skinless, boneless chicken breast, cut into ½-inch pieces
1 tablespoon low-sodium soy sauce
1 tablespoon dry sherry
1 tablespoon cornstarch
½ teaspoon toasted sesame oil
¼ teaspoon freshly ground pepper
1 tablespoon canola oil
3 (¼-inch) slices peeled fresh ginger
4 garlic cloves, peeled and crushed
1 large red bell pepper, cut into 1-inch pieces
¼ teaspoon crushed red pepper
2 tablespoons hoisin sauce
¼ cup low-sodium chicken broth
¼ cup dry-roasted peanuts

1. Combine the chicken pieces, soy sauce, sherry, cornstarch, sesame oil, and ground pepper in a medium bowl.
2. Heat the canola oil in a large nonstick skillet over medium-high heat. Add the sliced ginger and crushed garlic, and stir-fry for 1 minute. Add the chicken mixture in an even layer, but do not stir for 1 minute. Stir-fry the chicken mixture for 4 minutes, or until the chicken is browned. Stir in the bell pepper pieces and crushed red pepper, and cook for 1 minute. Add the hoisin sauce and low-sodium chicken broth, and stir-fry for an additional 2 minutes, or until the chicken pieces are cooked through and the bell pepper pieces are crisp-tender. Stir in the peanuts.

PER SERVING (about 1 cup): Calories 261; Fat 10g (sat 1g, mono 5g, poly 3g); Protein 29g; Carbohydrate 12g; Fiber 2g; Cholesterol 66mg; Iron 1mg; Sodium 459mg; Calcium 30mg

HOT-AND-SOUR SOUP

prep: 30 minutes • **soak:** 15 minutes
• **cook:** 10 minutes • **serves** 4

4 dried Chinese (or shiitake) mushrooms
¼ cup tree ears, optional
4 cups canned chicken broth
5 tablespoons rice wine vinegar
¼ cup lean pork (from a center-cut pork chop),
   cut into julienne strips
1 block firm tofu (about 4 ounces), rinsed and
   cut into ¼-inch cubes (about ¾ cup)
⅓ cup matchstick-cut canned bamboo shoots,
   rinsed and drained
2 tablespoons cornstarch
1 large egg, well-beaten
1 teaspoon toasted sesame oil
¼ teaspoon ground white pepper
⅛ teaspoon granulated sugar
2 tablespoons chopped scallions

1. In a small bowl, soak mushrooms in ½ cup
hot water for 15 minutes. Drain and squeeze dry;
reserve soaking liquid. Cut off and discard stems;
slice caps thinly. In a small bowl, soak tree ears (if
using) in ½ cup hot water for 30 minutes. Drain;
squeeze dry. Remove any hard spots, and roughly
chop tree ears. Discard the soaking liquid.
2. In a large saucepan, combine broth, 1 cup water,
vinegar, and reserved mushroom liquid; bring to a
boil over high heat. Add pork, mushrooms, tree
ears, tofu, and bamboo shoots.
3. In a small bowl, whisk together the cornstarch
and 3 tablespoons cold water. When soup returns
to a boil, stir in cornstarch, stirring constantly until
soup is just thickened (about 30 seconds). Stir in
egg, and remove from heat. Stir in the oil, white
pepper, sugar, and scallions.

PER SERVING (about 1¼ cups): Calories 167; Fat 7g (sat 2g,
mono 2g, poly 1g); Protein 13g; Carbohydrate 14g; Fiber 1g;
Cholesterol 70mg; Iron 1mg; Sodium 318mg; Calcium 57mg

BRAISED LAMB STEW WITH GINGER

prep: 15 minutes • **cook:** 55 minutes • **serves** 4

1 pound lamb stew meat
2 tablespoons cornstarch
1 tablespoon low-sodium soy sauce
1 tablespoon dry sherry
¼ teaspoon freshly ground black pepper
6 dried shiitake mushrooms
1 tablespoon canola oil
2 tablespoons peeled, minced fresh ginger
3 garlic cloves, minced
3 cups fat-free, less-sodium chicken broth
1⅓ cups sliced carrot
2 tablespoons oyster sauce
¼ cup chopped fresh cilantro
4 cups hot cooked rice noodles

1. Combine first 5 ingredients (through pepper)
in a bowl.
2. Combine ½ cup boiling water and mushrooms
in a bowl. Let stand 15 minutes; drain, reserving
the soaking liquid. Discard stems; thinly slice caps.
3. Heat oil in a large nonstick skillet over medium-
high heat. Add ginger and garlic; sauté 30 seconds.
Add lamb mixture; sauté 4 minutes. Stir in broth;
bring to a boil. Cover and reduce heat; simmer
40 minutes. Uncover and bring to a boil; add carrot, mushrooms, and reserved liquid. Cook 5 minutes, or until slightly thick. Add oyster sauce and
cilantro; serve with rice noodles.

PER SERVING (1 cup stew and 1 cup noodles): Calories 451; Fat 10g
(sat 2g, mono 5g, poly 2g); Protein 28g; Carbohydrate 59g; Fiber 4g;
Cholesterol 74mg; Iron 3mg; Sodium 650mg; Calcium 37mg

CANTONESE SPINACH WITH GARLIC

prep: 10 minutes • **cook:** 13 minutes • **serves** 4

2 tablespoons canola oil
8 medium garlic cloves, peeled and crushed
1 pound prewashed baby spinach
1 tablespoon rice wine
¾ teaspoon sugar
¾ teaspoon salt

1. Heat oil in a wok or nonstick skillet over medium heat. Add garlic; cook 3 minutes, stirring constantly. Add half of spinach; stir-fry 1 minute. Add remaining spinach; stir-fry 1 minute. Add wine, sugar, and salt; stir-fry 1 minute.

PER SERVING (½ cup): Calories 92; Fat 7g (sat 1g, mono 4g, poly 2g); Protein 2g; Carbohydrate 6g; Fiber 2g; Cholesterol 0mg; Iron 1mg; Sodium 589mg; Calcium 77mg

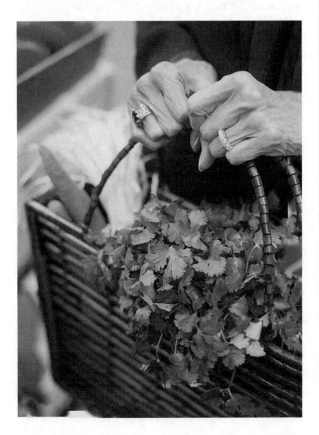

Sushi: A Raw Deal for Dieters?

Sushi used to be relatively straightforward: raw fish, rice, seaweed. The recipe echoes the healthy habits of seasoned dieters, wrapped up in one delicious package. But like many ethnic foods favored by American palates, new variations of sushi have been added and old ones tinkered with—especially portion size. Such creativity can mean inventive new flavors, but it can also mean significantly higher calories.

In the last 10 years, the number of sushi restaurants in the United States has boomed to about 6,000, and that doesn't include supermarket sushi or non-Japanese venues that serve California rolls in addition to other fare, according to Kunio Yasutake, chairman of the Washington, D.C., Sushi Society.

Sushi is a great alternative to typical fast food as long as you keep your portions in check, advises Leslie Bonci, R.D., director of sportsmedicine nutrition at the University of Pittsburgh Medical Center. About six pieces should tide you over for lunch. Splurge on 8 to 10 pieces for dinner and maybe a cup of soup.

And choose wisely. "Keep it simple," Bonci says. She advises eating fewer nontraditional selections, such as bagel rolls or tempura rolls, as well as such high-cal sides as inari (fried bean curd pockets stuffed with rice). Here are the highest calorie rolls on the market.

Nutrition Facts for the Highest-Calorie Rolls

- **California roll:** Imitation crabmeat, cucumber, avocado, sesame seeds, and rice. Calories 290; Fat 5g (sat 1g); Protein 7g*
- **Tempura roll:** Deep-fried shrimp, masago (smelt eggs), cucumbers, eel sauce, and rice. Calories 603; Fat 13.2g (sat 5.4g); Protein 28.6g*
- **Bagel or cream cheese roll:** Cream cheese, cucumber, salmon, and rice. Calories 569; Fat 29.4g (sat 15g); Protein 23.1g*

per 9 pieces (about 1 serving)

183

A Spoonful of
Comfort

These home cures are so good, you'll want to make them even when you're not under the weather.

BY DOROTHY FOLTZ-GRAY • PHOTOGRAPHY BY RITA MAAS

For centuries, mothers around the world have turned to healing foods when their families are achy with colds or flushed with fever. Chinese women administer hot soups full of garlic or ginger to trounce colds; Italian grandmas offer dishes cooked in bianco (white and bland) for troubled stomachs; and Vietnamese moms spoon-feed vitamin-rich steamed vegetables to break fevers.

The home remedies that follow share the same objective: to restore good health. But don't think of them as bitter pills; most are so tasty, you'll want to eat them anytime. Although what drives sickness from the body is sometimes hard to pinpoint, the following recipes have one thing in common: the certainty of Mama's imprimatur, a medicine in itself.

CLEARING THE HEAD

What mother doesn't turn to hot broths to steam away stuffy noses? Hence the ubiquitous bowl of chicken soup, made with matzo balls, noodles, or rice. But food writer Nancy Harmon Jenkins's mother used to bring her homemade tomato soup, seasoned with garlic and basil, instead. "The

tomatoes had a lot of vitamin C," says Jenkins, author of the new cookbook *The Essential Mediterranean*. "For me, this soup is still the most restorative thing in the world." So are many of the dishes that follow. Dig in.

PEAR CONGEE

"In China, when someone is not feeling well, he or she is often given a rice congee," says Asian-food authority Nina Simonds, author of *A Spoonful of Ginger: Irresistible Health-Giving Recipes from Asian Kitchens*. A sly soul might even feign illness to earn this rice porridge with pears, poached in a fragrant syrup of sugar and spices (see page 187). With each creamy spoonful, the ginger eases lung congestion, and the cinnamon wards off bacterial infection.

SPICY CHICKEN-AND-RICE SOUP

Chicken soups do appear to fight colds, thanks to ingredients that have anti-inflammatory powers, say researchers at the University of Nebraska. In addition, the broth's heat stimulates the flow of mucus, soothing inflamed membranes; the liquid replaces lost fluids. Our warming Asian version, full of scallions, ginger, chilies, and garlic, possesses even more cold-fighting powers than Grandma's standard (see page 188). Compounds in raw scallions can soothe inflammation and act as an antihistamine to help clear sinuses. Ginger dilates constricted bronchial tubes, lessening congestion; it also helps fight viruses.

WARMING INDIAN TEA

"This is a classic in India," says Robert A. Barnett, author of *Tonics: More than 100 Recipes That Improve the Body and the Mind*. "You toast fennel seeds, peppercorns, and cloves; grind them; and then let them steep in hot water. The fennel settles the stomach, the pepper opens the nasal passages, and the cloves kill pain." And, of course, the spicy tea warms and rehydrates your entire body (see page 189).

SOOTHING COUGHS AND SORE THROATS

Food writer Pat Willard, author of *A Soothing Broth: Tonics, Custards, Soups, and Other Cure-Alls for Colds, Coughs, Upset Tummies, and Out-of-Sorts-Days*, swears by a potion that 19th-century preachers in the Midwest sipped to soothe throats made raspy from delivering sermons—ice-cold cider vinegar seasoned with a pinch of cayenne pepper. But for those who prefer more appetizing therapies, we offer the following.

Tea Thyme

Thyme is an antiseptic, antibacterial, and expectorant used for hundreds of years for sore throats or nagging coughs. "It can help reduce inflammation; relax throat muscles, and according to German studies, increase infection-fighting white blood cells.

Simmer a bunch of fresh thyme in 6 cups water for an hour, and you'll have a wonderful tea or stock for soup or risotto.

SWEET POTATO-AND-GINGER SOUP

"My grandmother boiled sweet potatoes cut in cubes with lots of ginger until the potatoes were very soft; then we sipped the broth and ate the potatoes," says Corinne Trang, author of the cookbook *Essentials of Asian Cuisine: Fundamentals and Favorite Recipes*. Grandma's cure makes sense: The abundant ginger blocks enzymes that trigger inflammation and pain; sweet potato is a powerful immune system recharger with a healthy dose of beta-carotene (see page 189).

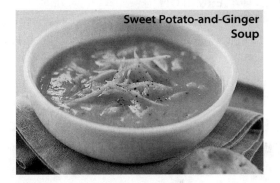

Sweet Potato-and-Ginger Soup

LEMON, HONEY, AND GINGER TEA

When Simonds has a sore throat, she sips a brew of hot water, lemon, honey, and fresh ginger. The hydrogen peroxide in the honey kills germs. Doctors don't know why, but it also reduces inflammation, as does ginger. According to Italian researchers at the University of Siena, lemon oil dulls pain.

FIGHTING FEVER

In Asia, the feverish mix up tonics of honeysuckle flowers and lotus-seed embryos. Since these curatives may be in short supply, here are a few others to try.

PORT-WINE JELLY

Willard says this cooling gelatin was a popular fever treatment during the 18th and 19th centuries. But it's so elegant, she has also served it for dessert at dinner parties. "It's cold, so it makes your feverish mouth feel better," she says. "And the port calms you down a bit."

STEAMED SQUASH AND RICE
"My mom liked to feed us steamed vegetables when we had a fever," says Mai Pham, author of *Pleasures of the Vietnamese Table* and owner of Lemon Grass Restaurant in Sacramento, California. "She would start a pot of rice and then add large chunks of winter squash. When the rice was done, so was the squash." To the comforting rice, the veggies add beta-carotene to help shore up weak immune systems.

ICED WATERMELON
Willard also offers this 19th-century approach to fevers: Cut watermelon into cubes, and chill. Add cracked ice and a little water, and eat with a spoon. The iced fruit and chilled liquid draw heat from the body and help replace lost fluids.

TAMING TUMMIES
Eating when you have an upset stomach may seem counterintuitive, but some foods can indeed quell disturbances. Incredibly, Jenkins notes, Middle Easterners and Italians drink strong, bitter coffee for this purpose, while Indians chew fennel seeds after meals to ease digestion. To us, though, the following alternatives somehow seem more appealing.

PEPPERMINT TEA
A handful of peppermint leaves, a couple of cloves, and a cinnamon stick steeped in 1 cup boiling water settle a swirling stomach. The compounds in peppermint oil help calm spasms in the intestinal tract and fight bacteria that may make you sick. Both peppermint and cinnamon reduce gastric distress.

CINNAMON ATOLE
Mexicans seek comfort in a thick, warm beverage called atole (see recipe at right), made from masa harina (corn flour) simmered with milk and a cinnamon stick, says restaurateur and cookbook author Rick Bayless. This drink is best for a patient who's on the upswing. Cinnamon helps calm nausea; the milk and masa offer nourishment.

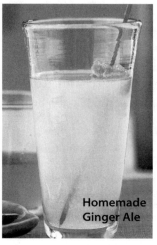

Homemade Ginger Ale

HOMEMADE GINGER ALE
We've teamed healing gingerroot with club soda to create a spicy drink that lots of moms, especially Middle Eastern ones, use to soothe stomachaches. According to Barnett, ginger stimulates intestinal muscles and the productions of digestive juices; it can also relieve stomach cramps and nausea (see page 189).

BOUNCING BACK
You know you're feeling better when your nose and appetite lead you back into the kitchen. Still, your energy and immunity probably aren't up to speed just yet. These dishes invigorate them both.

SPINACH-WATERCRESS GOMAE
A cup of spinach has about one-fourth the minimum dietary requirement of vitamin C and more than a third of the necessary daily dose of beta-carotene, both immune system boosters. Watercress is thought to cleanse the body of toxins and stimulate the liver to work more efficiently (see page 189).

SHIITAKE SUSHI
This mix of broiled shiitakes and sushi rice wrapped in nori (seaweed) may be just the thing if your party spirit is back but your stomach is lagging behind. Mushrooms are valued in the East for their flavor and their health benefits. Asians add them to home remedies or take them as dietary supplements. And some compounds derived from medicinal mushrooms are now being used in Asia and the United States as cancer drugs. The fungi in this recipe (see page 188) bolster immunity and help fight viruses; the easy-to-digest rice is good for a recuperating system.

Cold Comfort

The following recipes for home remedies can help cure what ails you.

PEAR CONGEE

prep: 15 minutes • **cook:** 2 hours • **serves** 14

Pears:
10 cups water
1½ cups sugar
 8 (⅛-inch-thick) slices unpeeled fresh ginger
 2 (3-inch) cinnamon sticks
¼ cup fresh lemon juice
 7 peeled Bosc pears, cored and cut into ½-inch-thick wedges

Congee:
 1 cup Arborio rice or other short-grain rice
 8 cups water
 1 teaspoon salt

1. To prepare pears, combine the first 4 ingredients (through cinnamon) in a Dutch oven; bring to a boil. Reduce heat to low; cook 30 minutes. Add the lemon juice and pears; bring to a boil. Reduce heat and simmer 15 minutes, or until the pears are tender. Remove pears with a slotted spoon, and set aside.
2. Strain the liquid through a sieve over a bowl, discarding solids. Set aside 3 cups cooking liquid; discard leftover liquid. Pour reserved liquid into a small saucepan. Bring to a boil, and cook until reduced to ⅔ cup (about 15 minutes).
3. To prepare congee, rinse rice under cold water; drain. Combine rice, water, and salt in a heavy saucepan; bring to a boil. Partially cover, reduce heat, and simmer 1 hour, stirring occasionally. Serve topped with pears and sugar syrup.
Recipe adapted from A Spoonful of Ginger: Irresistible Health-Giving Recipes from Asian Kitchens, *by Nina Simonds*

PER SERVING (¹/₂ cup congee, 4 pear slices, and 2 teaspoons syrup): Calories 199; Fat 1g; Protein 1g; Carbohydrate 49g; Fiber 3g; Cholesterol 0mg; Iron 1mg; Sodium 173mg; Calcium 20mg

CINNAMON ATOLE

prep: 5 minutes • **cook:** 20 minutes • **serves** 8

3½ cups warm water
⅔ cup masa harina
3½ cups whole milk
⅔ cup sugar
 1 (3-inch) cinnamon stick, plus additional for garnish

1. Place the water and masa harina in a blender, and process until smooth. Strain the masa mixture through a sieve into a large saucepan; discard the solids. Add milk, sugar, and a cinnamon stick, stirring mixture with a whisk. Cook over medium heat 20 minutes, or until mixture is slightly thick, stirring frequently.
Recipe adapted from Rick Bayless Mexico: One Plate at a Time, *by Rick Bayless*

PER SERVING (1 cup): Calories 168; Fat 4g (sat 2g, mono 1g, poly 0g); Protein 4g; Carbohydrate 29g; Fiber 1g; Cholesterol 15mg; Iron 1mg; Sodium 56mg; Calcium 143mg

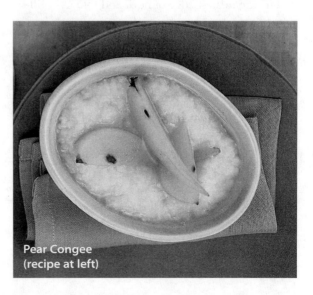

Pear Congee
(recipe at left)

SHIITAKE SUSHI

prep: 20 minutes • **cook:** 30 minutes • **serves** 5

1½ cups sushi rice or other short-grain rice
1½ cups water
 2 tablespoons seasoned rice vinegar
 5 cups thinly sliced shiitake mushroom caps
 1 tablespoon dark sesame oil
 5 nori (seaweed) sheets
½ cucumber, peeled, halved lengthwise, seeded,
   and julienne-cut into 10 strips
¼ cup pickled ginger
¼ cup low-sodium soy sauce
Wasabi paste to taste

1. Preheat broiler. Prepare rice and water according to package directions. Once rice has cooled, toss with vinegar. Set aside.
2. Combine shiitake mushroom caps and sesame oil in a large bowl, and toss well. Place mushroom caps on a baking sheet; broil 11 minutes, and cool.
3. Cut off top quarter of nori sheet along short end; place shiny side down on a sushi mat, with long end toward you. Pat ¾ cup rice over nori with moist hands, leaving a 1-inch border on one long end.
4. Arrange ¼ cup mushroom caps and 2 cucumber strips along top third of rice-covered nori.
5. Lift the nearest edge of nori, and fold over filling. Lift the bottom edge of the sushi mat; roll toward the top edge, pressing down firmly on sushi roll. Continue rolling to top edge; press mat to seal sushi roll. Let rest, seam side down, for 5 minutes. Repeat procedure with remaining ingredients. Slice each roll into 8 pieces. Garnish with ginger, soy sauce, and wasabi paste.
Recipe adapted from Tonics: More Than 100 Recipes That Improve the Body and the Mind, *by Robert A. Barnett*

PER SERVING (1 roll): Calories 296; Fat 3g (sat 1g, mono 1g, poly 1g); Protein 6g; Carbohydrate 62g; Fiber 4g; Cholesterol 0mg; Iron 3mg; Sodium 127mg; Calcium 127mg

SPICY CHICKEN-AND-RICE SOUP

prep: 10 minutes • **cook:** 1 hour, 25 minutes • **serves** 8

 4 cups water
 4 cups low-sodium, fat-free chicken broth
 2 chicken-breast halves (about 1 pound), skinned
¼ teaspoon sea salt
 2 teaspoons vegetable oil
¾ cup uncooked jasmine rice
 1 garlic clove, sliced
 1 tablespoon fish sauce
 1 tablespoon minced fresh ginger
¼ cup sliced green onions
 2 tablespoons chopped fresh cilantro
¼ teaspoon freshly ground black pepper
 2 teaspoons vegetable oil
¼ cup sliced shallots
Chili-garlic paste

1. Combine first 4 ingredients (through sea salt) in a large saucepan, and bring to a boil. Cover, reduce heat, and simmer 45 minutes, or until chicken is tender. Remove from heat. Remove chicken from broth; cool chicken 10 minutes. Remove and discard bones. Shred chicken into bite-size pieces. Skim fat from top of broth. Return chicken to broth.
2. Heat 2 teaspoons vegetable oil in a small non-stick skillet over medium heat. Add rice and garlic; sauté 3 minutes. Add rice mixture, fish sauce, and ginger to broth; bring to a boil. Cover, reduce heat, and simmer 25 minutes, or until rice is tender. Stir in green onions, cilantro, and pepper.
3. Heat 2 teaspoons vegetable oil in skillet over medium-high heat. Add the shallots, and sauté for 3 minutes, or until lightly browned. Sprinkle the shallots over soup. Serve with chili-garlic paste.
Recipe adapted from Pleasures of the Vietnamese Table, *by Mai Pham*

PER SERVING (1 cup): Calories 101; Fat 2g (sat 0g, mono 1g, poly 1g); Protein 3g; Carbohydrate 16g; Fiber 1g; Cholesterol 0mg; Iron 0mg; Sodium 477mg; Calcium 7mg

SWEET POTATO-AND-GINGER SOUP

prep: 15 minutes • **cook:** 30 minutes • **serves** 6

3 cups water
3 cups peeled, diced sweet potato
¼ cup julienne-cut peeled fresh ginger
2 tablespoons sugar
¾ teaspoon salt

1. Boil water in a large saucepan. Add remaining ingredients. Cover, reduce heat, and simmer 30 minutes. Place half of sweet potato mixture in a blender; process until smooth. Return to saucepan; cook over medium heat until thoroughly heated.
Recipe by Corinne Trang

PER SERVING (1 cup): Calories 89; Fat 0g; Protein 1g; Carbohydrate 21g; Fiber 2g; Cholesterol 0mg; Iron 0mg; Sodium 306mg; Calcium 18mg

SPINACH-WATERCRESS GOMAE

prep: 10 minutes • **cook:** 1 minute • **serves** 4

1 (10-ounce) package spinach, stems trimmed
1½ cups trimmed watercress (about 1 bunch)
2 tablespoons sesame seeds, toasted
2 tablespoons low-sodium soy sauce
2 teaspoons sugar

1. Cook spinach and watercress in boiling water for 1 minute; drain and rinse under cold water. Squeeze the remaining moisture from spinach mixture; chop.
2. Process sesame seeds in a coffee grinder until finely ground. Combine sesame seeds, soy sauce, and sugar in a bowl. Add spinach mixture; toss to coat.
Recipe adapted from Tonics: More Than 100 Recipes That Improve the Body and the Mind, *by Robert A. Barnett*

PER SERVING (½ cup): Calories 59; Fat 2g; Protein 3g; Carbohydrate 6g; Fiber 2g; Cholesterol 0mg; Iron 9mg; Sodium 328mg; Calcium 87mg

WARMING INDIAN TEA

prep: 5 minutes • **cook:** 8 minutes • **serves** 4

2 teaspoons fennel seeds
8 whole cloves
6 whole black peppercorns
4 cups boiling water

1. Heat a medium skillet over medium heat; add fennel seeds, cloves, and peppercorns. Cook for 3 minutes, or until lightly toasted, stirring constantly. Place the mixture in a spice or coffee grinder, and process until finely ground. Combine the spice mixture and water; let stand 5 minutes. Strain mixture through a fine sieve into cups, and discard solids.
Recipe adapted from Tonics: More Than 100 Recipes That Improve the Body and the Mind, *by Robert A. Barnett*

PER SERVING (¾ cup): Calories 6; Fat 0g; Protein 0g; Carbohydrate 1g; Fiber 1g; Cholesterol 0mg; Iron 0mg; Sodium 10mg; Calcium 20mg

HOMEMADE GINGER ALE

prep: 5 minutes • **cook:** 10 minutes • **serves** 12

1 cup sugar
1 cup peeled, sliced fresh ginger
1 cup water
12 cups club soda, chilled
12 lemon slices or candied ginger pieces

1. Combine the sugar, ginger, and water in a small saucepan over medium-high heat, and bring to a boil, stirring to dissolve sugar. Reduce heat, and simmer 10 minutes; strain through a fine sieve into a pitcher, and cool. Add the club soda; garnish with lemon or candied ginger.

PER SERVING (1 cup): Calories 72; Fat 0g; Protein 0g; Carbohydrate 19g; Fiber 0g; Cholesterol 0mg; Iron 0mg; Sodium 52mg; Calcium 16mg

Why the Meat Label Is a Must-Read

It's not just about animal rights. The way cattle, chickens, and pigs are raised can affect your health.

BY KERRI CONAN

The new organic-food labels must be doing their job. Since national standards took effect in October 2002, alternatives to mainstream food, marked with the government's green seal, shout out from every corner of the supermarket. Except the meat aisle, that is. It's become painfully obvious how little organic beef, pork, and chicken is available in stores.

Why? "Meat isn't as simple as carrots or cereal or dairy products," says Holly Givens, a spokeswoman for the Organic Trade Association (OTA), a group that represents organic-food growers and manufacturers. "It takes more time to raise organic livestock, and there are a lot more challenges."

To be certified by the U.S. Department of Agriculture

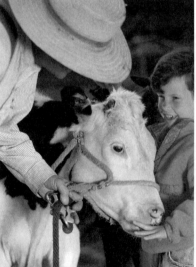

Concern about the health issues of meat are changing the way farmers raise animals.

(USDA), meat must come from sources that are raised on organic feed (which is free of genetically modified grain and antibiotics) and are not treated with hormones. Animals must also spend a specified amount of time outdoors, and ranchers are prohibited from using chemical pesticides or fertilizers on grazing fields. The cost in time and money of raising cattle, chickens, and pigs this way is one reason organic meat is more expensive than its conventionally produced counterpart.

MORE ORGANIC OPTIONS ON THEIR WAY TO MARKETS

The OTA expects production of organic meat and poultry to nearly triple every year through 2005. That doesn't mean people looking for natural alternatives are out of luck until then. Several beef, pork, and chicken producers address at least some of the major issues covered in the USDA's certification program—if you know what to look for on the label.

For starters, the word "natural" is not enough. By law, that only means that meat has been "minimally processed without additives." While food companies do have to state these qualifications (no artificial ingredients, no added colors, etc.) on labels, they are not legally required to spell out exactly how they raise livestock. You're better off looking for claims that address specific concerns: "hormone-free," "raised without antibiotics," or "fed with non-GMO grain." "Free-range" and "grass-fed" can be misleading, since they neither reveal exactly how much time animals have spent outside nor guarantee against exposure to drugs and pesticides.

WHY YOU SHOULD CARE

Should you be concerned about what's in your pork chops, hamburgers, and chicken wings (besides protein and fat, that is)? A growing number of health experts and groups—including the American Medical Association (AMA) and the World Health Organization (WHO)—think so. Even the National Cattlemen's Beef Association (NCBA), the Colorado-based trade body that represents cattle ranchers and beef producers, has begun looking into some of the farming practices of its members, including the use of growth hormones.

Of particular concern is the nontherapeutic use of antibiotics in beef, pork, and poultry production. The AMA is supporting legislation proposed by Sen. Edward Kennedy, D-Mass., that calls for more restrictions on the practice. Most animals raised for food in the United States receive regular doses of antibiotics in their feed or water to protect them from injury and diseases they might receive while being raised in crowded, confined conditions.

For instance, supermarket chickens known as broilers are tightly packed in a controlled indoor environment until they are about 7 weeks old; pigs usually spend their entire 6-month life span in similar conditions. Once cattle reach a certain size, they're moved from grazing fields into large pens called feedlots. Such conditions pose an increased risk of injury and illness. As a preventive measure, all of the animals, not just the sick ones, are given antibiotics. Another important consideration: These drugs accelerate growth, maximizing production so that meat gets to market cheaper and faster.

The cost in time and money of raising organic livestock is one reason it's more expensive than the conventionally produced counterpart.

BEYOND ANIMAL RIGHTS

According to recent medical studies, nontherapeutic dosing may exacerbate the growing problem of antibiotic-resistant bacteria, including such food-borne germs as salmonella and campylobacter, and also the bacteria that cause urinary-tract infections and pneumonia. This means that the once-powerful antimicrobial drugs commonly prescribed for these illnesses may no longer work as well as they used to. In fact, a study published in February 2003's *Journal of the American Medical Association* found that the effectiveness of ciprofloxacin—aka Cipro, which became a household word during the post–September 11 anthrax scares—has dropped as much as 13 percent in the last decade. Cipro is part of a family of antibiotics called fluoroquinolones, commonly given to such animals as chickens. While this research didn't specifically link antibiotic resistance to livestock, "the evidence is compelling that using antibiotics on animals contributes to resistance in humans," says John Quinn, M.D., professor of medicine at Rush Medical College in Chicago, and co-author of the study. "Human overuse is definitely a factor, too."

Such evidence has led WHO to repeatedly recommend that antibiotics used on humans not be prescribed to promote animal growth. Most developed countries in the world, except Canada and the United States, restrict this use.

THE GROWTH HORMONE DEBATE

Health experts in the United States and abroad are also raising alarms about growth hormones. Poultry farmers discontinued the drugs' use several decades ago, based on early concerns about their effects. (Because of the naturally rapid growth of pigs, pork producers do not need to use hormones.) But the practice remains standard in the beef industry. To help a cow or bull bulk up quickly with less feed, thus keeping costs low, producers routinely implant a pellet into its ear that releases a continual dose of hormones during certain periods of the animal's life.

These substances can find their way into water and soil, and residues can remain in meat. "It is reasonable for us to make the link between the increased incidence of certain cancers, such as those of the breast and prostate, to the increased amount of estrogen-like hormones in our environment," says Carlos Sonnenschein, M.D., a professor at Tufts University School of Medicine who has studied the effects of hormones on cancer growth for 25 years. "The most common sources for these are pesticides, plastics that shed synthetic estrogens, and the use of hormones in beef production." For now, the USDA says that hormone-treated beef is safe, provided cattle are drug-free for a given length of time before slaughter.

But the European Union (which includes France, the United Kingdom, Spain, Germany, and Italy) has banned imported American beef for more than a decade because of concerns about growth-hormone residues. The NCBA has been researching less aggressive hormone regimens, says Bo Reagan, Ph.D., the association's vice president of research. "I expect the use of growth hormones to go down as more of our members decide to export to Europe or tap the growing specialty niche here," he says.

ALTERNATIVES IN STORES NOW

Concern about these issues is bringing more choices to supermarkets and changing the way farmers raise animals. Fast-food companies, such as McDonald's and Burger King, now post information on their Web sites about how their suppliers treat

livestock, and the nation's largest poultry producer, Tyson, has introduced certified-organic chicken.

"People are worried that conventional ranching and farming methods are not resulting in the most nutritious foods," says Bill Niman, founder and president of Niman Ranch, a company that relies on a national network of small farms to produce its beef, lamb, and pork.

Chances are, you've seen some of these items in your supermarket. Gourmet grocers and natural-food stores usually carry organic meats. "If the meat tastes good, customers will come back for more," says Theo Weening, a buyer for the Whole Foods Market chain. "And more demand means lower prices." ∎

Where to Find It

Some of the country's best beef, pork, chicken, and lamb is right in your own backyard. For local producers, try these online guides.
- The U.S. Department of Agriculture's Guide to Farmers' Markets (www.ams.usda.gov/farmersmarkets/)
- FoodRoutes Network (www.foodroutes.org/localfood)
- Local Harvest (www.localharvest.org)
- The Organic Trade Association (www.ota.com; click on "The Organic Pages Online")
- Eat Wild (www.eatwild.com/products/index.html)

Take advantage of national brands. If your favorite store doesn't stock these brands, put in a request. Many are also available by mail order.
- Coleman Natural Products (www.colemannatural.com)
- Laura's Lean Beef (www.laurasleanbeef.com)
- Nature's Farm Chicken from Tyson (www.naturesfarm-organic.com)
- Niman Ranch (www.nimanranch.com)
- Organic Valley (www.organicvalley.com)
- Petaluma Poultry (www.petalumapoultry.com)
- Springer Mountain Farms (www.springermountainfarms.com)

Can Lunch Meat Make You Sick?

Beware of dangerous bacteria that could be lurking at your deli.

BY KERRI CONAN

Uncle Sam wants you to take responsibility for food safety, especially if you're pregnant, elderly, or affected by a compromised immune system. Ever since the recent outbreak of listeriosis—a foodborne disease that killed eight people, caused three women to either miscarry or deliver stillborn babies, and made another 42 people sick—the U.S. Department of Agriculture (USDA) has been stressing strict guidelines for those at risk: Reheat all deli meat until steaming hot and completely avoid feta, Brie, blue cheese, chilled smoked seafood (like salmon), or anything made from unpasteurized milk.

Problem is, these products carry no warning labels. In fact, all that ham, chicken, and turkey claims to be ready to eat. But if you fall into one of the high-risk categories and decide to grab a sandwich on the run, you'd better ask someone to pop it in the microwave.

"When was the last time you fried your bologna?" asks Carol Tucker Foreman, director of the Food Policy Institute at the Consumer Federation of America (CFA), an advocacy group. "The message is totally misleading, because precooked meats say they're USDA-approved."

Whether you're a germophobe or not, the fact is that listeriosis is life-threatening. Each year, about 2,500 cases result in 500 deaths, according to the Centers for Disease Control and Prevention. Fortunately, healthy and nonpregnant people are rarely affected, and once children are old enough to eat solid food, their immune systems are strong enough to fend off the *Listeria monocytogenes* bacterium.

Listeria is associated with flulike symptoms and digestive distress. In advanced cases, it can cause encephalitis or meningitis. Even with treatment, listeriosis can kill. A pregnant woman may harbor the disease and unknowingly pass it along to her unborn child without ever showing signs of infection.

Listeria occurs naturally in soil, water, and animals. Unlike other foodborne bugs, such as *E. coli* and salmonella, it multiplies in cold temperatures. So a product that leaves the manufacturer contaminated with even minuscule amounts of the organism might develop a dangerous colony while it sits on the refrigerated shelf. Tainted products can spread listeria to deli cases, coolers, drains, and kitchens, where it continues to grow unless all surfaces are thoroughly cleaned. Furthermore, someone who eats infected food might not show signs of listeriosis for weeks. All of these factors make the source tough to trace.

Meat processors are subject to rules set forth by the Food Safety Inspection Service (FSIS) division of the USDA. According to FSIS spokesman Steven Cohen, about 10,000 samples are randomly tested each year, and many companies perform voluntary screening. In 2002, there were 34 product recalls because of listeria, more than in 2001 or 2000; however, the incidence of listeriosis in the United States actually declined by 35 percent between 1996 and 2001. While new government directives encourage manufacturers to perform tests for the germ, it could be years before the USDA makes testing mandatory.

Consumer advocates, such as the CFA, are pushing the food industry and government agencies to be more diligent sooner; they accuse the USDA of stalling on rules that should have been put in place years ago. At the very least, Foreman says, products should be labeled with appropriate warnings.

The New Eggs

Are the latest designer eggs all they're cracked up to be?

BY WAYNE KALYN

Call me old-fashioned or just time-crunched, but I long for the days when shopping for eggs was simply a matter of deciding between brown or white, large or extra-large. Those days are gone with the emergence of the so-called designer eggs, which, according to manufacturers, are more natural, better-tasting and, in some cases, heart-friendlier than their commercially produced cousins. But now you need a scorecard to help sort through the array of offerings: free-range, cage-free, organic, lower-cholesterol, vegetarian-grain-fed, even the impressive omega-3–enhanced. How to choose?

While omega-3-enhanced and lower-cholesterol eggs have an advantage over their kin—namely, the potential to reduce your risk of heart disease—how do the other newfangled varieties stack up nutritionally against traditional eggs? We examined five designer types in all to find out how well they live up to their health claims.

CAGE-FREE EGGS

Although some research has shown that these may be bigger and their yolks heavier than those of conventional eggs, the hen's diet, not its living space, usually determines the level of nutrients in the final product. What's more, cage-free doesn't guarantee that the egg contains no antibiotics (which are rarely used by commercial egg farmers anyway) or that the hens' diet is free of so-called "meat meal," made from the remains of dead animals.

If one of your main interests—apart from pure nutrition—is that the hens whose eggs you're eating are treated humanely, cage-free is no guarantee. These birds can be as tightly packed and poorly cared for as their caged sisters, essentially corralled together in big poultry houses or barns, and they may never see the outside at all. Look for the phrase "free-farmed" on the carton, which guarantees the chickens are raised with care.

FREE-RANGE EGGS

Free-range hens can roam outdoors and eat a more natural, varied diet of bugs and plants as well as standard feed. But that doesn't necessarily mean that these eggs are healthier. There's nothing barring the company from giving the hens meat meal or feed that contains pesticides. On the other hand, the more eclectic diet may make for a more nutritious egg. According to clinical nutritionist Virginia Worthington of Washington, D.C., free-range eggs are naturally higher in omega-3 fatty acids than regular eggs; plus, they might be higher in vitamin D.

> ### Keep Them Fresh
> Whatever type of egg you choose to buy, store it in its original carton on a shelf inside the refrigerator, not in the egg cups on the door. This prevents the eggs from losing moisture and gas, as well as absorbing food odors.

ORGANIC EGGS

Eggs carrying this designation come from birds that are fed an organic, all-vegetarian diet free of antibiotics and pesticides, according to the federal government's National Organic Program rules. Humane-minded egg eaters will also be glad to know that organic hens aren't caged and, by law, must have access to the outdoors when weather permits. Sounds great, but does all this result in a food that's higher in vitamins, minerals, and protein? Findings from the few studies that have been conducted are inconclusive, but, like free-range hens, chickens that dine on nature likely lay more healthful eggs.

OMEGA-3-ENRICHED EGGS

For the many Americans who aren't getting their twice-weekly servings of fatty fish, omega-3-enriched eggs can help by offering an extra hedge against heart disease. Egg farmers increase omega-3 levels by feeding their hens grain rich in these substances. The outcome? An egg that can contain between 100 milligrams and 350 milligrams of omega-3s (a mere fraction of what's in a 3-ounce serving of salmon), as well as higher levels of vitamin E (a nutrient that helps preserve the fatty acids) than those in standard eggs. Look for the "organic" label on omega-3–enhanced eggs to make sure that pesticides and antibiotics aren't part of the package.

OMEGA-3-ENRICHED/
LOWER-CHOLESTEROL EGGS

Hens that produce these nutrition-enhanced eggs are fed all-vegetarian grain fortified with vitamin E. Eggland's Best uses a formula that includes sea kelp and alfalfa meal in addition to the usual soy and corn. This yields an egg that is higher in omega-3s (about 100 milligrams per egg), 25 percent lower in saturated fat, and 35 milligrams lower in cholesterol than common eggs. Look for "organic" on the carton to avoid chemical toxins or "all-vegetarian feed" to make sure the hens haven't eaten meat meal. (When hard-boiling lower-cholesterol eggs, cook them an extra two minutes to ensure desired firmness.)

What Price an Egg?

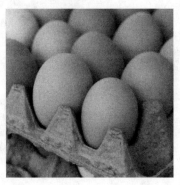

A harsh reality to consider when buying eggs: Hens on large commercial farms don't have much of a life. They're so tightly packed in cages (about half the size of a magazine page) that they can't move freely or stretch their wings. Even more disturbing, laying hens are debeaked so they don't hurt each other and are periodically starved, a practice that extends their egg-laying careers. Unfortunately, the birds at some designer-egg farms have a similarly bleak existence.

Some mild winds of change are ruffling industry feathers, though. Because there is no legislation governing the raising of farm animals in the United States, the United Egg Producers (UEP), an umbrella organization that represents most U.S. egg farmers, has tried to fill the void. The UEP now recommends that each bird be allotted 67 to 88 square inches of living space, instead of the current 48 to 54 square inches, and that birds be debeaked at a much younger age, when it's less painful. The UEP has also funded projects examining alternatives to starvation, though legislation mandating these new methods hasn't yet been adopted.

But some producers do treat their animals less harshly than others. The American Humane Association recently issued a new certification called "Free-Farmed." Egg companies that use this label (look for it on the carton) guarantee that their chickens have been treated humanely before, during, and after the laying cycle.

A Grain Of
TRUTH

Not all breads are created equal. We slice through the misconceptions to find the healthiest of all.

BY DARYN ELLER

Eating bread all by its lonesome or as tasty bookends for ham and cheese is the easiest way to get more grains into your diet. Better yet, it's the easiest way to get more *whole* grains into your diet—a significant distinction. Unlike their refined and processed cousins, whole-grain breads offer more nutrition per bite.

Such loaves come complete with the plant's germ and fiber-rich bran; a lode of B vitamins; the minerals zinc, magnesium, and chromium; and the antioxidants vitamin E and selenium. They're also rich in phytochemicals ranging from lignans, which may protect against cancer, to heart-healthy saponins and intestine-friendly oligosaccharides. These breads are even hedges against diabetes. Because whole grains are digested slowly, they stabilize blood sugar and prevent overproduction of insulin, both of which can lower your risk of Type 2 diabetes.

Does all this mean you should ban white bread from your diet? The squishy slices many of us grew up on do have some dietary value. But you shouldn't overdo it.

For the greatest health perks, experts suggest eating a range of whole-grain breads during the course of a month. "Each whole grain has its own portfolio of healthy properties," says Joanne Slavin, R.D., Ph.D, a professor of nutrition at the University of Minnesota. "So it's a good idea to eat a variety of them."

Look for these foolproof clues to help you distinguish whole-grain bread from its refined-flour relatives. Check the wrapper for the words "rich in whole grains" or "whole-grain" listed first in the ingredients—if it comes after yeast and sugar (which are used in small amounts), then it's not a major player. Additionally, make sure that each slice has at least 2 grams of fiber. Another test is to hold the whole-grain loaf in your hands. If it feels dense and compact and you can see visible kernels, then it's a keeper.

To find out how your favorite type stacks up nutritionally, check out our Q and A. But before you buy, take a close look at the label so you know you're getting the best out of your bread.

196

How healthy is your bread?
★★★★ as good as it gets
★★★ a cut above average
★★ OK in our book
★ could be better

WONDERING ABOUT BREAD?

We answer the most telling and compelling questions about your daily loaf.

Q: **I've always heard white bread is a nutritional zero. Does it have any redeeming qualities?**

A: Although the fiber, phytochemicals, and trace minerals have all been refined out, white bread isn't completely without merit. Enriched with iron and B vitamins, including folic acid (which helps prevent birth defects), white bread is often fortified with calcium, plus cellulose to add bulk. (This tacked-on fiber—sometimes as much as 5 grams in two slices—isn't as good for you as that which other breads contain naturally.)
Health score: ★

Q: **Isn't wheat bread really just white bread with a tan?**

A: This may be your biggest nutritional phony. Although wheat bread contains about 25 percent whole-grain flour, it can't compete with the real thing in terms of fiber (it has only about ½ to 1 gram per slice). As with white bread, the phytochemicals and antioxidants have been refined out, but it is enriched with the same nutrients.
Health score: ★½

Q: **When it comes to sourdough, does heavy mean healthy?**

A: Don't be fooled by the heft of sourdough—it comes from the starter used in the baking process, not from whole grains. Although some specialty bakers do make whole-grain versions, sourdoughs are no healthier than wheat or white breads. Enjoy the flavor, but vary your choice occasionally with a whole-grain bread.
Health score: ★½

Q: **Aren't all rye breads the same?**

A: Much of the soft rye in stores contains little whole grain. Thin, dense loaves do contain it, as do some made locally (ask at your bakery). Whole-grain rye contains lignans, which the body converts to enterolactone, an estrogen-like molecule that may lower the risk of breast cancer. Also look for caraway seeds on the ingredient list. They contain limonene and small amounts of perillyl alcohol, both potential cancer fighters.
Health score: ★★½ (if it contains whole-grain rye)

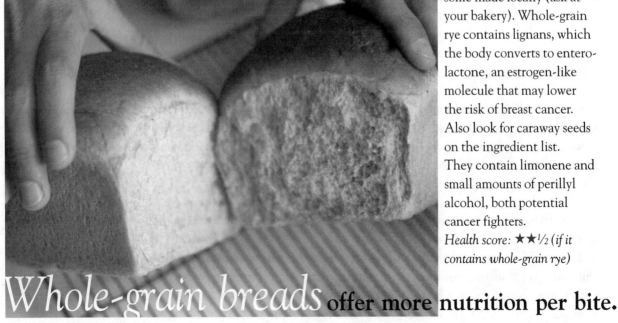

Whole-grain breads offer more nutrition per bite.

Q: **Pumpernickel's better for you because it's dark, right?**

A: Not necessarily. The deep hue of most store-bought selections comes from molasses or caramel coloring, and most pumps contain nothing more than refined wheat flour. True pumpernickel has a grainy texture, 1 to 2 grams of fiber per slice, and whole-grain rye flour. Like rye bread, whole-grain pumpernickel is available at grocery stores or at your local bakery.
Health score: ★★★ *(if it's made with whole-grain rye)*

Q: **Does raisin bread have a nutritional edge over white bread?**

A: While raisins do contain potassium (which may lower blood pressure and stroke risks) and iron, most raisin breads are made with refined flour. Look hard enough, though, and you'll find some varieties made with whole-wheat flour that contains high-quality fiber. An even better choice is a loaf that also contains nuts, which provide vitamin E and healthful monounsaturated fat.
Health score: ★★ *(three stars if it's made with whole wheat and contains nuts)*

Q: **Just what is it about whole wheat that's so great?**

A: For starters, phytic acid, a powerful antioxidant; flavonoids; and oligosaccharides, indigestible compounds that may improve bowel health and immune function. This bread contains 2 to 4 grams of insoluble fiber per slice, which may lower your risks of colon and breast cancer, as well as several bowel diseases. Don't mistake regular wheat bread for whole wheat: Make sure "whole wheat" is on the wrapper and at the top of the ingredient list.
Health score: ★★★½

Q: **Are sprouted-wheat and cracked-wheat breads even better than whole wheat?**

A: In a way. They contain the same amount of fiber. But some experts suggest that the antioxidants in sprouted- and cracked-wheat breads—vitamin E, selenium, phytic acid, and flavonoids—may be more easily absorbed by the body than those in whole wheat, because the grains are broken down into a more digestible form. Found in natural-foods stores or in the freezer cases of large supermarkets, these breads list whole-grain flour as the first ingredient. To get the full effect of antioxidants, look for finely milled varieties; the antioxidants in coarser-grain types aren't as easily absorbed, but they do a better job of maintaining blood sugar and preventing constipation.
Health score: ★★★★

Q: **What health attributes do the different grains in multigrain bread bring to the party?**

A: Each whole grain possesses its own complement of phytochemicals. In theory, the more grains, the more types of nutrients—and benefits—you get. There are multigrain wanna-bes, however, that contain mostly refined wheat flour and very little of the other grains. Even if they say 7-, 9-, or, the most impressive of all, 12-grain, you should still look for "whole-grain" at the top of the ingredient list and make sure that each slice has at least 2 grams of fiber.
Health score: ★★★★ *(depending on amounts of whole grains and fiber)*

Q: **What exactly will flaxseed bread do for me?**

A: It's a concentrated source of lignans, soluble and insoluble fiber, and heart-protective alpha-linolenic acid. You can usually find this nutty, crusty bread at natural-foods stores or in the frozen sections of larger markets. Again, be sure that "flaxseed" appears near the top of the ingredient list.
Health score: ★★★★

Now that you know about the good things each variety offers, here are a couple of quick storage tips. If you tend to finish a loaf in less than a week, keep it unrefrigerated in a dark, dry place like a bread box. If it lasts you a week or more, freeze half of it to keep the bread's phytochemicals and other nutrients from losing their potency. ■

The Mediterranean Diet Full Story

At first it seemed that researchers had pinpointed exactly why the Mediterranean diet, known to protect against cardiac disease, is so successful: wine and omega-3-packed fish. Now, a Spanish study has found that fiber may be the beneficial ingredient. People on this diet who ate the most fiber were 86 percent less likely to suffer from heart trouble than those who avoided it.

Before inhaling a bran muffin, though, we sought an expert's advice. "Americans read something like this study and think, 'OK, I'm going to load up on fiber,'" says Kathleen Putnam, M.S., C.D., a nutrition educator at Swedish Medical Center in Seattle. "The people on the diet probably are getting fiber from the beans, grains, and other things they're eating. But they're consuming vitamins, minerals, nutrients, and phytochemicals in those foods, too." As Putnam points out, the same high-fiber folks may be walking to the market, cooking up fresh foods at home, and dealing with less stress—all of which make for a healthier heart. No one disputes that fiber helps your heart by lowering cholesterol, but before you change your life based on one study, look at the whole picture.

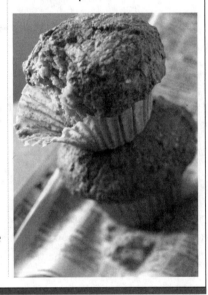

The Sugar Buzz

MYTH: Too much candy will leave little Freddie bouncing off the walls.

REALITY: Relax, Mom. According to a Duke University study, sugar doesn't cause high-wired kids or mood swings. Researchers believe the myth of the sugar high is rooted in treats coated with caffeine-charged chocolate. If you're over age 5 and looking to get a buzz without the calories, warm up with a cup of tea.

The Fat That Lingers

Sure, exercise burns fat, but that doesn't mean you can snack on Krispy Kreme doughnuts with impunity after a hard workout. What's important is the type of fat you ingest: A small-scale study from the University of Wisconsin-Madison recently concluded that what your killer aerobics class burns off is mostly monounsaturated fat (the good kind)—not the saturated goop found in fast food and, of course, those melt-in-your-mouth doughnuts. You'll eventually start burning bad fat as well, but you'll burn the good fat faster—which is a great way to help keep your weight in check. So to quell those postworkout hunger pangs, reach for a handful of nuts instead of giving in to a junk-food craving.

Protect Yourself from Pepper

The aftereffects of chopping a hot chili pepper can be painfully memorable (ever try to remove a contact lens after mincing a jalapeño?). The incendiary quality comes from capsaicin, the antioxidant that produces peppers' unmistakable heat. To protect your skin while you chop, wear rubber gloves or slide plastic sandwich bags over your hands. Afterward, wash your cutting board thoroughly with soap and water to avoid adding unwanted heat to other foods.

Salads
Hit the Grill

RECIPES BY SUSIE LILLY OTT

GRILLED SCALLOPS WITH LEMON-CHICKPEA SALAD

1 (15½-ounce) can chickpeas, rinsed and drained
Minced garlic clove
1 stalk celery, chopped
Chopped fresh flat-leaf parsley
Fresh lemon juice
Extra-virgin olive oil
½ pound sea scallops, rinsed and patted dry
4 cups baby spinach

1. Preheat grill to high. Combine chickpeas, garlic, celery, and ⅓ cup parsley with 2 tablespoons lemon juice and 1 tablespoon oil. Drizzle scallops with 2 teaspoons oil and 1 tablespoon juice. Toss and season with salt and pepper.
2. Grill scallops 2 to 3 minutes per side, or until firm to the touch.
3. Toss spinach with 1 tablespoon *each* of juice and olive oil; top with chickpea mixture and scallops. Serves 4.

PER SERVING (about 2 cups): Calories 170; Fat 8g (sat 1g, mono 3g, poly 1g); Protein 11g; Carbohydrate 19g; Fiber 4g; Cholesterol 12mg; Iron 2mg; Sodium 310mg; Calcium 60mg

CHICKEN-AND-CORNBREAD SALAD WITH LIME

4 cups cornbread, cut into large cubes
Fresh lime juice
Extra-virgin olive oil
Ground cumin
3 (6-ounce) skinless, boneless chicken-breast halves
Chopped tomato
Chopped red onion
1 romaine heart, chopped

1. Preheat grill to high. Preheat oven to 350°. Toast cornbread 10 minutes.
2. Whisk together 2 tablespoons juice, 2 tablespoons olive oil, and 1½ teaspoons cumin. Brush 1 tablespoon mixture on chicken; season with salt and pepper.
3. Grill 5 minutes per side; slice. Toss cornbread, 1½ cups tomato, ¾ cup onion, and romaine with dressing. Season with salt and pepper. Top with chicken. Serves 4.

PER SERVING (about 2½ cups): Calories 390; Fat 14g (sat 1g, mono 10g, poly 3g); Protein 30g; Carbohydrate 34g; Fiber 4g; Cholesterol 94mg; Iron 4mg; Sodium 760mg; Calcium 153mg

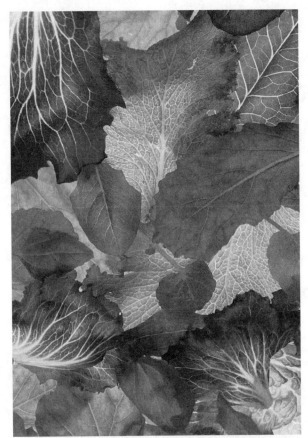

Leafy greens meet some of your favorite grilled foods to make these three tasty main-course meals.

GRILLED MUSHROOM-AND-ASPARAGUS SALAD

Balsamic vinegar
Extra-virgin olive oil
  2 minced garlic cloves
Fresh lemon juice
Dijon mustard
  1 bunch asparagus, trimmed
  8 baby portobello mushrooms, or 4 large
  8 cups mesclun salad greens

1. Preheat the grill to high. Whisk ¼ cup vinegar, 3 tablespoons oil, garlic, 2 teaspoons *each* juice and mustard, and a pinch *each* of salt and pepper.
2. Place asparagus and mushrooms in a zip-top plastic bag with half of dressing; marinate 15 minutes.
3. Grill asparagus 5 minutes. Grill mushrooms, gill sides down, for 4 minutes; turn. Grill 7 more minutes. Slice thickly. Toss greens with vegetables and dressing. Serve warm. Serves 4.

PER SERVING (about 2 cups): Calories 173; Fat 11g (sat 2g, mono 8g, poly 1g); Protein 7g; Carbohydrate 14g; Fiber 6g; Cholesterol 0mg; Iron 3mg; Sodium 387mg; Calcium 100mg

Are You a Supertaster?

If you avoid bitter vegetables like the plague, you might fit in this category. Women who dislike broccoli, Brussels sprouts, and dark, leafy greens because they taste ultrabitter live in a more vivid sensory world than others, according to researchers. For nearly three decades, Linda Bartoshuk, Ph.D., professor of otolaryngology in the surgery department at Yale University School of Medicine, has studied "supertasters"—those who experience flavors, especially bitterness, more intensely than the rest of us. About a quarter of the population are supertasters, Bartoshuk says, and most of them are women.

Consequently, many people with hypersensitive taste buds abstain from the same foods they should be eating more of. Dark green vegetables are abundant in vitamins, minerals, fiber, and good (read: complex) carbohydrates. They're also rich in such phytochemicals as beta-carotene and sulforaphanes, which cause the body to produce enzymes that ward off cancer-causing agents and prevent malignant cells from spreading. Diets lacking these substances may leave supertasters susceptible to certain diseases, especially lung, breast, and cervical cancers.

Fortunately, women tend to lose their perception of bitterness after menopause. Until then, a pinch of sugar, a squeeze of lemon, and a drizzle of extra-virgin olive oil can counter the acrid edge of certain vegetables.

Perfect Your Pasta

Check out *Health* Food and Nutrition Editor Susie Quick's recipe for a healthier version of everyone's favorite carb.

I'm a little weary of pasta. It never seems as satisfying as what you get in a good Italian restaurant. But this easy dinner, which includes almost as many vegetables as noodles, is awfully good. And it's one of the healthiest pasta dishes you can make.

When you make a simple meal with just a few ingredients, be sure everything that goes into it is at its best. For instance, buy a head of fresh garlic and choose fast-cooking fresh pasta rather than dry. If you can't find prewashed, bagged arugula or nice bunches, grab a bag of sturdier baby spinach instead. This dish includes a number of food groups, so you don't need anything on the side, except maybe garlic bread. And wine. It's in that other food group: the fun one.

LINGUINE WITH WALNUTS AND ARUGULA

prep: 15 minutes • **cook:** 8 minutes • **serves** 6

¾ cup drained, chopped sun-dried tomato halves packed in oil
1 tablespoon olive oil
6 garlic cloves, thinly sliced
¼ teaspoon crushed red pepper
12 cups trimmed arugula (about 8 ounces or 1½ [5-ounce] packages)
2 teaspoons fresh lemon juice
9 ounces fresh uncooked linguine
⅓ cup (1½ ounces) grated fresh Parmesan, plus more, if desired
1 cup (4 ounces) chopped walnuts, toasted

1. Put a large pot of water on to boil for the pasta. Place the sun-dried tomatoes in a small bowl with ½ cup very hot water. Let sit 5 minutes; drain and set aside.
2. In a large nonstick skillet, heat the olive oil over medium flame. Add the garlic and crushed red pepper, and sauté 30 seconds. Remove from heat. Add the arugula and lemon juice to the skillet, and toss to coat.
3. When the water boils, add 2 teaspoons salt and the linguine. Cook for 3 minutes, or until al dente. Reserve ¼ cup of the hot pasta water. Drain the linguine quickly, and add it to the skillet along with the arugula mixture. Toss with the Parmesan cheese, drained sun-dried tomatoes, salt, and freshly ground black pepper to taste, adding just enough of the pasta water to melt the Parmesan cheese. Transfer to warm pasta bowls, and top generously with the walnuts. Grate some additional Parmesan cheese over the top, if desired.

PER SERVING (about 1⅓ cups): Calories 494; Fat 18g (mono 5g, poly 10g, sat 3g); Protein 17g; Cholesterol 4g; Carbohydrate 66g; Fiber 6g; Iron 4mg; Sodium 235mg; Calcium 192mg

This recipe was adapted from Quick Simple Food.

This is a paradigm of vegetarian virtue that even your meat-loving friends will enjoy. Everyone I've ever served it to practically begs me for the recipe.

Learn to Love Lentils

We spill the beans about our favorite quick-cooking legumes.

BY LORI LONGBOTHAM

What they are:

These small, flat shrub seeds cook quickly and, unlike most dried beans, don't require presoaking in water. The larger brown kind are great for soups. Little green *lentilles du Puy*, from the Puy region of southern France, are by far the best choice for salads (as in the recipe here) because they stay firm after cooking. Lentils also come in black and red varieties.

Health benefits:

Lentils are packed with protein, complex carbohydrates, and fiber; they also contain calcium, vitamin B, and iron. More slowly digested than other high-fiber foods, these legumes leave you feeling fuller longer.

Where to find them:

Brown (and sometimes green) lentils are available at most grocery stores with the dried beans. For other types of lentils, try natural-foods stores, such as Whole Foods Market, or online sources such as www.chefshop.com.

Some ideas:

- Drizzle cooked green lentils with extra-virgin olive oil, lemon juice, and salt. Serve alongside roast salmon, duck, or grilled sausages.
- Combine prepared lentils with shredded Cheddar to make meat-free "burgers"; cook in a skillet.
- Simmer red lentils with onions; blend with cumin, cayenne, curry powder, and garlic. Puree and serve as a dip for carrots or pita bread.

LENTIL SALAD

prep: 10 minutes • **cook:** 20 minutes • **serves** 6

Vinaigrette:

2 tablespoons balsamic vinegar
1 tablespoon minced capers, drained
1 garlic clove, minced
2 tablespoons extra-virgin olive oil

Salad:

1⅓ cups petite green or brown lentils
2 bay leaves
½ cup finely chopped celery, with some leaves
½ cup finely chopped red onion
¼ cup chopped fresh flat-leaf parsley
½ teaspoon salt
12 cherry tomatoes, halved
¼ cup chopped fresh chives, divided
4 cups trimmed watercress

1. To prepare vinaigrette, whisk together all ingredients. Add salt and black pepper to taste.
2. To prepare salad, combine 4 cups water, lentils, and bay leaves in a saucepan; bring to a boil. Reduce heat; simmer 18 to 20 minutes. Drain; discard bay leaves. Stir together lentils, celery, onion, parsley, and salt. Add tomatoes and 2 tablespoons chives. Drizzle with vinaigrette; toss to coat. Divide watercress among 6 plates; top with ¾ cup lentil mixture. Top with remaining 2 tablespoons chives.

PER SERVING (about 1½ cups salad): Calories 208; Fat 5g (sat 1g, mono 3g, poly 1g); Cholesterol 0mg; Protein 11g; Carbohydrate 31g; Fiber 8g; Iron 3mg; Sodium 210mg; Calcium 86mg

STEAK
Sensibly

Health Food and Nutrition Editor Susie Quick shares
a delicious reason not to ban beef from your diet.

Red meat is a red flag for many people who care about eating healthfully. But if you have it only occasionally and in reasonably small portions, it's a flavorful source of protein, zinc, and iron, and the best source of certain B vitamins.

Saturated fat is something that everyone should watch for, but meat's benefits outweigh its downsides when you take a sensible approach. I eat it about once a week; I seek out beef that's been raised without antibiotics and growth hormones. Many more markets are stocking this alternative nowadays, so it's no longer the rarity it once was.

I like to serve these easy steak tacos instead of fatty T-bones for a change of pace. I serve them with the simplest guacamole, which cushions the chili's heat. A cooling cucumber-and-yogurt salad rounds out the meal, along with thick-sliced beefsteak tomatoes fresh from your local farmers' market.

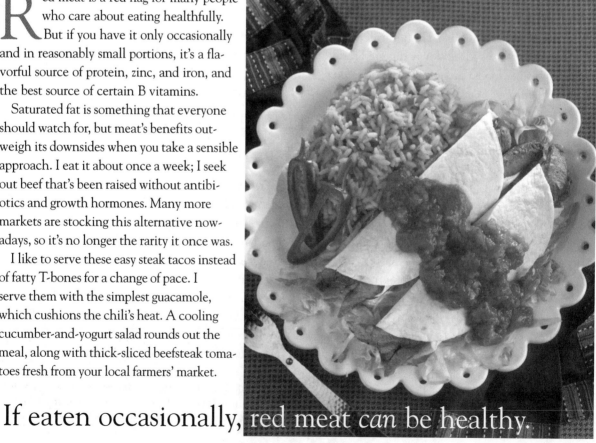

If eaten occasionally, red meat *can* be healthy.

STEAK TACOS WITH SIMPLE GUACAMOLE

prep: 20 minutes • **marinate:** 1 to 24 hours
cook: 10 minutes • **serves** 6

Most of the fat in this recipe is the good-for-you monounsaturated kind in the avocado.

Steak:

3 teaspoons vegetable oil, divided
2 teaspoons dried Mexican oregano
½ teaspoon kosher salt
½ teaspoon cayenne pepper
¼ teaspoon black pepper
2 garlic cloves, minced (or pressed through a garlic press)
1 (1½-pound) flank steak, fat trimmed
3 cups vertically sliced onion (about 2 medium onions)
2 cups red and yellow bell pepper strips (about 2 large peppers)
2 jalapeño peppers (or 1 serrano pepper), halved lengthwise and thinly sliced, with seeds

Guacamole:

2 ripe avocados, peeled and seeded
1 garlic clove, minced (or pressed through a garlic press)
2 teaspoons fresh lime juice
Kosher salt to taste

Tacos:

12 (6-inch) flour tortillas, warmed

1. To prepare steak, combine 1 teaspoon oil and next 5 ingredients (through garlic) in a bowl. Rub steak with garlic-oil mixture; place in a large zip-top plastic bag. Seal; marinate in the refrigerator 1 hour, or overnight.
2. Lightly spray the rack of an outdoor grill with cooking spray. Heat to medium-high.
3. Heat remaining 2 teaspoons oil in a large nonstick skillet over medium-high heat. Add onion, bell pepper, and jalapeño; sauté 5 minutes. Keep warm.

4. Place the steak on the grill, and cook 4 minutes on each side (without turning) for medium, or to desired degree of doneness. Let stand 10 minutes on a cutting board before slicing crosswise into ⅓-inch-thick slices.
5. To prepare guacamole, combine all ingredients in a small bowl, and mix well, mashing with a pestle or fork until mixture is chunky.
6. Heat the tortillas in a covered casserole in a 300° oven until warm and pliable. Place a small amount of meat in each tortilla; top with the onion-pepper mixture and guacamole.

PER SERVING (serving size: 2 tortillas, ⅓ cup meat, ⅔ cup onion mixture, and 2 tablespoons guacamole): Calories 490; Fat 19g (sat 6g, mono 10g, poly 2g); Cholesterol 54mg; Protein 30g; Carbohydrate 48g; Fiber 7g; Iron 5mg; Sodium 535mg; Calcium 116mg

Why Strawberries Are Sweet for Your Heart

Tasting a strawberry in spring proves that produce is best when it's in season—for strawberries, that means May and June in most places. You'll want to eat even more of them when you hear this:

Preliminary results of a clinical trial conducted by Gene Spiller, Ph.D., of the Sphera Foundation in Los Altos, California, suggest that eating eight or nine strawberries a day promotes heart and circulatory health by reducing artery-damaging inflammation, which leads to heart disease. Spiller's findings back up other studies confirming the anti-inflammatory properties of berries. Researchers credit this benefit to strawberries' antioxidants (vitamin C, ellagic acid, and anthocyanins). Berries have the highest antioxidant levels of any fresh fruit, and a new study from the University of California, Davis, finds that organic strawberries are packed with even more disease-fighting power than conventionally grown ones.

The New Look of Teatime

Asian-inspired bubble tea is like a grown-up milk shake with a healthy twist—or maybe the Chinese answer to the smoothie.

BY NANCY DAVIDSON

In its simplest form, ultratrendy bubble tea is a mixture of black tea, milk or nondairy creamer, and sugar syrup poured over large tapioca balls that look like marbles. ("Bubble" refers to both the foam on top and the chewy beads resting at the bottom of the glass).

Tea connoisseurs might scoff at the jumbo straw that is a signature part of the presentation or the sensation of simultaneously drinking tea and chewing pieces of tapioca just a tad smaller and softer than gummi bears. Apparently, though, a lot of people like having something to chew on as they sip. Boba tea, as the beverage is sometimes called, has bubbled over and beyond its Chinatown beginnings and is set to become the next chai, or maybe even the next Frappuccino.

Bubble drinks lack the caffeine jolt of a latte. The kick they offer to a health-conscious public

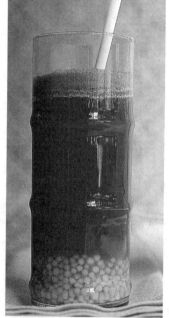

intrigued by all things Asian is a hefty dose of flavonoids—powerful antioxidants that help neutralize disease-promoting free radicals, which can damage cells. The latest studies show that these substances in tea may reduce the risk of colon cancer in women and can help protect against heart attack and stroke. Less-processed green and white teas contain the highest levels of some flavonoids, but everyday black tea has them, too.

Bubble tea began as an after-school treat for children in Taiwan during the mid-1980s. It became a hit with teens and then migrated to other Asian countries. A few years ago, bubble drinks made their way to America, and long lines began to form outside small booths and cafés in the Chinatowns of major cities on both coasts.

The foamy potables (about $2.50 each) are more widely available now, in the food courts of shopping malls, as well as Eastern-themed cafés and juice bars, where blenders are at a constant roar. Once the province of young Asian hipsters, bubble tea has become big business. "In large cities, people are more open to new things," observes restaurateur Steven Pyun, whose Sago Tea Café franchise started two years ago and is still growing. "The amount of tea-making supplies coming into the United States now is exploding."

Bubble drinks come in flavors and colors that put Baskin-Robbins ice cream to shame: They're frothy pink, green, purple, and orange; they taste of taro, coconut, ginger, lavender, and coffee. The pearls that seem to dance at the bottom of the glass are made with tapioca flour, which comes from the root of the cassava plant (think of the beads as larger versions of those used in tapioca pudding). Some are white, and others are tinted with green tea, but black *sago* tapioca, which gets its hue from caramel, is most common. Before cooking, the pellets resemble kibble; afterward, they become soft, like an al dente Jell-O. The starchy pebbles deliver pure enjoyment, offering little nutritional value.

But you'll get pleasure, flavonoids, *and* lots of vitamins if you make your bubble drink with fresh fruit. Drinks that contain milk add calcium to the list of benefits. Plenty of options exist for the lactose-intolerant, though (many people of Asian descent have trouble digesting dairy). Most bubble-tea bars offer almond, soy, or coconut milk, as well as nondairy creamer.

Labeling these drinks as health food may be pushing it: Flavonoids, vitamins, and calcium notwithstanding, the sugar content in some bubble teas can be sky-high. Consider the beverage a refreshing treat that's healthier for you than a diet soda or a fat-laden milk shake. Even better, consider it a great excuse for a party. Several companies sell home kits, complete with teas, tapioca pearls, flavor powders, and fat straws. To make your own, see our recipes and sources.

Nancy Davidson is a freelance food and travel writer based in New York City.

TAPIOCA PEARLS FOR BUBBLE TEA

makes: about 2 cups

6 cups cold water
1 cup tapioca pearls
½ cup Sugar Syrup (see recipe on page 208)

1. Boil water in medium saucepan. Add the tapioca; return to a boil. Reduce heat, cover, and boil gently 30 minutes. Remove from heat. Let tapioca sit 25 minutes in water, covered. Drain and rinse in a colander under cool running water. Pour Sugar Syrup over tapioca; use within 4 to 5 hours.

Variation for make-ahead tapioca:
1. Bring water to a boil in a medium saucepan. Add tapioca; return to a boil. Reduce heat, cover, and simmer gently 20 minutes. Remove from heat; let sit 15 minutes, covered. Drain and rinse in a colander beneath cool running water. Add Sugar Syrup; place in sealed container. Refrigerate until ready to use.
2. For tea, bring a medium saucepan of water to a boil (use a 4-to-1 ratio of water to tapioca), and add tapioca (¼ cup per serving). Boil 1 to 3 minutes, or until soft. Rinse and cover with Sugar Syrup to taste. Add tea mixture of choice (see our recipe for Bubble Milk Tea on page 208).
Note: Precooked tapioca should be used within 3 days, or it will get mushy.

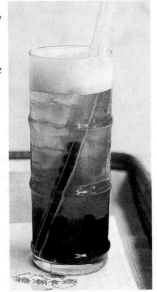

PER SERVING (¼ cup):
Calories 80; Fat 0g; Protein 0g;
Carbohydrate 19g; Fiber 0g;
Iron 0mg; Sodium 40mg;
Calcium 0mg

SUGAR SYRUP

makes: about 2 cups

1 cup granulated sugar
1 cup dark brown sugar
2 cups water

1. Place all the ingredients in a medium saucepan. Stir over medium-high heat until mixture begins to simmer. Remove from heat; cool and refrigerate until ready to serve. (The syrup will keep for up to a month in a tightly sealed container.)

PER SERVING (2 tablespoons): Calories 50; Fat 0g; Protein 0g; Carbohydrate 13g; Fiber 0g; Iron 0mg; Sodium 3mg; Calcium 6mg

FRUIT BUBBLE DRINK

makes: about 1 serving

1 cup crushed ice
1 cup sliced fresh fruit (such as mango, papaya, or watermelon)
1 tablespoon Sugar Syrup (more or less to taste; see recipe above)
½ cup milk (or soy, almond, rice, or light coconut milk)
¼ cup Tapioca Pearls (see recipe on page 207)

1. Place the ice, fruit, syrup, and milk in a blender; puree until smooth. Pour pearls into a tall glass. Pour fruit mixture over pearls, and serve with a fat straw.

PER SERVING (about 12 ounces): Calories 181; Fat 2g (sat 1g, mono 1g, poly 0g); Protein 5g; Carbohydrate 38g; Fiber 3g; Iron 0mg; Sodium 105mg; Calcium 167mg

BUBBLE MILK TEA

makes: about 1 serving

¾ cup brewed tea (such as black, green, chai, or jasmine)
1 cup ice cubes
2 tablespoons Sugar Syrup (more or less to taste; see recipe at left)
½ cup milk (or soy, almond, or rice milk)
¼ cup Tapioca Pearls (see recipe on page 207)

1. Combine the tea, ice, syrup, and milk in a blender or cocktail shaker; blend or shake until frothy. Place pearls in a tall glass. Pour tea mixture over pearls, and serve with a fat straw.

PER SERVING (about 12 ounces): Calories 230; Fat 1g (sat 1g, mono 0g, poly 0g); Protein 4g; Carbohydrate 79g; Fiber 0g; Iron 0mg; Sodium 107mg; Calcium 150mg

Recipes adapted from Sweet-n-Tart Restaurant in New York City.

Make Your Own

You can find ingredients for bubble tea at some larger Asian markets in major cities. Or contact one of the following distributors.

- Bubble Tea Supply (call 877-869-2622 or visit www.bubbleteasupply.com) offers a starter kit including tapioca pearls, flavor powders, teas, and straws for $35.
- Ten Ren Tea Company (call 877-898-0858 or visit www.tenren.com) carries supplies and teas.
- Bruce&Clark (fax 604-263-7006 or visit www.bubbleteastore.com) sells complete party kits; prices start at $31.95.

Bubble drinks come in flavors and colors that put Baskin-Robbins ice cream to shame.

Did You Say "Tomato"?

Here are five essentials for enjoying summer's favorite fruit.

It doesn't get any better than juicy, fresh-picked tomatoes. Eat an abundance of them with a wee bit of oil, and you'll also be savoring nature's best source of lycopene, the antioxidant that not only fights heart disease but could also help prevent osteoporosis, according to pre-liminary research at the University of Toronto.

All told, several thousand tomato varieties are available to home and professional growers. Right now, farmers' markets are bursting with a kaleidoscope of them, particu-larly popular heirloom types. You can prepare tomatoes a zillion ways, but we only have room to list five of our favorites. We like them ...

Coddled: Roll a basketful of cherry tomatoes around in a nonstick skillet over low heat, drizzling with a touch of extra-virgin olive oil. Serve over grilled fish.

Deviled: Split a beefsteak, top with egg salad, and broil until golden.

Whirred: Load up a blender and liquefy. Press the pulp through a strainer with a wooden spoon for the best tomato juice ever.

Intensified: Now take that juice and simmer over medium heat until it's syrupy. Let cool; whisk in some olive oil and a pinch of salt and pepper to create a velvety vinaigrette.

Spiced: For a bright citrus flavor in your next salsa, try green tomatoes that are just beginning to turn red.

Q + A

AFTER-WORKOUT MARGARITAS

Why do I feel such a big buzz when I drink a margarita after I work out?

The alcohol might be going right to your head for a couple of reasons, says Nancy Clark, R.D., director of nutrition services at SportsMedicine Associates in Brookline, Massachusetts, and author of *Nancy Clark's Sports Nutrition Guidebook*. Do you usually exercise after work, then head out for drinks? If so, you proba-bly haven't eaten since lunch, and an empty stomach absorbs alcohol quickly. Or you may be dehydrated, and your body is using whatever you're drinking to replenish fluids you lose as you sweat. So unless you enjoy being a cheap date, be sure to drink plenty of water during your workout and have another glass before you order. And to help block the buzz, get a burrito, too.

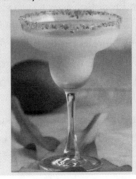

Take This Dietary Supplement with Caution ... *It Could Make You Sterile*

The dietary supplement chromium picolinate may damage your genes and make you infertile, according to a report published in the Proceedings of the *National Academy of Sciences*. Many weight-loss products contain the supplement, which fans say supercharges metabolism and helps people slim down. (In the same study, chromium chloride, which is found in many multivitamins, did not pose a risk.) Before you stop taking it, though, keep in mind that this research was done in a lab; stay tuned for results of studies in humans.

Give HEMP a Chance

This controversial seed is great for your heart and skin.

BY ALISA BLACKWOOD

Cereals, snack bars, and other foods made with a seed that's full of concentrated nutrients for your heart and skin are in danger of being pulled from the food supply forever. Hemp seeds rival soy in protein content and are a potent source of essential fatty acids (EFAs), vitamin E, and antioxidants. But nutrition buffs aren't the only ones noticing hemp—legal circles are buzzing, too. That's because hemp comes from the same plant species as marijuana.

Even though edible hemp seeds contain little to no THC, the psychoactive component their cousin is infamous for, the U.S. Drug Enforcement Administration (DEA) says any amount of the substance in food is illegal. The small but determined hemp industry has sued the DEA, countering that hemp foods cannot elicit druglike effects. In June 2003, the 9th U.S. Circuit Court of Appeals in San Francisco rejected the agency's ban, saying the government did not follow procedure when it first announced the rule. Until the court decides on the constitutionality of the prohibition, hemp foods can still be legally imported, sold, and consumed in the United States.

Curiosity about these foods continues to grow. Makers, such as Nutiva and Nature's Path, have added hemp seeds to such products as bars, frozen waffles, and granola. At home, hemp oil can be used to make salad dressings, while the seeds can be eaten plain as a snack or toasted and sprinkled atop casseroles and salads.

Their concentration of EFAs makes hemp oil and seeds unique, says Ellen J. Fried, who teaches food law at New York University's Department of Nutrition, Food Studies, and Public Health. These fats are necessary for normal brain and heart function, as well as healthy bones, skin, and hair. Since your body doesn't produce EFAs naturally, you have to get them from the foods that contain them: salmon, walnuts, spinach, flaxseed—or hemp.

> People are buzzing about hemp. It comes from the same plant species as marijuana, but it's loaded with good nutrients.

Hemp seeds are also a direct source of gamma-linolenic acid (GLA), an omega-6 fatty acid that plays an important role in regulating blood pressure and inflammation, says Cynthia Sass, R.D., a spokeswoman for the American Dietetic Association. GLA may also improve skin conditions, such as eczema, Fried says.

Sass says that while hemp's nutrient profile is positive, further research is still needed to determine if eating it actually has a significant impact on health. ■

Could the Atkins Diet Be Safer Than You Thought?

BY ALISA BLACKWOOD

It's been the party line among most nutritionists and medical experts: The Atkins diet may help you lose weight, but it can't be good for you. How could a regimen that allows unlimited high-fat foods, such as bacon, and eschews high-carb foods, including certain fruits and vegetables, be healthy? But a funny thing happened not long ago. Researchers tested this popular plan, and the results suggest that Atkins might not be so bad after all.

The two studies, both of which were published in the *New England Journal of Medicine*, compared volunteers on the low-carbohydrate Atkins diet to others following a low-fat, high-carbohydrate program. Gary Foster, Ph.D., clinical director of the Weight and Eating Disorders Program at the University of Pennsylvania and lead researcher on one of the studies, says the scientists expected to learn that the diet was unhealthy, thus ending the debate. But once the trial was completed, Atkins followers had higher levels of HDL (good) cholesterol and lower levels of triglycerides than the other dieters (both groups dropped the same number of pounds). Foster doesn't know what caused the change in those blood fats, but he says it must have had something to do with cutting carbs. "The results showed not only that there were no harmful effects, but that there were a couple of positive ones," Foster says.

This was the first controlled trial of the Atkins diet, and it followed participants for one year. Despite the positive findings in Foster's study, the medical community isn't ready to give its seal of approval. Many registered dietitians and doctors still refuse to recommend the plan because its followers may potentially consume too much saturated fat and not enough fruits and vegetables.

Dieters in the study were asked simply to follow the program (but not record what they ate) as laid out in *Dr. Atkins' New Diet Revolution*. That means a meal could consist of 50- to 60-percent fat, compared with the 30 percent recommended by most health experts. High-fat diets have been linked to colorectal cancer, among other forms of the disease. The Atkins diet is also high in protein, too much of which can strain the kidneys and liver over time.

In summer 2003, Foster and his colleagues began a five-year study to explore the diet's long-term effects. But if you want to lose weight now, five years is a long time to wait. So here are ways to do the high-protein, low-carb thing and eat healthfully, too.

Choose low-fat meats. Keep saturated-fat intake to around 10 percent of total daily calories. Buy such lean cuts of pork and red meat as loin and round.

Favor good fats. Some of the best protein sources are high in healthy omega-3 acids and monounsaturated fats. Salmon and other fatty fishes are optimal choices; a handful of almonds or walnuts makes a great high-protein snack.

Don't cut out vegetables. Atkins devotees might be tempted to overdo the meat, but such veggies as spinach, kale, green beans, and salad greens are all options listed on sample menus in *Dr. Atkins' New Diet Revolution.* ■

School Lunch
Gets an Overhaul

See how one woman really *can* make a difference.

BY MAUREEN KENNEDY • PHOTOGRAPH BY CAREN ALPERT

Like many moms, 36-year-old *Health* reader Karen LeFurgy of Mill Valley, California, tries to steer her three children away from junk food. But in summer 2002, when her son Alec was about to enter preschool, LeFurgy realized feeding him healthy meals at home was one thing; encouraging him to eat right at school would be another.

Ring Mountain Day School doesn't have a cafeteria, so parents took turns delivering take-out foods, such as burritos, pizza, and Chinese, for the school's 200 students. LeFurgy says she doesn't mind her kids eating these meals on occasion, but not every day. She worried that even if she did pack a lunch, Alec might start to crave what his classmates were snacking on. "If he saw a fried egg roll, I was afraid he would say, 'I want that, too,' " LeFurgy says.

Her solution: making sure all the kids, not just Alec, would have healthy options. With the principal's blessing, she researched alternatives to takeout.

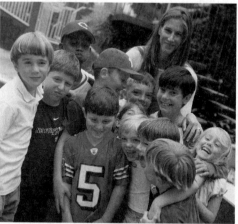

The lunch bunch: Karen LeFurgy helped these kids appreciate the fresh flavors of healthy food.

The logical place to start was her local grocery, Whole Foods Market, which specializes in organic and natural products. LeFurgy got lucky on her first try: The store's catering service helped assemble sample menus featuring such items as turkey burgers and meatballs, pizza with organic tomato sauce, and organic produce and milk. LeFurgy and the school asked parents how much they were willing to pay and set up taste testings. Within a month, LeFurgy had successfully initiated the new lunch program at Ring Mountain. The meals, which Whole Foods delivers to the school, cost $4.90 apiece (compared with $4 each for the take-out lunches).

Some parents were skeptical at first. "My concern was that my kids weren't going to eat it because my house is junk-food central," says Ruth Epstein, 40, mother of Ring Mountain students Max, 9, and Alex, 6. Foods that earned a thumbs-down from kids were quickly tweaked, and now, less than one year into the program, a full 70 percent of Ring Mountain students are signed on.

Granted, what's happened at Ring Mountain is the result of hard work and organization. But efforts like LeFurgy's exemplify what nutritionists and public-health advocates say is critical to stemming the alarming rate of childhood obesity. The number of overweight kids has tripled over the past 30 years because today's children are less physically active and have poorer eating habits, says Mary McKenna, Ph.D., a nutritionist at the U.S. Centers for Disease Control and Prevention in Atlanta.

"Never before in our history have kids been suffering from completely preventable diseases that come from their diets," says Antonia Demas, Ph.D., a nutritionist and head of the nonprofit Food Studies Institute in Trumansburg, New York, a group that has created nutrition curricula for more than 100 public schools, most of them in low-income neighborhoods. "I think schools have an obligation to serve healthy food."

Private schools like Ring Mountain have considerable latitude in menus and pricing. But public schools, which feed students through the federal government's National School Lunch Program, are more financially constrained because they must provide free and reduced-price meals to children from low-income families. Such lunches usually cost about $2.50 each.

To be eligible for the program, cafeterias are required to prepare meals containing one-third of the recommended dietary allowance for protein, iron, and other nutrients, and no more than 30 percent of calories from fat. While the amount of fat in lunches is declining, a typical meal still clocks in at 35 percent of calories from fat, according to a 2001 U.S. Department of Agriculture (USDA) survey of more than 1,000 public schools.

Even more troublesome to health experts than plate lunches are such à la carte selections as chips, sodas, ice cream, burgers, and pizza, which aren't required to meet nutritional standards. "You want your children to make their own decisions, but when it's a matter of buying a nice big cookie or the school lunch, it may be tough for them to make the healthier choice," says Karen Cullen, Ph.D., R.D., assistant professor at Baylor College of Medicine's Children's Nutrition Research Center in Houston.

Erik Peterson, a spokesman for the American School Food Service Association, which represents 55,000 school-cafeteria managers nationwide, says these extras are a financial necessity. "School food service is a business," he says. "They have to generate their own income, pay for staff, be self-sustaining." If kids eat off campus or bring their own lunches, cafeterias risk going into the red, he says. In addition, many schools rely on revenue from vending machines to buy uniforms, textbooks, and other items.

> Efforts like LeFurgy's exemplify what nutritionists and public-health advocates say is critical to stemming the alarming rate of childhood obesity.

Nutrition advocates say that parents can lead the way in making changes, whether it's encouraging their children's schools to offer healthier à la carte items or relying less on burgers and more on fresh produce.

Many parents are rallying behind the USDA's Fresh/Dried Fruit and Vegetable Pilot Project, which provided free produce to 100 public and private elementary, middle, and high schools during the last school year. The goal was to find out if kids would choose healthy snacks over junk food. Implemented in schools throughout Indiana, Iowa, Michigan, and Ohio, and on the Zuni Indian Reservation in New Mexico, it was so successful that lawmakers may expand it nationwide.

"Some children were telling their parents about what they had tried that day and requesting their favorites at home," says economist Jean Buzby, lead author of the program's report to Congress.

Teaching children about nutrition should be a priority.
Kids will eat healthy food if they are educated about it.

—Antonia Demas, Ph.D.

While the future of the USDA project is uncertain, small groups around the country are making changes to school lunch menus. In Berkeley, California, for example, parents successfully fought to make organic offerings available to their kids, while parents in Broward County, Florida, convinced school administrators to sell bottled water in elementary schools.

Demas says education should also be part of the recipe. "Teaching children about nutrition should be a priority," she says. "Kids will eat healthy food if they are educated about it."

LeFurgy agrees. In fact, at Ring Mountain Day School, nutrition is integrated into lesson plans. But more importantly, students are learning firsthand that healthful food can taste good. Among the most popular menu items are maple-glazed carrots and steamed broccoli, LeFurgy says.

In fact, the meals are such a hit, both kids and parents have asked that the program continue for the next school year. "Now, it's perfectly natural for students to expect warm carrots with baked chicken nuggets and broccoli with a burrito," LeFurgy says. "If only it were that easy to feed them at home." ■

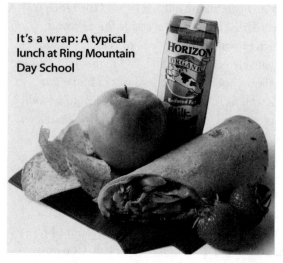

It's a wrap: A typical lunch at Ring Mountain Day School

How to Help Your Kids Eat Better

Think changing your child's eating habits is too daunting? Even the busiest moms can take these simple steps.

Get kids cooking. It creates a healthy appetite for good food. Let your kids peel vegetables or tear up lettuce for a salad, says Mary McKenna, Ph.D., a nutritionist at the U.S. Centers for Disease Control and Prevention in Atlanta.

Don't use food as a reward. "You want to keep food in its place and not create an emotional or psychological connection to it," McKenna says. For example, don't give your children treats to praise them for being good or to comfort them. This will help stop kids from overeating when they're upset.

Talk to other parents. Making changes to school-lunch menus is easier if parents join together. Too busy to make phone calls? Get organized online. "We could never have gotten our committee going without E-mail," says San Francisco mom Dana Woldow. She and other parents and teachers successfully ousted junk food from the cafeteria at Aptos Middle School. "There was no way we could have met face-to-face and accommodated everyone's schedules."

Make breakfast and dinner healthy. Face it: You can't totally control what your kids eat during school hours. But having nutritious meals at home might encourage them to make better choices when they're making decisions. "Repetition is key," McKenna says. "The more we eat healthy food, the more we will enjoy it."

Saving Summer Flavors

The best way to preserve fresh summer produce is in the freezer. Try these simple steps. Start with just-picked farm-stand fruits and vegetables, and prepare the same day.

Wash and trim. Prep food as if you were cooking it now. Remove all stems; core tomatoes and strawberries; string snap peas and green beans, and remove the tips; shuck and silk corn.

Tray-freeze berries and sliced fruit. Place whole berries; peeled, sliced peaches; or unpeeled, sliced nectarines onto cookie sheets. Pop them into the freezer for a couple of hours, then package tightly. This way, you can pull out individual pieces when needed. Tossing

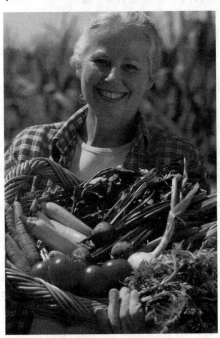

fruit first in a syrup of half sugar and half water (or even just sprinkling lightly with sugar) helps preserve flavor and prevents browning.

Blanch most vegetables. Boil in unsalted water, microwave, or steam for about half the usual cooking time; plunge into ice water. Freeze corn on the cob without blanching and use within three months. Freeze tomatoes whole without blanching; they skin and seed easily when thawed for quick sauces and salsas.

Pack tightly. Air is food's worst enemy. Use wraps and containers designed for freezer use; fill, leaving ½ inch of space for expansion. Push remaining air out of bags before sealing. "Burp" plastic containers.

Thaw right. Freezing stops the growth of foodborne bacteria but doesn't kill them. Cook frozen food directly from the freezer; or thaw it in the fridge and plan to eat it quickly.

Expect some mush. Formerly frozen fruits and veggies may taste like summer, but their crunch is generally gone for good. Plan to use most produce in cooked dishes within six months.

Q + A

KEEP EATING FRUIT

I love fruit, but I've heard that eating too much can lead to Parkinson's disease. How can that be?

Despite recent headlines, eat up. What started the buzz was a study tracking some 8,000 Japanese-American men over 38 years. The researchers found that subjects who ate three or more daily servings of fruit had a higher risk of developing Parkinson's than their counterparts who ate one serving or less a day. Experts have different theories on why the participants' odds increased: A handful of past studies have suggested a connection between high intake of vitamin C and Parkinson's, but the author of this particular study believes one likely culprit might be pesticides on the fruit. More research is needed; meanwhile, keep some perspective: Parkinson's is a fairly uncommon disease, affecting only about 1 percent of people over age 60 and fewer younger people. You are far more likely to be stricken by heart disease, stroke, diabetes, or cancer than by Parkinson's. And speaking of these more common illnesses, solid evidence indicates that you can reduce your risk of them by loading up on fruit. To be on the safe side, of course, always make sure it's well-washed.

How to Cook Simple

Health's Food and Nutrition Editor Susie Quick shares her secrets for creating fast, healthy, and delicious meals at home.

When I first got married, I would get home from a full day of work and prepare what I considered a proper dinner. I stuffed a duck with figs. I composed a chilled seafood terrine layered with the colors of the Italian flag. I served courses on weeknights, for God's sake. Good thing my husband didn't arrive home until the moon was high. One night, as I placed his plate before him, he looked up at me woefully and asked, "Soufflé ... again?"

I cooked this way for years because I believed that food could be delicious only through hours of effort. But as life got busier (and I shed the high-maintenance husband), my cooking style evolved. I learned how to cook simply, with a sense of discovery and enjoyment. The fact that the foods I loved happened to be good for me was an added blessing.

I know many people today have similar issues. The idea of heating up a frozen dinner or ordering pizza too many times a week goes against the desire to serve their families wholesome dishes that taste great.

There is a middle ground between frozen dinners and four-course meals: Just think simple. These timesaving secrets will get you in and out of the kitchen with a fantastic, healthy meal in no time.

QUICK SIMPLE SECRETS

EDIT, EDIT, EDIT.
Most people think of their kitchens as storage areas for wedding presents they might use someday. Look at yours the way you do your clothes closet and apply some of the same rules.
- Toss out any gadgets you haven't used in a year.
- Likewise, pare down the stuff in your cabinets and drawers. Be brutal!
- Box up never-used appliances and pans. Put them in the garage or give them away.
- Place appliances and favorite tools near the work area where you chop and prep.

GET ONE PAN THAT DOES EVERYTHING.
Choose a heavy 12-inch nonstick skillet with an ovenproof handle and lid. Use it for sautéing, stir-frying, braising—even roasting a chicken.

ORGANIZE YOUR CABINETS.

- Place your spices (divided up for savory or sweet dishes) on a lazy Susan for easy access.
- If you only bake on special occasions, store products for that purpose on a high shelf.
- Keep like items (such as canned goods and noodles) together, with labels facing out, so that you can grab and go.

PURGE YOUR PANTRY AND FRIDGE.

- Toss out old cereals and grains after two months (they tend to turn rancid after a while).
- Donate canned goods that you're probably never going to use; toss items older than two years.
- Open the spice jars and take a whiff—if a seasoning lacks a pungent aroma, pitch it (most last six months to a year, with a few exceptions).
- Empty the refrigerator door's collection of vintage condiments. Keep only the ones that are fresh and that you use regularly.

CUT BACK TO THREE KNIVES.

Do you fish through a drawer full of knives before you find the one you want? Stick to these must-haves. (Keep them sharpened for faster chopping and buy the best you can afford—they'll last a lifetime.)
- 8-inch chef's knife (It will fit most women's hands comfortably.)
- 8-inch serrated bread knife
- 4-inch paring knife

CREATE A "FLAVOR TRAY."

Place everyday items—like olive oil, vinegar, salt, pepper, crushed red pepper, and a favorite herb—on a tray near the stove (but not so close that they'll get hot). And use them!

SHOP SIMPLE.

Not just for the obsessive organizer: Create a permanent shopping checklist. Include the foods you buy all the time and arrange items according to the layout of your favorite supermarket. This way, anyone—not just you—can go to the store to pick up what you need (and get the brands you like).

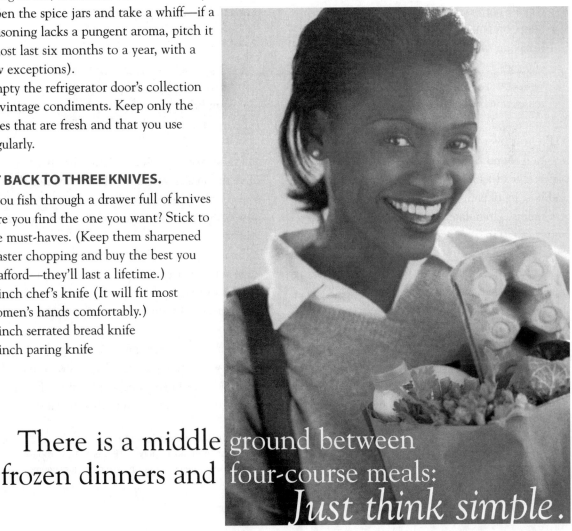

There is a middle ground between frozen dinners and four-course meals: *Just think simple.*

SIMPLE BUTTER CAKE

prep: 15 minutes • **cook:** 25 minutes • **serves** 4

This cake is as versatile as it is buttery. Serve with sweetened strawberries and whipped cream; or make cupcakes, and top with your favorite frosting. To cut fat and calories, use reduced-fat milk in the batter, and skip the butter in Step 4.

8 tablespoons unsalted butter, softened and divided
¾ cup granulated sugar
2 large eggs, at room temperature
1 teaspoon vanilla extract
1 cup all-purpose flour
1 teaspoon baking powder
¼ teaspoon salt
⅓ cup plus 1 tablespoon whole milk, at room temperature
1 teaspoon powdered sugar

1. Preheat oven to 350°. Cover the bottom of a 9-inch round cake pan with parchment or wax paper; spread 1 tablespoon butter over the sides and bottom of pan.
2. Combine granulated sugar and 6 tablespoons butter in a stand-up mixer; beat at medium-high speed 5 minutes, or until fluffy. Add eggs and vanilla; beat until combined. Sift together flour, baking powder, and salt. With mixer on its lowest speed, add flour mixture and milk alternately to butter mixture, scraping and mixing just until combined.
3. Scrape batter into prepared pan. Bake at 350° for 25 minutes, or until a wooden pick inserted in the center comes out clean. Cool on a rack for 5 minutes. Invert pan onto rack, and remove paper from cake. Invert again onto rack; cool completely.
4. Spread remaining 1 tablespoon butter over the top and sides of cake. Dust with powdered sugar. Cut the cake in half crosswise, and place one half on top of the other. Cut into 4 wedges, and serve.

PER SERVING (1 slice): Calories 520; Fat 24g (sat 15g, mono 8g, poly 1g); Protein 7g; Carbohydrate 64g; Cholesterol 170mg; Iron 2mg; Sodium 314mg; Calcium 120mg

ASPARAGUS WITH PROSCIUTTO-BACON AND EGGS

prep: 10 minutes • **cook:** 15 minutes • **serves** 4

Baking prosciutto makes it crisp like bacon, sans the fat. Crumble it over salads and vegetables, or add it to scrambled eggs.

2 teaspoons extra-virgin olive oil
3 ounces thinly sliced prosciutto
1 pound thin asparagus
2 large hard-boiled eggs, coarsely chopped

1. Preheat oven to 400°. Lightly brush 1 teaspoon olive oil on a large baking sheet. Arrange the prosciutto in a single layer on the prepared sheet. Bake at 400° for 10 minutes, or until crisp. Cool the prosciutto, and crumble into large pieces.
2. Snap off the tough ends of the asparagus. Fill a large skillet with 2 inches of water, and bring to a boil. Add 1 teaspoon salt and asparagus. Cook the asparagus for 3 minutes, or until crisp-tender, and drain.
3. Arrange the asparagus on a serving platter. Drizzle with the remaining 1 teaspoon olive oil. Sprinkle with salt and pepper to taste. Top the asparagus with the eggs and the prosciutto.

PER SERVING (one-fourth of the asparagus mixture): Calories 136; Fat 8g (sat 2g, mono 3g, poly 1g); Protein 11g; Carbohydrate 5g; Fiber 2g; Cholesterol 125mg; Iron 1mg; Sodium 440mg; Calcium 37mg

TURKISH MEAT LOAF

prep: 10 minutes • **cook:** 50 minutes • **serves** 6

This is the ultimate in meat loaves (it's good without the eggs, too). Serve hot with mashed potatoes or cold on a slice of crusty bread with hearty mustard.

1 slice white bread
¾ pound ground turkey
¾ pound ground pork
1 cup grated carrot
¼ cup grated fresh onion
½ cup chopped fresh flat-leaf parsley
3 tablespoons whole milk
2 teaspoons curry powder
1 teaspoon salt
¼ teaspoon freshly ground black pepper
1 large egg, beaten
1 garlic clove, minced
2 large hard-boiled eggs, shells removed
3 bacon slices

1. Preheat the oven to 400°. Place the bread in a food processor, and pulse 5 times, or until fine crumbs measure ½ cup. Combine breadcrumbs and the next 11 ingredients (through garlic) in a large bowl, and mix thoroughly. Place half of the meat mixture into a 9-inch glass loaf dish. Arrange the

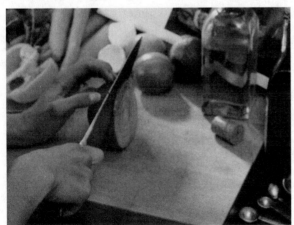

You really need only three knives but keep them sharpened for faster chopping.

hard-boiled eggs, end to end, on top. Spread remaining meat mixture over the eggs. Lay the bacon slices lengthwise across the top of the loaf.
2. Bake at 400° for 50 minutes, or until the juices run clear. Let the meat loaf stand for about 10 minutes. Drain off any liquid before slicing.

PER SERVING (about 2 slices): Calories 395; Fat 26g (sat 10g, mono 12g, poly 4g); Protein 24g; Carbohydrate 6g; Fiber 1g; Cholesterol 194mg; Iron 3mg; Sodium 628mg; Calcium 91mg

BASIC VINAIGRETTE

prep: 5 minutes • **makes:** ¹/₃ cup

One of the best things you can do for your health is to make your own dressing and keep it on hand for lots of fresh salads. This way, you'll know it's made from natural ingredients, without all the preservatives and stabilizers in bottled dressings. Plus, it tastes infinitely better. This is my favorite. Rice-wine vinegar is less acidic than others, so you can use more vinegar and less oil. If you wish, add a couple of teaspoons of finely minced fresh herbs, or substitute a different-flavored vinegar.

3 tablespoons seasoned rice-wine vinegar
1 tablespoon fresh lemon juice
½ teaspoon Dijon mustard
¼ teaspoon salt
¼ teaspoon freshly ground black pepper
1 garlic clove, minced
¼ cup extra-virgin olive oil

1. Combine first 6 ingredients (through garlic) in a small bowl; stir well with a whisk. Slowly pour olive oil into bowl, stirring constantly.

PER SERVING (1 tablespoon): Calories 65; Fat 7g (sat 1g, mono 5g, poly 1g); Protein 0g; Carbohydrate 1g; Fiber 0g; Cholesterol 0mg; Iron 0mg; Sodium 192mg; Calcium 2mg

FARFALLE WITH ZUCCHINI AND LEMON-CREAM SAUCE

prep: 15 minutes • **cook:** 10 minutes • **serves** 6

Letting the cheeses come to room temperature ensures a creamy sauce.

1½ cups whole-milk ricotta, at room temperature
½ cup (3½ ounces) mascarpone cheese, at room temperature
⅓ cup (1½ ounces) grated fresh Parmesan cheese
2 tablespoons finely grated lemon rind
¼ cup fresh chopped basil leaves
1 pound uncooked farfalle (bow-tie pasta)
2 tablespoons extra-virgin olive oil
4 cups thinly sliced zucchini
6 garlic cloves, thinly sliced

1. Combine the first 5 ingredients (through basil) in a large bowl.
2. Cook pasta according to package directions. Drain, reserving ½ cup cooking liquid.
3. Heat the oil in a large nonstick skillet. Add zucchini and garlic; sauté 4 minutes, or until zucchini is crisp-tender. Sprinkle zucchini with ½ teaspoon salt and ¼ teaspoon pepper.
4. Stir in ¼ cup of the reserved cooking liquid into cheese mixture. Add hot pasta, zucchini mixture, ½ teaspoon salt, and ¼ teaspoon pepper to cheese mixture. Toss gently. If necessary, add a few tablespoons of the cooking liquid to the mixture to make it creamy. Serve immediately.

PER SERVING (2 cups pasta mixture): Calories 536; Fat 18g (sat 11g, mono 6g, poly 1g); Protein 22g; Carbohydrate 63g; Fiber 4g; Cholesterol 56mg; Iron 3mg; Sodium 538mg; Calcium 245mg

MAHIMAHI MASALA KABOBS WITH MANGO RAITA

prep: 35 minutes • **cook:** 5 minutes • **serves** 4 to 6

Small cubes of fish (or meat) for kabobs soak up flavors fast. Fifteen minutes at room temperature is just enough time for them to marinate.

Equipment:
12 (12-inch) thin wooden skewers
Kabobs:
1½ pounds mahimahi, cut into 1½-inch cubes
2 teaspoons garam masala
1 tablespoon fresh lime juice
2 tablespoons extra-virgin olive oil
½ teaspoon salt
Raita:
1½ cups peeled, cubed ripe mango
½ cup plain yogurt
1 tablespoon chopped fresh mint
1 tablespoon honey
1 red serrano chile, coarsely chopped
¼ cup sliced scallions

1. Soak skewers in warm water 20 minutes.
2. To prepare kabobs, combine ingredients in a bowl, and toss well. Marinate 15 minutes.
3. To prepare raita, combine the ingredients in a food processor. Pulse 2 times, or until mango is finely chopped. Chill until ready to serve.
4. Thread 4 or 5 fish cubes onto each skewer.
5. Preheat grill to medium-high. Grill kabobs 2 minutes on each side, or until done. Sprinkle with scallions and additional mint. Serve with raita.

PER SERVING (2 kabobs and ¼ cup raita): Calories 143; Fat 6g (sat 1g, mono 4g, poly 0g); Protein 22g; Carbohydrate 12g; Fiber 1g; Cholesterol 85mg; Iron 2mg; Sodium 305mg; Calcium 53mg

CHOPPED SPRING SALAD WITH LIME-MINT VINAIGRETTE

prep: 15 minutes • **serves** 6

Any vegetable can be substituted in or excluded from this recipe without messing it up. Just keep in mind that salad doesn't have to start with lettuce. Take a look in your refrigerator for chopped leftovers, such as potatoes, string beans, and celery; then toss them together in a bowl with a little vinaigrette. Add chunks of grilled chicken or tuna for more protein, if you wish.

4 cups watercress
1½ cups thinly sliced fennel bulb (about 1 medium bulb)
1½ cups flat-leaf parsley
1 cup haricots verts, steamed until tender
¾ cup thinly sliced radishes
⅓ cup chopped scallions
2 peeled, diced avocados (about 1 cup)
2 large hard-boiled eggs
2 tablespoons thinly sliced fresh mint
4 tablespoons extra-virgin olive oil
2 tablespoons fresh lime juice
Salt and pepper to taste

1. Combine the first 9 ingredients (through mint) in a large bowl.
2. Whisk the remaining ingredients in a small bowl. Drizzle dressing over salad; toss gently.

PER SERVING (1½ cups): Calories 177; Fat 15g (sat 2g, mono 10g, poly 2g); Protein 4g; Carbohydrate 7g; Fiber 3.4g; Cholesterol 71mg; Iron 2mg; Sodium 59mg; Calcium 83mg

Toss out cereals after two months, spices after six months; purge items in the fridge more often than that.

CURRIED TOMATOES AND TOFU

prep: 10 minutes • **cook:** 6 minutes • **serves** 5

Even people who say they hate bean curd really like this tangy, slightly sweet curry. It's best made with fresh tomatoes (you can use cherry tomatoes as well). Serve with yellow saffron-flavored rice.

2 teaspoons olive oil
1 tablespoon peeled, grated fresh ginger
2 garlic cloves, minced
1 pound firm tofu, drained and cubed
3 cups seeded, chopped tomatoes
3 tablespoons bottled chili sauce, such as Heinz
2 teaspoons Madras curry powder
1½ teaspoons sugar
½ teaspoon salt
¼ teaspoon freshly ground black pepper

1. Heat the oil in a large nonstick skillet over medium heat. Add ginger and garlic, and stir-fry 30 seconds. Add tofu and remaining ingredients, and stir-fry 5 minutes, or until thoroughly heated.

PER SERVING (1 cup): Calories 151; Fat 4g (sat 1g, mono 1g, poly 0g); Protein 11g; Carbohydrate 11g; Fiber 2.5g; Cholesterol 0mg; Iron 3mg; Sodium 543mg; Calcium 112mg

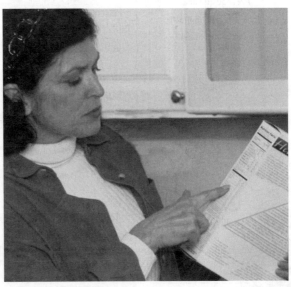

vital *stats*

80
Percentage of Americans who celebrate FATHER'S DAY

50
Percentage of Father's Day CARDS bought by CHILDREN for their dads

18
Percentage bought by WIVES for their husbands

$113.80
Average amount spent on a Father's Day gift

$90.70
Average amount spent on a Mother's Day gift

25
Average age of a FIRST-TIME MOM in the United States in 2000

21.4
Average AGE in 1970

22
Average age of a first-time mom in MISSISSIPPI in 2000

27.8
Average age in MASSACHUSETTS

22
Percentage of Americans in 1950 who got up before 6 a.m. on Saturdays

10
Percentage who do now

67
Percentage of baby boomers who cited HEALTH-CARE COSTS as a major retirement concern in 2002

39
Percentage who did in 2001

24
Percentage of women who POSTPONED RECEIVING MEDICAL CARE in 2002 because of the expense

16
Percentage of MEN who did

21
Percentage of women who DIDN'T FILL A PRESCRIPTION in 2002 because of the expense

13
Percentage of men who didn't

48
Percentage of women who take VITAMINS every day

32
Percentage of MEN who do

64
Percentage of Americans who are OVERWEIGHT or obese

55
Percentage of those Americans who are at least 25 POUNDS overweight

25
Estimated percentage of overweight or obese CATS AND DOGS

1
Rank of WEIGHT among top health issues of women ages 35 to 54

2
Rank of ARTHRITIS or any kind of rheumatism

3
Rank of MIGRAINES

$20.3 BILLION
Amount Americans spent in 2002 to rent or buy DVDs or VIDEOTAPES

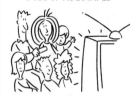

$12.2 BILLION
Amount spent on GYM memberships

1.5 MILLION
Number of American women who are ABUSED by their partners each year

20
Percentage who get a RESTRAINING order

80
Percent less likely a battered woman is to be abused again within a year if she gets a PERMANENT RESTRAINING ORDER against a violent partner

---

17
Percentage of Americans who say they are in EXCELLENT HEALTH

31
Percentage of those Americans who smoke

36
Percentage of those Americans who never exercise

Sources:
Hallmark, International Mass Retail Association, Gallup Poll, Allstate, Kaiser Family Foundation, National Center for Health Statistics, CDC, University of Minnesota College of Veterinary Medicine, Solucient, *The Journal of the American Medical Association*, DVD Entertainment Group, International Health, Racquet & Sportsclub Association, Oxford Health Plans/Magnet Communications/Central Marketing Inc.
—Reported by Laura Riccobono

chapter 5

fitness

reap the benefits of exercise

Discover Your
Body-Specific
Workout Prescription

Experts show you the best exercise plan for your individual fitness profile.

BY MARTICA K. HEANER

Forget about ectomorphs, mesomorphs, apples, pears, and rulers. These typical descriptions of physical types aren't all that useful when you're talking about real women and men with real bodies. But chances are, you do fit a particular profile that reflects your level of muscle tone, fat, and activity (or lack thereof). With the help of top fitness pros, we've identified the four most common real-world types and custom-designed fitness prescriptions that will help you address your individual needs. Here are their secrets to making your body its best.

TRIM & FRAIL

You look fit, and rightly so, because you log hours walking, running, or performing other cardio activities. But you're not very strong, and some body parts jiggle more than you'd like. "You can hit a physical and psychological plateau by doing the same type of cardio workout over and over," says Christa Bache, M.A., owner of Dellbach Personal

Training Studio in New York City. "Women like this often know they should do more resistance training, but they're afraid of bulking up." That won't happen, though, Bache says.

FITNESS RX:

Get creative with cardio. Stick to 30-minute cardio workouts three to five days per week. Consider including at least one routine that uses your upper and lower body, such as swimming or kickboxing. To get more out of your running, walking, cycling, or elliptical-training sessions, try an interval workout, which alternates high- and low-intensity segments. (See chart on page 226 for a sample regimen.)
Build muscle. Lift two to three days a week, skipping a day in between. "Remember that your muscles should feel fatigued after about 15 reps," Bache says. Vary your workout by mixing upper- and lower-body moves, such as squats, then lateral raises, followed by lunges, then triceps extensions.

STARTING FROM SCRATCH

You may be a bit exercise-shy because you haven't moved much lately. "So you need to do something gentle to begin with and push a little more the fitter you become," says Scott Cole, a Palm Springs, California-based fitness expert. You'll probably see faster results than a regular exerciser would. But don't overdo it. "You may start off gung-ho and expect to see huge results in a few days, get disappointed, and go back to couch-potato behavior," Cole says.

FITNESS RX:

Develop stability. Start by increasing body awareness and a sense of balance. Try a mind/body discipline, such as Tai Chi, Pilates, yoga, or free-form dance classes that focus on balance, agility, and flexibility (look for names like Nia, DanceKinetics, and YogaRhythmics). "Tai Chi helps you loosen up your joints and feel centered. Once you learn how to move with more grace, you'll feel more comfortable lifting weights or trying a fitness class," Cole says.

Get flexible. Improve your range of motion by incorporating regular feel-good stretches, especially for those notoriously stiff spots, such as your lower back, hamstrings, and chest. Before stretching deeply, warm up with a brisk walk until you begin to sweat a little.

Concentrate on cardio. Get used to moving your whole body with walking or water-aerobics classes, or hop on an elliptical trainer, a step machine, a stationary bike, or a treadmill. "Start slowly and work at a low intensity," Cole says. For four to six weeks, aim for a 20- to 40-minute session every other day, allowing your body a day to recover. Then increase the speed, frequency, or duration of your workout as you become fitter and more at ease with exercise. But avoid pushing too hard. "You should feel energized after each session. If you feel brutalized, you did too much," Cole says. Later, when you're ready, ease into resistance training to tone and burn more calories.

Keep it simple. The last thing you need to do is crush your confidence, so stick to activities you know you can do. (Walking, for instance, is great for beginners.)

When you've developed a base fitness level, move up to workouts that demand more skill and stamina.

Get outdoors. "Go to a park or walk in your neighborhood," Cole says. Connecting with nature may lighten your mental load, no matter how fit you are.

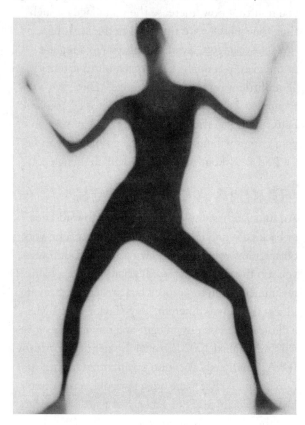

STRONG & SOFT

You put in time at the gym, but you've still got more padding than you'd like. To get more sculpted, fine-tune your strategy. "It's not that what you're doing isn't working," says Hugo Diez, group exercise manager for the Reebok Sports Club in New York City. "To get leaner, you need to eat a little less and jump-start your routine to expend more calories."

FITNESS RX:

Wake up your muscles. Strive for variety to stay challenged, Diez says. If you're walking four miles, try jogging one of them, or do an interval workout. (See chart on page 226.) If you're already taking Spinning classes, add kickboxing.

Rev up your resistance. You might have shied away from heavier weights because you already feel a little hefty, but lifting light may not give you the body-shaping results—or the metabolic boost—you need. If a set of 15 reps feels pretty easy at the weight you're lifting now, increase the poundage enough that your muscles are tired before the 10th rep.

Fine-tune your focus. Even though you're a regular at the gym, you might be slacking off in intensity. "Find little ways to make a change," Diez says. Example: Wear more formfitting clothes. "You look better than you think, and seeing signs of tone in your curves will motivate you to push a little more." Or find a workout partner who will challenge you.

MAKING A COMEBACK

An injury, a nasty cold, or a tendency toward knee or back pain might have put a damper on your workouts. Unless you merge slowly back into your routine, you run the risk of relapse. "It's hard to give a blanket recommendation for a specific approach, since every illness or injury is different," says Taylor Isaacs, M.S., a clinical exercise physiologist and physical therapist who was named 2002 Personal Trainer of the Year by IDEA, a national education organization for fitness professionals. "But there are a few golden rules to go by when you're ready to get active again." The first: Get the OK from your doctor.

FITNESS RX:

Don't skimp on rest. Skipping a workout altogether is sometimes the best solution on those days when you're feeling tired, sore, worked-over, burned-out, or unfocused. "Being in a sleep-deprived state will impair your healing and your energy levels, so make sure that you stay well-rested for maximum rejuvenation," Isaacs says.

No pain, all gain. Whenever you perform an activity, constantly evaluate how you feel. On a scale of 0 (pain-free) to 10 (excruciating), keep your pain level at 4 or less. If the pain registers any higher, decrease the intensity of your workout or switch to an activity that's more comfortable, Isaacs says.

For instance, if you have a bad knee and walking on the treadmill makes it worse, try non-weight-bearing exercises, such as swimming or using the elliptical trainer. "Go around the injury rather than trying to work through pain," Isaacs says.

Move as freely as you can. "Aim to move all of your joints, especially weak ones, through their full pain-free range of motion," he says.

Chill. Putting ice on an injured area for 10 minutes after exercising can aid the healing process by decreasing inflammation. "Avoid taking aspirin or a painkiller before a workout," Isaacs says. "It may mask the signals that you need to take it easy." If you were in super shape before, you may find being less fit especially hard to accept. "Remind yourself that you've had a setback. You need to take it easy before you can play at full strength again," Isaacs says. ▪

Martica K. Heaner, M.A., an exercise physiologist and fitness trainer, is the author of Cross-Training for Dummies.

Aerobic Interval Workout for One 30-Minute Session

Minutes	Intensity	RPE*
1 to 4	Warm-up	2 or 3
5 to 6	Moderate	4 or 5
7	Hard	6 or 7
8 to 9	Moderate	4 or 5
10	Hard	6 or 7
11 to 12	Moderate	4 or 5
13	Hard	6 or 7
14 to 15	Moderate	4 or 5
16	Hard	6 or 7
17 to 18	Moderate	4 or 5
19	Hard	6, 7, or 8
20 to 21	Moderate	4 or 5
22	Hard	6, 7, or 8
23 to 24	Moderate	4 or 5
25	Hard	6, 7, or 8
26 to 30	Cooldown	2 or 3

Rate of Perceived Exertion (RPE)

0–1 little or no exertion	6–7 very vigorous
2–3 moderate (warm-up and cooldown intensity)	8–9 panting, lungs on fire
4–5 stronger, breaking a sweat	10 maximum effort

How to Deal with Bad Manners at the Gym

The gym is one of the few places where adults are forced to share (besides the office break room), and we're just not good at it. We hog mirror space, leave wet towels on the floor, and sweat all over the StairMaster with no regard for the unlucky sap next in line. "Paying for membership makes some of us think we own the gym," says Peter Post, great-grandson of etiquette legend Emily Post and director of the Emily Post Institute in Burlington, Vermont. Here are his recommendations for dealing with uncouth behavior at the health club.

THE OFFENDER	WHAT YOU'D LOVE TO SAY …	WHAT POST WOULD SAY …
The marathon man, oblivious to the 30-minute time limit on the treadmill	"Thirty minutes is when the big hand moves from the 12 to the 6. Get it?"	"I'm sorry to interrupt you, but I've been waiting 40 minutes for this machine. Would you mind finishing up so I can use it?"
The oblivious woman in the weight room lounging on the leg-extension machine like it's a La-Z-Boy	"May I get you a drink? A pillow for your feet, perhaps?"	People are so self-absorbed at the gym, they may not even see you standing there. So try asking, "Are you still using that?" or "Would you mind if I get in a few reps?"
The foul-smelling guy using the bench press	"Ever heard of something called deodorant?"	Don't even go there. "The situation's too personal for direct confrontation," Post says. So just use a machine at the other end of the room.
The short, hairy man strutting around the gym, turning on the smarm—uh, charm: "Hey, baby. Lemme buy you a protein drink."	"Can you go back into the hole you just crawled out of?"	Unless you want to pass him your number, make it clear that you aren't interested: "No, thanks. I'd just like to concentrate on my workout."
Your personal trainer, who's just asked what kind of lingerie you like	"A nursing bra and a girdle. Why do you ask?"	In private, tell him (or her) that you expect more professional behavior. If there's no change, switch trainers and tell management why.
The jerk who rains putrid sweat on every machine, then walks away, leaving you to clean up the mess	"Do I look like a maid to you?"	"I'd like to make them lick it clean," Post jokes, "but with repeat offenders, they're probably slobs at home, too." Ask management to enforce the wipe-down rule.
The woman who stakes out the same territory each time in aerobics class—go near it, and she snaps like a guard dog.	"You paying rent on that property, or are you buying?"	"You can't just give her the boot for no reason," Post says. So chill. Exercise where you want to and don't let her or her issues disturb your workout.
The irate woman screaming into her cell phone at her boyfriend after seeing him at a party with someone else	"Just forget about him, girl. He's obviously got commitment issues."	"You shouldn't be having loud conversations about personal matters," Post says. But confronting her won't help, so just move away. If the problem persists, let management handle it.

How Much Exercise Do You Really Need?

The newest guidelines say you need to spend an hour a day to get—and stay—fit. Before you panic, read on.

BY DIMITY McDOWELL

When you're dealing with housework, office work, and the kids' homework, getting in a daily shot of exercise is a real accomplishment. So in fall 2002, when the National Academies' Institute of Medicine (IOM) released guidelines that recommended a full hour-long workout seven days a week, it made people feel like forgetting biceps curls completely and curling up on the couch instead.

"It was horrible," says Tim Church, M.D., Ph.D., medical director at the Cooper Institute in Dallas, who is currently studying how exercise affects cardiovascular risk factors in postmenopausal women. "Some of my study participants were in tears, thinking the work they'd done was worth nothing." The IOM, which doesn't differentiate between aerobic activity and weight training in its paper, counts leisurely cycling, golfing without a cart (and who does that?), walking three to four miles, gardening, raking, mopping, and

The new "rules" are more focused on weight-loss and obesity than overall health benefits.

vacuuming toward your daily tally. For more vigorous efforts—such as jogging, playing squash, or chopping wood—about 30 minutes most days of the week will suffice.

What the news accounts failed to tell you was that the source of the guidelines, a report titled *Dietary Reference Intakes for Energy, Carbohydrate, Fiber, Fat, Fatty Acids, Cholesterol, Protein, and Amino Acids*, is primarily a nutrition document—only one of the 14 chapters deals chiefly with exercise. Furthermore, the recs are more focused on weight loss and maintenance than they are on the health benefits that physical activity yields, such as reducing the risks of heart disease, premature death, depression, and other conditions.

"The intent of the report was to help our nation win the battle against obesity. It found that individuals who move for an hour or more every day are most successful in maintaining a normal body weight," explains Cedric X. Bryant, Ph.D., chief exercise physiologist for the American Council on Exercise, who has studied the effects of strength training on women of all ages. "But it was not intended to minimize the surgeon general's recommendations of 30 minutes most days of the week. What they wanted to let people know is that while some exercise is better than none, more is better than some."

Not only are the IOM's guidelines double those recommended by the surgeon general in 1996, but they also exceed the American College of Sports Medicine's suggestions: cardio 20 to 60 minutes, three to five days a week, plus weight and flexibility training two to three days a week. "There are definitely mixed messages out there," admits Richard Cotton, chief exercise physiologist for MyExercisePlan.com, a Web site that helps users develop personalized fitness programs.

So, where does that leave you? For most people, a combination of cardiovascular activity and weight training that adds up to 30 minutes a day, five days

Three Success Stories

Think finding the time and energy to achieve 150 minutes (30 minutes times 5) of exercise a week is impossible? Check out the routines of these three women who've figured out how to squeeze physical activity into their busy lives (and note that they're not all hitting the gym every day, either).

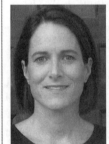

Maura Burke Vanderzon, 41
Stay-at-home mom, Chevy Chase, Maryland
<u>Weekly fitness routine:</u> Attends indoor-cycling or body-sculpting classes three or four days a week; also goes walking a couple of miles with her 1-year-old most days of the week.
<u>Total time per week:</u> 255 to 360 minutes
<u>What she says:</u> "My child keeps me really busy, so I'm constantly moving. When I can't get to the gym, I just go for a longer walk so I can still get my exercise."

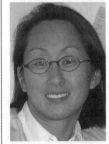

Linda Wong, 33
Systems manager, San Francisco
<u>Weekly fitness routine:</u> Runs 45 minutes twice a week, with 15 minutes of weight lifting afterward; uses elliptical trainer two days a week, with 15 minutes of lifting afterward; indoor-cycles once a week.
<u>Total time per week:</u> 300 minutes
<u>What she says:</u> "Doing weights makes a huge difference. I injured my knees in lacrosse, and weight training has allowed me to strengthen them and keep running."

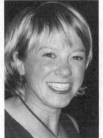

Deborah Pleva, 31
Public-affairs manager, Portland, Oregon
<u>Weekly fitness routine:</u> Uses StairMaster or elliptical trainer three to four times a week; weight-trains two to three times a week; does yard work (such as gardening) on a regular basis.
<u>Total time per week:</u> 180 to 270 minutes
<u>What she says:</u> "I'm working with a personal trainer who has me on an intense routine. I feel like I'm doing a lot."

a week, is plenty—both to maintain general health and keep your weight in check. But if you're looking to lose a few pounds or you have only a few minutes to spare, you will need to tweak your routine just a little bit.

Using expert advice, we've simplified the new guidelines and organized them according to your potential goals. If you're new to exercise, start slowly and build up gradually to your target. And remember: You can divide each day's total into 10- or 15-minute segments.

TO MAINTAIN WEIGHT/GENERAL HEALTH:

<u>Cardio:</u> Do 30 minutes of moderate exercise, such as walking or riding a stationary bike, a minimum of three days a week.
<u>Strength training:</u> Do one set of 8 to 10 exercises that hits all the major muscle groups (any basic gym circuit or home dumbbell program will do), two to three days a week. If you're postmenopausal,

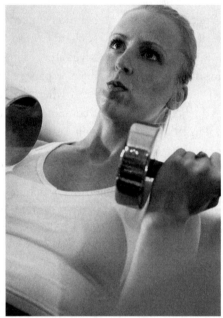

For most people, a combination of cardiovascular activity and weight training, 30 minutes a day, five days a week, is enough exercise.

aim for three days to stave off bone loss. Use enough weight that you're able to do only 8 to 12 reps of each move.

If you've faithfully followed this plan for three months but your pants are getting tight, switch to the guidelines that follow.

TO LOSE WEIGHT:

<u>Cardio:</u> Aim for 45 minutes of moderate exercise, four to five days a week.
<u>Strength training:</u> Do one set of 8 to 10 exercises that works all the major muscle groups (again, any basic gym circuit or home dumbbell program will do), two to three days a week. If you're postmenopausal, try for three days a week. As with the preceding program, use enough weight that you're able to do only 8 to 12 reps of each move.
<u>Watch your diet:</u> Exercise is only half of the weight-loss equation—you will also need to cut back on calories and monitor what you eat. ■

Q + A   WHEN YOU'RE TOO SICK TO WORK OUT

I think I'm coming down with a cold. Should I skip my usual workouts?

If you have a runny nose, a sore throat, a dry cough, or the sneezes—in other words, you have above-the-neck symptoms—it's fine to break a sweat, says ear, nose, and

throat specialist Mark Deutsch, M.D. Hitting either the gym or the great outdoors is fine (working out in cold weather should be OK unless you're prone to asthma or bronchitis). But you'll want to take some precautions. Before you begin, make sure you're well-hydrated. Start slowly and keep

your workout within your usual limits. "However, don't exercise if you have a fever," Deutsch cautions. "You don't want to push your body temperature up if you're already having trouble regulating it." That said, there isn't any shame in taking a break from your normal routine while you're sick.

Exercise and Drugs: Mix with Caution

Prescription and over-the-counter drugs can treat what ails you, but they may also throw your coordination, breathing, heart rate, and blood pressure off-kilter during a workout, explains Mark Chamberlain, Pharm.D., an expert on medications and exercise at the University of Maryland, Baltimore. He and Taylor Isaacs, a clinical exercise physiologist at California State University at Northridge, offer sound advice on how drugs can affect your workout—and what to do about it.

CONDITIONS	MEDICATIONS	WORKOUT WARNINGS	RX FOR EXERCISE
Allergies, Sinusitis	Diphenhydramine (Benadryl) or other antihistamines	May cause drowsiness or dizziness, impair coordination, or slow reaction time.	Avoid moves and equipment that will throw you off balance. Try seated cardio activities, such as indoor cycling and rowing, or equipment with handrails, such as stairsteppers and elliptical trainers.
Anxiety	Alprazolam (Xanax)	May make you drowsy and affect your coordination; side effects generally taper off in a few weeks.	Take a pass on complicated moves, such as highly choreographed dance and aerobics routines. Try seated cardio equipment until you've adjusted to your medicine.
Asthma	Theophylline (Uniphyl)	May cause dangerous heart-rate increases if you have high blood pressure or heart disease. Good choices for active people are albuterol (Proventil) and montelukast (Singulair).	Ask your doctor if an alternative would be appropriate. Have her approve your workout and adjust your drug dosage, if necessary. Avoid extreme heat and cold. Warm up at least 10 minutes, then cool down gradually. Always keep your bronchodilator on hand.
Colds	Pseudoephedrine (Sudafed, Triaminic)	May raise your temperature and heart rate to risky levels if you work out in extreme heat or have high blood pressure or heart disease.	Don't work out if you have an elevated temperature, severe congestion, or serious chronic health problems. Otherwise, drink water before, during, and after exercising. Scale back workout length and intensity.
Depression	Sertraline (Zoloft), fluoxetine (Prozac, Sarafem)	May cause drowsiness, nausea, or stomach upset that usually resolves in a few weeks.	Avoid working out until your stomach settles. If the drowsiness continues, stick to seated cardio equipment, such as indoor cycles and rowing machines.
Diabetes	Glyburide (Micronase), repaglinide (Prandin), insulin, others that lower blood sugar	Intense activity may cause fainting or dizziness. If you are insulin-dependent, ask about adjusting your dosage.	Never work out on an empty stomach; eat a high-carbohydrate, high-fiber snack, such as half a peanut-butter sandwich on multigrain bread, 30 to 60 minutes beforehand.

fitness falsehoods

Science writer Gina Kolata speaks out about exercise myths.

BY FRAN SMITH

If exercise is addictive, *New York Times* science writer Gina Kolata is a junkie. She started running in the days before running shoes. She signed up for aerobics when the look was *Flashdance*. Now the award-winning journalist and mother of two is a Spinning fanatic, sweating through at least four intense classes a week.

Three years ago, Kolata bought a heart-rate monitor to track her progress—and was astonished. Stationary cycling elevated her heart-beat well beyond the targets listed on every machine in the gym. It made her start to question the evidence for much of the lore in the workout world.

The result of her investigation, recently published, is *Ultimate Fitness: The Quest for Truth About Exercise and Health,* in which Kolata casts a skeptical eye on the history, culture, business, and science of fitness. Whether you exercise to lose weight, stay fit, or live longer, you'll be surprised by what Kolata has to say.

> After buying a heart-rate monitor, Kolata noticed that stationary cycling elevated her heartbeat well beyond the targets listed on machines in the gym. It made her question the evidence for much of the lore in the workout world.

Q: You write that the benefits of exercise have been oversold. Can you explain?

A: People think they're going to get thin. They'll look better, but most people won't lose substantial amounts of weight unless they do a lot of intense exercise. Even then, you have to watch your diet. People also think exercise will protect them from osteoporosis, but no experimental evidence shows that exercise reduces fracture rates. But we do know it improves stability and makes a bone-breaking fall less likely. People think that exercise will do one thing after another for their health, but there's no evidence that it happens. Or we know it *doesn't* happen.

Q: Doesn't exercise protect the heart?

A: I believed the more you exercised, the better your heart would be. But you get the most benefit when you go from doing almost nothing to doing a little bit—a brisk half-hour walk five days a week. It's not moseying around the mall, but it's not running, either.

Q: Then why exercise more?

A: You really feel good, energized. You have body confidence. You never have to say, "I can't carry this grocery bag" or "I can't climb these stairs." And I do think you look better. Your waist looks smaller if you broaden your back. Your thighs don't shake when you walk.

Q: What else surprised you?

A: I think of myself as a skeptic, and even I bought the myths. I thought if you added muscle you could eat more, since muscle is metabolically more active than fat. It turns out that the added muscle doesn't burn very many calories compared with the total metabolic needs of your body.

Q: Why do you trash the notion of the fat-burning zone?

A: You see machines that have charts to show you the fat-burning or weight-loss zone. The idea is that to burn the most fat, you should work at a fairly low heart rate—not be breathing hard. But that's a myth. It's true that when you're working at a low intensity, your muscles burn more fat. When you work harder, your muscles burn more sugar. But they burn it faster, so you use more calories. It's calories in versus calories out if you want to lose weight.

Q: Did you change your exercise regimen as a result of your research?

A: I work out a lot harder. ◼

The Truth About Toning

Myth: If you want to tone—not bulk up—you should do lots of repetitions with light weights.

Reality: That may be the conventional wisdom, but it's wrong, says Cedric Bryant, Ph.D., chief exercise physiologist for the American Council on Exercise. "The best way to develop tone or definition is to allow the muscle you have to become visible by losing the fat surrounding it," he says. The smart strategy is to choose a weight you can lift at least eight times but that tires you out before you reach 15 (we're not talking single-pounders here). Lifting alone, though, won't get you toned: Calorie-burning aerobic exercises and a little restraint at mealtime will help, too.

Tone Your Muscles While Watching TV

Staring at the tube burns barely more calories than sleeping. To make TV watching more conducive to fitness, Linda J. Buch and Seth Anne Snider-Copley created *The Commercial Break Workout: Trim and Tone Two Minutes at a Time.* Try this move next time there's a pause in your favorite show.

   Sofa squat: Sit up in your chair with your abdominal muscles tight, head neutral, and chest lifted (avoid arching your back). With your feet shoulder-width apart, lean forward slightly and exhale as you push through your heels to a standing position. Using the muscles in your legs to control your descent, inhale as you slowly sit. Keep your knees directly above your ankles. Repeat this exercise throughout the entire commercial break.

Use Exercise to Sharpen Your Memory

Researchers at New York University School of Medicine say that a good workout can help your body process glucose more efficiently, which helps keep those brain cells buzzing. So what's the best memory booster, according to the researchers? Try weight lifting, which tones muscles and helps move glucose into tissues.

Slow Workout, *Fast* Results

Slow-speed strength training promises to build muscles in no time. Does it deliver?

BY LORI SETO

I f you lunch at a drive-through, instant-message instead of E-mail, and "read" books on tape, you'll relish the timesaving possibilities of slow-speed strength training. The pitch: total fitness in just one or two 20-minute workouts a week, with no warming up, stretching, or cardio required. But is this approach a gimmick or a godsend?

In truth, it's a little of both—and it's nothing new. Extolled in such recent books as *The Slow Burn Fitness Revolution and Power of 10: The Once-a-Week Slow Motion Fitness Revolution,* the technique, which involves lifting heavy weights at about one-third of the usual speed for a single set, actually dates from 1927. The logic goes like this: The key to overall fitness is building muscle mass, and strength training is a far better way to do that than aerobic exercise. Lifting weights in slow motion is the most efficient strength-training technique, because it's the fastest path to muscle fatigue (the point at which you can't move another inch).

That last claim is undeniably true, although a program of overall fitness that excludes cardio is questionable. Dramatically slowing down a movement and letting one flow into the next without

pause eliminates momentum, so your muscles do all the work. Try it with the amount of weight you normally use, and you'll find that you tire out in fewer repetitions.

Those who love it may get a high from the extreme effort and sense of accomplishment, but most folks would equate it with legalized torture.

Pushing your muscles to their limit in one set saves time, but it probably doesn't build muscle as well as two or three sets at normal speed. Chances are, you'll have to lift lighter weights in order to do a slow-speed set correctly. "In any strength-training regimen, you need to lift at least 50 percent of the maximum amount you can handle in one rep to improve strength and muscle size," says Gary R. Hunter, Ph.D., who researches the effects of weight training on muscle growth. For instance, if the most you could lift in one rep is 40 pounds, you'd need to use 20 pounds for your biceps curls—more than you probably can handle at such a slow pace. A professor of human studies and nutrition sciences at the University of Alabama at Birmingham, Hunter has found that most people can lift 25 to 30 percent—or

10 to 12 pounds, using our example—if they're doing a slow-speed workout correctly. That will give you some strength gains, but not as much improvement as you'd see with a traditional regimen.

Even that so-so outcome may be hard to achieve. While the aforementioned books include at-home workouts, sticking to a slow-speed routine is tough without a trainer to keep you in line. The intensity makes it hard not to hold your breath, break form, and scream obscenities. Consider the slow-speed motto: Success is failure—muscle failure. That means your muscles shake and burn on the edge of total fatigue. Wayne Westcott, Ph.D., fitness-research director at the South Shore YMCA in

Strength in Numbers
Training the superslow way isn't for sissies.
Crunch the numbers below to see if this workout is right for you.

Strength-training method	Traditional weight machine/free weights	Slow-speed
Days per week	3	2 for beginners, 1 for the more experienced
Time required per session	35 minutes	20 minutes
# of exercises	8 to 10	6 to 8
# of sets	2	1
# of reps	8 to 12	6
Length of a single rep	7 seconds (with pause)	20 excruciating seconds (no pause)
Break between sets	30 to 60 seconds (more if a celebrity-gossip magazine is within reach)	About a minute or so (can be extended by faking an ankle sprain)
Amount of weight	At least 50% of maximum	Whatever turns you into a quivering mess in 6 reps
Importance of trainer	Low	High, due to intensity of exercise (which makes proper form and breathing extraimportant) and comparatively weak willpower of the average gym-goer
Trainer cost	$45 per hour	$45 per half-hour
Postworkout soreness	Medium, manageable	High, but it's a "good" pain (if you have masochistic tendencies, that is) that shouldn't last more than 2 or 3 days
Grimace factor	Low	High (this will feel like the longest 20 minutes of your life)

Quincy, Massachusetts, says that only 2 of the 65 people he's introduced to the method have stayed with it. Those who love it may get a high from the extreme effort and sense of accomplishment, but most folks would equate it with legalized torture.

What about slow-speed's claims that more muscle is the best way to optimal fitness—and that everything else, even flexibility and cardiovascular work, is unnecessary? Because the reduced speed eases you into each exercise gradually, you could technically drop the warm-ups and stretching—though doing them anyway might enhance your results. In a study of people lifting at regular speed, Westcott observed a 19-percent strength advantage in those who stretched versus those who didn't. And although strength training does beat aerobic exercise for building muscle mass, cardio offers its own benefits. "It delivers more oxygen to the muscles and uses more muscles at one time, so it's a better way to reduce your risk for heart disease, lower your blood pressure, and keep your cholesterol in check," says Walter Thompson, Ph.D., professor of kinesiology and health at Georgia State University. "If your goal is to lose weight, cardio burns more calories for most people." In other words, whether you emphasize one or the other depends on your goals—but both are necessary.

In the end, "what's important is that you exercise," Thompson says. "If you enjoy the slow-speed method and will actually do it, you'll gain some strength benefits." So if such a program fits your personality, pocketbook (you'll need that trainer), and pain threshold, go for it. But remember: It's just one part of the total fitness package. ▧

Lori Seto is a New York City–based writer and avid gym rat.

Q + A   WEIGHT LIFTING AND WEIGHT GAIN

About a month ago, I started lifting weights twice a week. Could my new muscles be responsible for my recent weight gain?

Unfortunately, those extra pounds are probably more belly than bicep. "If you believe the infomercials, you can gain 30 pounds of muscle in six weeks," says William Kraemer, Ph.D., professor of kinesiology at the University of Connecticut and editor in chief of the *Journal of Strength & Conditioning Research.* In reality, though, it would take at least eight weeks of progressive heavy lifting three times a week to see a muscle-related difference in your weight, and even then it would be only a couple of pounds. Is it possible that you are eating more because you feel you deserve a substantial snack after your workout? If so, make sure you're not wolfing down more calories than you're burning at the gym.

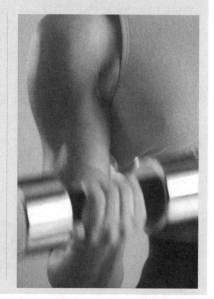

Who Trained Your Personal Trainer?

Before trusting someone to shape your routine—and your body—find out how that person learned the craft.

BY MARTY MUNSON

Beverly James, a public relations director in Atlanta, still has nightmares about the trainer who pushed her so hard three years ago that she almost fainted while using the biceps-curl machine. "I started to slide down to the floor. He told me to get up and looked around, embarrassed," she says. "I felt like I could have died in that gym and he would only be concerned about what people thought of him. I'd wondered if he was working me too hard, but I ignored my instincts."

You'd never let someone operate on you if that person hadn't graduated from medical school, right? Well, a personal trainer won't be coming at you with a scalpel, but if she's incompetent, she could do serious damage. Checking her credentials before you sign up is worth the effort, but you need to do more than verify that she's earned an official-looking piece of paper.

More than 300 groups certify personal trainers, but there are no state or federal licensing standards. If a trainer has earned a certification from one of the national groups listed at right, you can be certain that she has passed a rigorous written test on fundamentals, such as safety, anatomy, ethics, and creating a basic workout.

If you have more specific needs or goals, consider finding a trainer with a specialized background. For instance, if you're recovering from an injury, you might do best with a trainer certified by the American College of Sports Medicine (ACSM).

> Trust your instincts. It's your money, your time, and your body.

The ACSM requires a college degree or an equivalent amount of experience in a health-related field. If you are interested in pushing your athletic ability to a new level—you want to run a marathon, for instance—consider a trainer certified by the National Strength and Conditioning Association, which has been the key player in certifying coaches and athletic trainers since the 1970s.

Still, passing even the toughest test doesn't guarantee that a trainer will be good. Before you hit the weight room with a new one, talk with her. Walk away if she doesn't ask about your medical history or if she makes outlandish promises about fast weight loss or spot reducing. Ask for references, and contact them.

Finally, you should always trust your instincts. If a trainer is annoying or uninspiring, give someone else a try. After all, it's your money, your time, and your body. ◼

Find a Pro

American Council on Exercise
800-825-3636 or www.acefitness.org

American College of Sports Medicine
317-637-9200, x138, or www.acsm.org

Aerobics and Fitness Association of America
877-968-7263 or www.afaa.com

National Strength & Conditioning Association
800-815-6826 or www.nsca-lift.org

The Shorter, Smarter Workout

Discover how circuit workouts can shape you up in a flash.

BY TRACY TEARE

Total-body workout in 30 minutes? Sounds too good to be true, but time-starved women all over America are discovering that they don't need to carve out an hour or more to fit in fitness. The key is circuit training, which alternates strength moves with short bursts of aerobic exercise that keep your heart rate up.

Although the concept isn't new, it's enjoying a surge in popularity. Witness Curves International (800-848-1096 or www.curvesinternational.com), a chain of more than 5,000 fitness centers in the United States and abroad that owes its explosive growth since 1992 to its signature 30-minute circuit workouts. Other fitness firms have since followed Curves' lead: Pro Fit Enterprises (888-604-2244 or www.pacecircuittraining.com), which makes the PACE (Programmed Aerobic/Anaerobic/ Accommodating Circuit Exercise) equipment used in similar programs, operates 2,000 circuit centers in women's clubs, plus others in coed clubs. Pro Fit also plans to set up centers for kids ages 8 to 12, says president Rande LaDue.

"I was stunned that you don't have to spend an hour and a half to get a good workout," says Curves devotee Teressa Everett, 36, of Kinston, North Carolina. Since it's quick (she goes on her lunch hour with time to spare) and effective (she's lost more than 100 pounds since April 2001), she's stuck with it.

To do the Curves circuit, you start on one of the raised foam pads called "recovery stations" and march, hop, or do whatever it takes to boost your heart rate. Then a recorded voice cues you to move to the

Not only do you get both cardio and strength work in one neat package, but the fast pace and variety motivate you and help you avoid mental and physical plateaus.

resistance machine next to you. The device, which uses hydraulics instead of weights, adjusts to each person's fitness level—the more energy you exert, the more resistance it provides. After a minute, the voice prompts you to go to the next cardio station, and so on. You can get the same effect in a typical health club or at home, only without the automated prompts to move you through the workout.

"Circuit training is so efficient; that's why busy people love it," says Michael Wood, a certified strength and conditioning specialist and director of Sports Performance Group, a fitness-consulting company in North Attleboro, Massachusetts. Not only do you get both cardio and strength work in one neat package, but the fast pace and variety motivate you and help you avoid mental and physical plateaus. "You're doing something different every minute or two, and the possibilities are endless," Wood says.

Circuits aren't exactly perfect, though. If you try to put your own workout together at a gym or at home, space and access to equipment can pose problems. And because circuit training doesn't score big on flexibility, it's wise to stretch after your workout.

For fans, these downsides pale compared with the challenge and convenience of this ultraefficient, dynamic way to work out. See for yourself by trying one of the routines below.

2 Simple Circuits

We consulted with trainer Michael Wood and *Health* Contributing Editor Petra Kolber to put together two 30-minute circuit workouts: one for home or any place equipment is limited, and one for the gym. Start with a warm-up, then do a slow set of the first strength exercise (it should take about 60 seconds). Quickly move on to a 30- to 60-second burst of cardio, then start the next strength move. Alternate strength and cardio until you finish the circuit, then cool down.

HOME CIRCUIT

The challenge: Cardio in a confined space, without equipment
The remedy: Keep it simple—jump rope, run in place, do jumping jacks.
The props: Dumbbells, stairs, a jump rope

The routine:
1. Cardio warm-up (5 to 8 minutes)
2. Squats (10 to 12 reps)
3. Double dumbbell rows (10 to 12 reps)
4. Push-ups (10 to 12 reps)
5. Hover and Hold (10 to 12 reps; see BodyWork, page 241)
6. Dumbbell side raises (10 to 12 reps)
7. Seated V (10 to 12 reps; see Bodywork, page 240)
8. Lunge with Cross Chop (10 to 12 reps; see BodyWork, page 241)
9. Biceps curls/overhead presses (10 to 12 reps)
10. Repeat circuit, or do cardio cooldown (3 to 5 minutes)

GYM CIRCUIT

The challenge: Quick access to the required gym machines
The remedy: Go at nonpeak hours or substitute free-weight exercises.
The props: Standard weight-training equipment found in most gyms.

The routine:
1. Cardio warm-up (5 to 8 minutes)
2. Leg extensions (10 to 12 reps)
3. Leg curls (10 to 12 reps)
4. Lat pulldowns or seated rows (10 to 12 reps)
5. Triceps pushdowns (10 to 12 reps)
6. Bench presses or chest flies (10 to 12 reps)
7. Crunches (10 to 12 reps)
8. Side dumbbell raises (10 to 12 reps)
9. Military presses (10 to 12 reps)
10. Biceps curls (10 to 12 reps)
11. Back extensions (10 to 12 reps)
12. Repeat circuit, or do cardio cooldown (3 to 5 minutes)

BODYWORK

A Fast Workout to Help You *Slim Down*

Trim your waistline and your workout with these easy moves.

BY PETRA KOLBER • PHOTOGRAPHY BY DAVID MARTINEZ

If your schedule's packed and you need a workout that works, we've developed one you can do in 30 minutes or less.

These three moves are part of our fast-paced circuit routine on page 239, which combines cardio and strength training to save time, stave off boredom, and crush fitness plateaus. And they hit just about every muscle you've got.

While the Seated V focuses on your abdominal and back muscles, the Hover and Hold works your upper body, and the Lunge with Cross Chop targets your lower body.

We put these three exercises into the circuit, but you can also quickly and easily incorporate any or all of them into your own program.

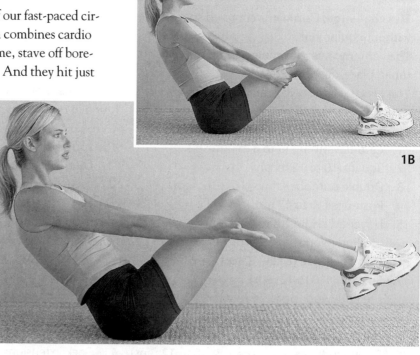

1A

1B

SEATED V

1A. Sit with your knees bent and abs tight. Maintain the natural curve of your spine as you hinge back from your hips.

1B. Extend your arms in front of you, then lift your legs off the floor slightly. Return to the starting position and repeat.

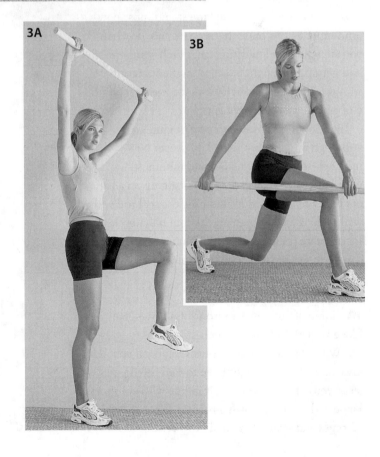

HOVER AND HOLD

2A. Lie facedown on the floor, keeping your knees bent slightly and your hands under your shoulders.

2B. Push up onto your knees. Use your abs to keep your back straight and look at the floor beyond your fingertips to keep your head from dropping. Slowly return to the starting position. Repeat 10 to 12 times.

<u>Trainer tip:</u> For more of a challenge, lift your knees off the floor into the plank position; hold and release.

LUNGE WITH CROSS CHOP

3A. With your feet hip distance apart, hold a wooden dowel in both hands (a broom handle or towel will work as well). Raise your left knee to hip level and lift your arms overhead.

3B. Take a long step back with your left foot and lower your left knee toward the floor. At the same time, draw the dowel down and across the front of your body. (To further challenge yourself, follow the dowel with your head.) Pause and return to starting position. Repeat 10 to 12 times, and switch legs. ■

Petra Kolber is a contributing editor. She is also a Reebok University master trainer and group fitness manager of Equinox in West Hollywood.

BODYWORK

Build a Better Butt

Here's a quick routine sure to tighten your tush.

BY PETRA KOLBER • PHOTOGRAPHY BY DAVID MARTINEZ

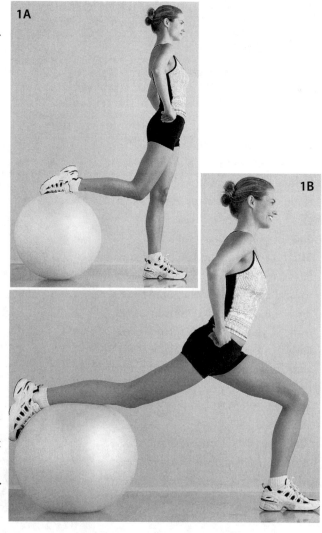

1A

1B

Some things are hard to hide. One of them is a great butt. Another one is a flabby butt. If yours falls into the latter category, it's better to use your glutes to your advantage than to chalk them up as a "problem area." Your gluteus maximus is one of the largest and most powerful muscles you have. It's a prime mover when you step out of a low-slung car, climb stairs, walk, and get up from a chair. Smart and consistent strength training can help displace the fat behind you with firmer and stronger glutes.

Traditional butt moves target the glute max and thigh muscles, but to call up deeper butt muscles—the gluteus medius and minimus—do your squats single-legged while balancing on a ball or chair. Steadying yourself during the ball roll and wall squat uses your back and abdominal muscles. Incorporate these exercises into your routine twice a week to see and feel changes in about eight weeks.

SINGLE-LEG SQUAT

1A. Stand about 2 feet in front of a fitness ball. Place your right foot on the ball.
1B. With your weight on the left foot, bend your left knee and lower your right knee toward the floor as far as you can while keeping it in line with your toes. Pause and return to starting position. Repeat 8 to 12 times and switch legs. Build to 3 sets.

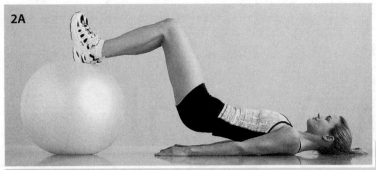

BALL ROLL

2A. Lie on your back with your knees bent and heels resting on a fitness ball. Raise your butt a few inches off the floor.

2B. Slide your heels away from you by extending your legs, keeping your back straight and your shoulders relaxed. Pause and return to starting position. Build to 3 sets of 8 to 12 repetitions.

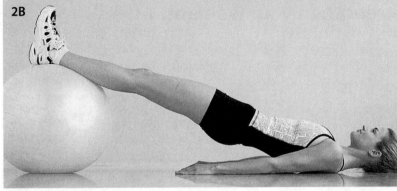

WALL SQUAT

3A. Stand with your back to a wall, resting your butt against a fitness ball. Your feet should be hip distance apart and about 2 feet away from the wall.

3B. Slowly roll your hips downward until your thighs are parallel with the floor. Pause and return to starting position. Build to 3 sets of 8 to 12 repetitions. ▨

Petra Kolber is a Contributing Editor and a Reebok University master trainer. You can reach her at her Web site (PetraKolber.com).

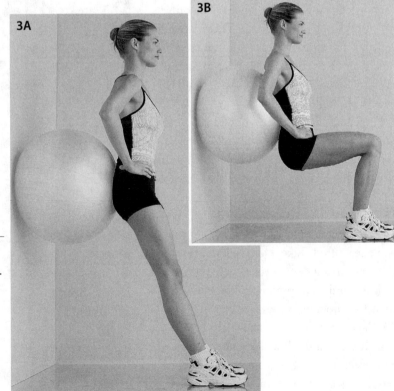

BODYWORK BODYWORK BODYWORK BODYWORK BODYWORK BODYWORK BODYWORK BODYWORK BODYWORK BODYWORK BODYWORK BODYWO

BODY WORK

Hip Appeal

Shape and strengthen your womanly assets.

BY PETRA KOLBER • PHOTOGRAPHY BY DAVID MARTINEZ

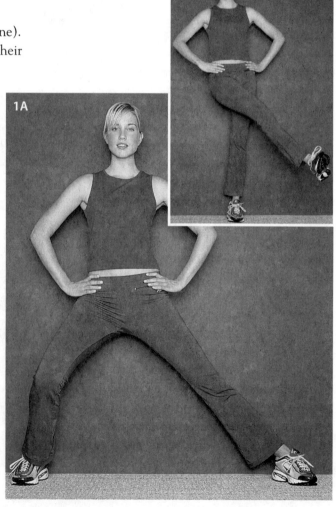

Hips endure some serious indignities. They've inspired terms like broad and BAM ("big-assed marine"—ask G.I. Jane). And lots of women consider them the bane of their existence.

It's time to show your hips some love and acknowledge their power, since you're only as strong and mobile as they are. These moves target your hips three-dimensionally, increasing fundamental strength for lunges and jumps, stability for quick direction changes, and balance with single-legged moves.

Three sets of each exercise—12 to 15 reps per side, three times a week—will produce results you'll start to feel in your stride after about three weeks and see in the mirror after about six weeks.

LUNGE AND CROSS

1A. Stand with your feet together, abs tight, and chest lifted. Take a long sideward step with your right leg. Keeping your knee in line with your toe and your spine straight, bend your right leg into a lunge position.

1B. Pause; push off with your right foot, straighten (but don't lock) your right knee, and sweep right leg in front of left. Then return to starting position. Complete one set, then switch sides.

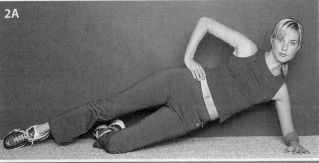

SIDE LEG RAISE

2A. Lie on your left side, holding your abdominal muscles tight, and prop yourself up on your left forearm, with your hips facing forward. Lift your left hip and fully extend your right leg while bending your left leg perpendicular to it.

2B. Keeping your abdominals tight, lift your right leg until it's parallel to the floor (don't shrug your shoulders). Pause and return to the starting position. Complete one set, then switch sides.

BRIDGE AND LEG EXTENSION

3A. Lie on your back with your left knee bent and your right leg extended. Place your hands at your sides, with your palms facing down.

3B. Keeping your right leg straight, contract your left glute and press through your left heel to raise your hips. Pause, then lower. Complete one set, then switch sides.

Petra Kolber is a Contributing Editor and Reebok University master trainer. She can be reached at our Web site (Health.com) or hers (PetraKolber.com).

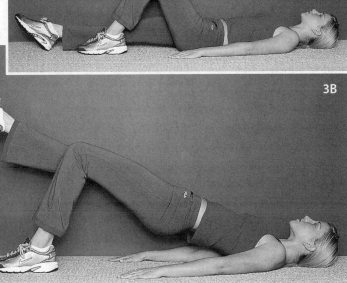

BODYWORK

3 Moves to Flat Abs

This multimuscle workout tightens your middle like no crunch can.

BY PETRA KOLBER • PHOTOGRAPHY BY DAVID MARTINEZ

Most people use their rectus abdominis, or crunch muscles, only when they raise their weary bodies out of bed. From then on, all the abs, not to mention the lower back, come into play, stabilizing you as you twist, reach, stand, walk, and run. So why spend all your time concentrating on muscles that you single out just once a day?

These moves put not only the rectus but the internal and external obliques to work, as well as the transversus abdominis—the innermost wall of muscle in your abdomen. Using all groups at once results in less workout time. Who couldn't use a few spare minutes?

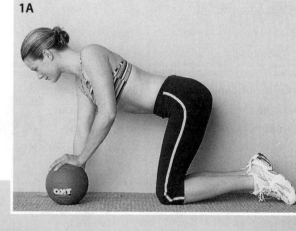

1A

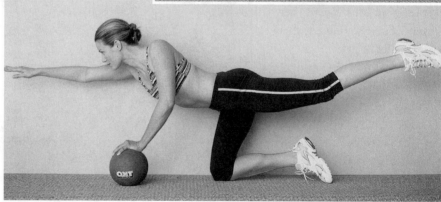

1B

QUADRUPED

1A. Kneel with your shoulders over your hands and your hips over your knees, keeping your weight evenly distributed. For more of a challenge, place a ball under your left hand.

1B. While contracting your abs, extend your right arm in front of you and your left leg behind you. Pause and return to the starting position. Repeat 8 to 12 times and switch sides. Build to 3 sets.

Trainer tip: Any kind of ball will do. Add one or more of these moves to your crunch routine, and you should see and feel a difference in four to six weeks.

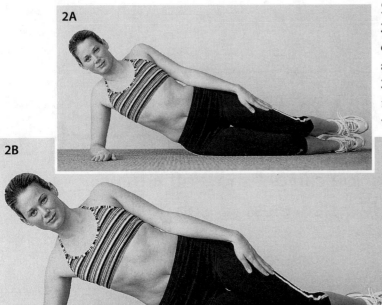

2A

2B

SIDE PLANK

2A. Lie on your right side, propped up on your elbow, with your knees bent and hips in line with each other.

2B. Keeping your abs tight; your neck in a relaxed, neutral position; and your shoulders down, lift your hips off the floor. Pause and return to the starting position. Repeat 8 to 12 times and switch sides. Build to 3 sets.

BALL REACH

3A. Stand on your left leg, with your knee slightly bent. Hold a ball at chest height.

3B. Keeping your abs tight, extend both arms up and out to the left. At the same time, extend your right leg behind you. Contract your abs to return to the starting position. Repeat 8 to 12 times and switch sides. Build to 3 sets.

<u>Trainer tip:</u> We've used a medicine ball for this exercise, but any ball will add a focal point or element of stability to the move. ▪

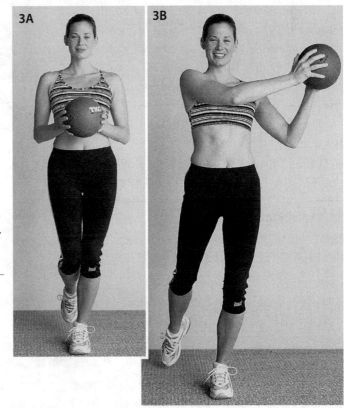

3A

3B

Petra Kolber is a Contributing Editor. Her new workout videos, Ready Step Go! *and* Breathe II, *are available at her Web site (PetraKolber.com).*

BODYWORK BODYWORK BODYWORK BODYWORK BODYWORK BODYWORK BODYWORK BODYWORK BODYWORK BODYWORK

BODY WORK

Toning Your Triceps

Here's how you can get show-off arms and never fear sleeveless season again.

BY PETRA KOLBER • PHOTOGRAPHY BY DAVID MARTINEZ

If you're stressing over upper-arm jiggle (or "bat wings," as some call it), don't. The triceps, three-part muscles that run along the back of each arm from the elbow to the shoulder, are at ease when you wave, point, or perform similar motions, so it's natural for them to swing a little.

Anatomy doesn't excuse a general lack of tone here, though. With the right exercises, you can minimize wobble while you maximize strength—loose triceps (the largest muscle group of the arm) don't justify running for the cover of a cardigan.

These simple moves hit the triceps from every angle. Do one or two of them, two to three days per week, alternating regularly to keep your routine challenging. You should see results in four to six weeks (rest at least a day between workouts.) Shoot for 1 to 3 sets of 8 to 12 repetitions.

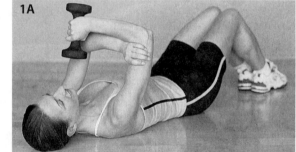

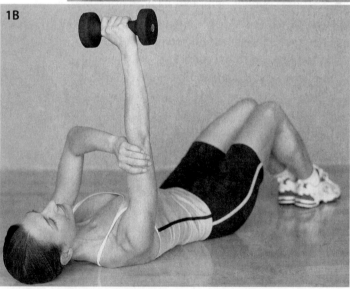

TRICEPS EXTENSION

1A. Lie on your back with a weight in your right hand. Extend your right arm up and steady it with your left hand.

1B. Keeping your right elbow directly above your shoulder, slowly bend it and draw your right hand toward your left shoulder. Contract your triceps to return to the starting position.

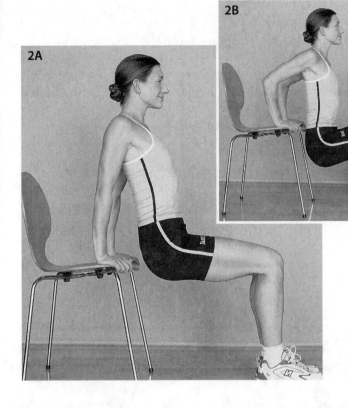

TRICEPS DIP

2A. Sit on the edge of a chair with your hands shoulder-width apart and fingers facing forward. Slide your hips off the seat by walking yourself forward until your knees are bent at a 90-degree angle.
2B. Keeping your shoulders down and elbows pointing behind you, lower your hips. Return to the starting position.

TRICEPS PUSH-UP

3A. Kneel, with your hands under your shoulders, knees in line with hips, and abdominals pulled in.
3B. Keeping your elbows close to your sides, lower your chest toward the floor. Pause, then return to the starting position. ▪

Petra Kolber is a contributing editor and Reebok University master trainer. She can be reached at our Web site (Health.com) or hers (PetraKolber.com).

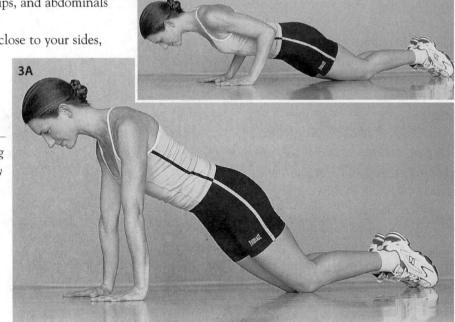

249

BODYWORK

Sexy Shoulders

Shape your shoulders with three easy moves (they'll make you stronger, too).

BY PETRA KOLBER • PHOTOGRAPHY BY DAVID MARTINEZ

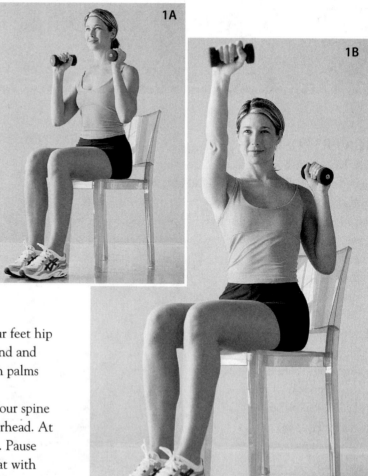

You appreciate shoulder strength when you hoist your carry-on into an overhead bin or stand for 30 minutes trying to hail a cab. Luckily, the same exercises that build your muscles can give you show-off shoulders as well.

These muscles are delicate, though, so start off with weights no heavier than 5 pounds. Work toward three sets of each exercise before adding weight. Doing this routine two or three times a week for six to eight weeks can make your shoulders look almost as good as they perform.

ARM RAISE WITH TORSO TWIST

1A. Sit on a chair or fitness ball with your feet hip distance apart. Hold a weight in each hand and bring your hands to shoulder height, with palms facing each other.

1B. Keeping your abdominals tight and your spine long, exhale and raise your right arm overhead. At the same time, turn your body to the left. Pause and return to the starting position. Repeat with the opposite arm. Build to 3 sets of 8 to 12 reps.

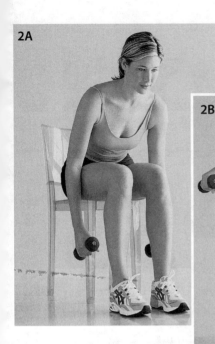

REAR-DELTOID SQUEEZE

2A. Sit on a chair and hinge forward from your hips (or lie facedown with a fitness ball under your abdomen). With your abdominal muscles tight and your spine long, hold a weight in each hand and let your arms rest at your sides.

2B. Without lifting your gaze from the floor, think of squeezing your shoulder blades together as you raise both arms to shoulder height. Pause and return to the starting position. Build to 3 sets of 8 to 12 repetitions.

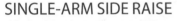

SINGLE-ARM SIDE RAISE

3A. Sit with your feet hip distance apart. Hold a weight in each hand and let your arms rest at your sides.

3B. Raise your right arm to shoulder height as you flex your foot and extend your left leg. Pause and return to the starting position. Repeat with the opposite arm and leg. Build to 3 sets of 8 to 12 repetitions. ▧

Petra Kolber is a contributing editor and a Reebok University master trainer. You can reach her at her Web site (PetraKolber.com).

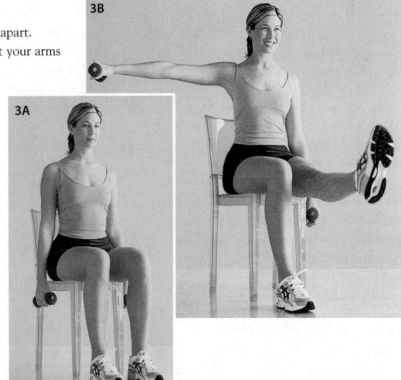

BODYWORK BODYWORK BODYWORK BODYWORK BODYWORK BODYWORK BODYWORK BODYWORK BODYWORK BODYWORK BODYWORK BODYWORK BODYWORK BODYWORK BODYWORK BODYWORK BODYWORK BODYWORK BODYWORK

Dressing for Fitness

A former fashion writer should always look her best—even when she's kayaking, rappelling, or trail-running.

BY PATRICIA JACOBS

Are you a pro?" the young Russian guy asked, grinning down at me. My face was still glistening after a two-hour bike ride from Manhattan to Coney Island, and I was stretched out on a boardwalk bench, tucking into a pile of Nathan's fries. I wondered if his expression was one of admiration or amusement.

I was training for my first adventure race—a sort of relay in which you mountain-bike, run, and kayak over miles of hellish terrain. I was also showing off my brand-new iridescent-green Stumpjumper bike, my fabulous black-and-yellow Pearl Izumi cleats, and my red Ralph Lauren jersey. And in my pocket was a tiny Topeak Alien tool kit so cool it would even make MacGyver jealous. I was so fly I probably could've taken on Lance Armstrong—or at least I looked like I could.

> I invested in shoes that kept me going despite wet feet and the occasional blister. For this, my Montrails beat my Manolos hands down.

This scenario was many miles and a decade away from my former fashionista days as a writer for the *New York Post*. Back then, my job was to clock the rise and fall of hemlines and search for the coolest clothes from Milan to Paris. However, in 2000, through a series of strange turns, I found myself accepting an invitation to Borneo to write a story about the Eco-Challenge, one of the world's toughest adventure races. That meant trailing four-person coed teams for 12 days and 300 miles as they traversed disease-filled rivers and jungles teeming with leeches, malarial mosquitoes, and mud slides.

As I watched the racers, I noticed that no matter how tired, sweaty, battered, or bloodied they were, they always crossed the finish line exhilarated, like kids fresh from a dirt fight. After reporting from the sidelines, I was ready to play.

So I attended a fitness camp, where I learned such out-of-comfort-zone feats as biking along mountain curves and walking tightropes. I completed a minitriathlon, in which I walked half of the three-mile run. I loved every single minute of it.

Then I joined an adventure-racing club, full of other folks to kayak and rappel off trees with. I took up trail running. I also learned to dress the part, in clothes that wick away sweat, protect in a downpour, and help you stay cool even in a heat wave. I invested in shoes that kept me going despite wet feet and the occasional blister. For this, my Montrails beat my Manolos hands down.

My Chanel bracelet studded with gold Cs is the single luxury item I wear amongst the gear. It isn't very practical, but apparently most racers have a talisman. I still covet Gucci, Dior, Marc, and Prada. But I also revere Suunto, Columbia, Salomon, and Patagonia. Though Jamin Puech makes a to-die-for purse, it does nada for a deep-down body thirst compared with a cool drink from a Camelbak.

Resting on that Coney Island bench, refueled for the ride home, my body pleaded with me to take the subway. But my inner racer summoned me back onto the bike.

Those Eco-Challengers are on to something. Adventure racing is a metaphor for the resiliency of the spirit: In spite of adversity, you can work harder and become stronger. The right clothes can help, too, even when they're full of sweat, bike grease, and the occasional leech. Looking at the Russian guy's smile, I decided it was one of admiration. And to answer his question: Why, yes, I am a pro. ■

London-born Patricia Jacobs bikes, writes, and paints in New York City.

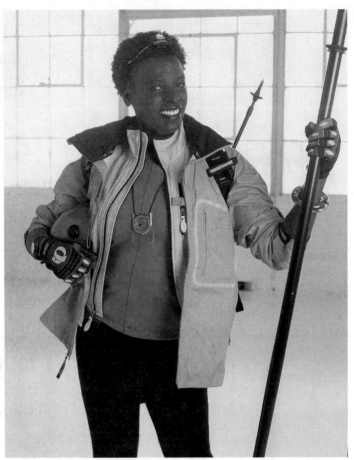

I was so fly I could've taken on Lance Armstrong—or at least I looked like I could.

Be Your Own Personal Trainer

Assuming you're not the type of person who shows up for a workout only if someone's counting on you, it's possible to save money by thinking of your personal trainer as a teacher instead of a gym pal. Pay attention to her suggestions, and when you feel comfortable (expect it to take about two to three weeks), do your workout alone: A recent study found that women who go solo with a routine they know well and who continue exercising consistently were able to maintain both strength gains and body-fat losses.

FUN
&FITNESS
do mix

One woman's hip-hop class challenges her body … and her self-image.

BY SHARON GOLDMAN EDRY

I stood in the back row of the studio, wearing my trusty black leggings and cropped white T-shirt. I was trying not to stare at the two dozen J. Lo and 'N Sync wanna-bes surrounding me, complete with tight abs, bare navels, and taut backsides. I had decided to put myself to the ultimate exercise test with a 4:30 p.m. hip-hop class at New York City's Broadway Dance Center, but as I watched the chorus of lithe young things stretch in preparation, I suddenly wondered if I was really the ultimate idiot. I was concerned that I'd need a paramedic before class was over.

> **I hadn't danced in years and had never really accepted my over-21 body.**

It wasn't always this way. When I was a kid, dancing was no sweat. Four days a week, from ages 6 to 16, I fairly flew to my local dance studio for hours of fun and freedom in ballet, jazz, or tap classes, where I would admire myself in the mirror, marveling at my thin, graceful body and its feats of flexibility. I used to be able to lift my right leg and put it behind my left ear—standing up!

But things have changed over the years—and not just the fact that my right leg and left ear haven't met since college. My stomach isn't as flat, my backside is a lot flatter, my top half is getting positively jiggly, and the backs of

254

my thighs are not-so-slowly turning into cottage cheese. I seriously needed to get my fitness act in gear. So, I thought, why not revisit my childhood passion? After dabbling in everything from Pilates and yoga to kickboxing and Spinning, I liked the idea of going back to something I was good at and had once enjoyed. On the other hand, I didn't want to get bored, so I passed on classes like beginner's ballet. I wanted to be with "real" dancers. Like me.

So that's how I ended up standing behind a row of hot bodies, wondering whether I'd lost my mind. The truth was, I hadn't danced at all for several years, had never taken a hip-hop class, and had never really accepted my over-21 body. I suffered a slight panic attack when the dance teacher, a petite African-American woman in a sports bra and low-rise tights, without an ounce of fat on her body, entered the room and turned up some thumping music. "I only have one rule," she shouted. "If you stop, I'll freak."

Pretty soon, I started to freak. Within five minutes of hip shaking and pelvis thrusting, I was huffing and puffing. Looking at myself in the mirror, I saw nothing that remotely resembled the dancer of yesteryear. I tripped over my own feet, and my face was getting redder and sweatier by the moment. I felt awkward and silly, but mostly I felt envious. *I used to look like them*, I thought. *I used to jump like that. I used to move like that....*

After 30 minutes, I was amazed that I'd survived. I even made it through the one-handed push-ups. (OK, I did cheat on those.) Then it dawned on me: That was only the warm-up. I was halfway to the door when I realized that I wasn't going to change my body—certainly not that day. What I needed to change was my mind-set. Who cares what the class teenyboppers thought of my less-than-firm rear and my pitiful moves? I was there to have a good time and get my heart rate up. And it was up—way up.

So I went back, banishing all negative thoughts as we began to work on some choreographed moves. I studiously avoided my reflection and kept my eyes either on the teacher or the pink-haired girl in front of me who seemed to know what she was doing. The next thing I knew, there were only 10 minutes left. I listened to the driving beat of the latest Janet Jackson tune and started to shake. And thrust. And shimmy. When I finished, no one in the room was sweatier or more red-faced than I—and no one wore a wider smile.

No, Ms. Jackson will never hire me as a backup dancer, and my stomach will never again see 16-year-old tautness. But I definitely got what I'd gone there for: a couple of hours of fun, freedom, and fitness. ■

Sharon Goldman Edry also writes for TV Guide, Self, *and the* New York Daily News.

Get Over Yourself

Beat the I-can't-do-this blues with these confidence boosters from Joan Price, author of *Yes, You CAN Get in Shape!*

Just show up. That's most important. Even if you're feeling weird in class, remember that you succeeded the moment you walked through the door.

Pick your own milestones. Don't compare yourself to the you of yesterday or to anyone else in the room.

Remember why you're there. Did you make the leap into a new activity because it inspires you or makes you feel good? Staying in touch with why you're there may help you feel less self-critical.

Bring a buddy. It'll help lighten the experience when you can laugh with—and at—each other and gossip about Ms. Firm Butt next to you.

Change your vocabulary. Instead of saying "I can't dance," for example, tell yourself, "I just haven't learned to dance yet." No matter what your new fitness challenge is, this trick can help change your self-defeating beliefs, Price says.

When Om Turns to OUCH!

Beware of these four most common yoga injuries.

BY MARTICA K. HEANER

With every new fitness trend comes a rush of fans—followed by a rash of injuries. In the '70s, gung-ho runners racked up miles and shinsplints. In the '80s, energized aerobicisers pounded their way to foot, ankle, knee, and back pain. In the '90s, enthusiastic Tae-Bo-style kicks and punches also knocked elbows, hips, and shoulders out of joint. The latest craze—yoga—may seem like a gentler pursuit, but don't be fooled. Its seemingly stress-free moves are straining as many bodies as they are soothing souls.

Yoga is no safer than a fitness class, according to Leslie Kaminoff, a yoga therapist who specializes in treating the aching bodies of both yoga novices and veteran teachers at The Breathing Project, his Manhattan studio. "What ups the injury rate is that the popular classes are often physically challenging types of yoga in which it's easy to push too hard."

If you've paid for a yoga class, your first instinct might be to get your money's worth and work through any pain, but don't. Instead, prevent strains by warming up thoroughly and stretching only as far as you feel comfortable, despite what an overzealous teacher or experienced classmate might say. Many yoga poses take years of practice to master. And don't forget that serious or chronic pain is your cue to call a sports physician or physical therapist.

We've listed four common yoga aches, ways to avoid them, and advice on when to see a doctor.

LOTUS LOCK

Description: Pain when you sharply bend or simultaneously bend and twist your knees at extreme angles, as in the lotus pose, in which you sit cross-legged with each foot hooked into the crook of the opposite leg

Cause: Any position that bends and twists at the knees—a painful combination for many people. "I've seen lots of torn cartilage from positions like the lotus that put excess torque on the joints," Kaminoff says.

Prevention: Avoid moves that bend or twist any joint past your comfort point. The lotus pose is often used in meditation. Instead, sit cross-legged with your legs folded loosely beneath you or meditate while standing, lying down, or sitting in a chair.

Other culprits: Extreme bent-knee positions, such as the child's pose, hero pose, and pigeon

When to seek help: Anytime your knee swells, hurts, won't bend as far as usual, or won't straighten completely

DOWNWARD DOG-ITIS

Description: Strain or inflammation of your wrist, elbow, or shoulder joints, caused by such poses as the downward-facing dog

Cause: The shoulders are designed for mobility, not brute strength. You're liable to strain your wrists, elbows, or shoulders if you perform long, strenuous sequences supporting your weight on your hands. "I've seen people who have thrown out their shoulder joints from the overextension of their arms during the downward dog," says Paul Juris, Ed.D., director of the Equinox Fitness Training Institute in Palm Desert, California.

Prevention: While you build your strength and stamina, limit the time you spend on your hands. If your wrists, elbows, and shoulders continue to hurt, avoid those poses altogether and see if your pain fades. Maintain good upper-back alignment when bearing weight on your hands by lowering your shoulders and drawing your shoulder blades together. Strengthening wrists and shoulders with light weights can help, too. Do three sets of 8 to 12 wrist curls and lateral raises three times a week.

Other culprits: Stressful arm moves, such as the plank pose, upward-facing dog, and handstands

When to seek help: If you feel numbness or pain in your hands or pain in the wrists, fingers, elbow, or shoulders

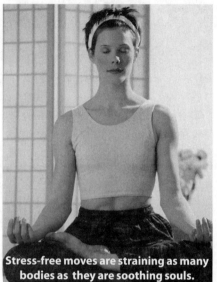

Stress-free moves are straining as many bodies as they are soothing souls.

INVERSION PERVERSIONS

Description: Neck or shoulder pain when too much weight is placed on your back while it's bent, as in the plow pose

Cause: "Herniated discs, chronic arthritis, and degenerative disc disease in the neck and lower back are the main injuries I see from yoga," says Stuart Kahn, M.D., director of the Spine Institute at Beth Israel Medical Center in New York City.

Prevention: "Avoid head and shoulder stands until you've spent several years building the flexibility to perform them," Kahn says. "When you do them, be extra-careful when rolling up into the position, as that's the most stressful part. Don't drop your legs over your head into the plow pose."

Other culprits: Neck-straining poses, such as shoulder stands, the camel, and headstands

When to seek help: If you experience severe or chronic pain in your neck or shoulders

SPINAL ZAP

Description: Low-back pain from vigorous or prolonged forward bends or twisting poses

Cause: Severe spinal bending or twisting, which can rupture discs or overstretch spinal ligaments

Prevention: Some yoga classes use the sun salutation to warm up, but that's a bad idea because it begins and ends with a standing forward bend. Before class, warm up on a cycle or treadmill. Do mobility exercises, such as shoulder and neck rolls as well as light stretches, before you attempt hard-core yoga postures. Also, strengthen and stabilize your abs and back with such poses as the boat and fitness-ball exercises.

Other culprits: Twists, such as the revolved triangle, and deep bending, as in seated forward bends

When to seek help: If you feel acute or chronic low-back pain ■

Q + A

WATCH OUT FOR LOCKED KNEES

My yoga instructor tells us to lock our knees in some standing poses, but my trainer says this is risky. Who's right?

Your trainer is correct. Maya Breuer, a certified yoga instructor and owner of Tomaya Studio in Providence, Rhode Island, says that locking your knees while standing can force the joints to bend backward slightly and increase your chance of injury. "I guide my students to gently lift their kneecaps, which engages the quadriceps without locking the knee," Breuer says.

Moving a Little Helps a Lot
New studies show small strides lead to big heart gains.

Trimming a few inches from your waistline isn't the only reason to exercise. Two recent studies have found that even moderate

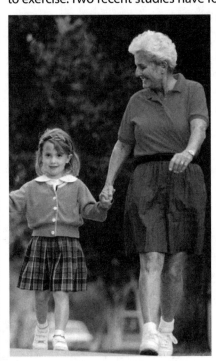

amounts of low-intensity activity can safeguard your heart, even if your weight doesn't budge. Duke University researchers discovered that walking just a couple of miles most days of the week can protect you from heart disease and stroke by transforming smaller, heavier—and more dangerous—cholesterol particles into larger, lighter ones that are less likely to clog arteries. A Cooper Institute study determined that performing any exercise can help lower C-reactive protein levels in your blood (high levels can put your heart in peril).

Q + A

STOP SWEATING THE WEIGHT CHARTS

Is body-mass index (BMI) a better way to tell if you're overweight than the old height-weight charts?

Both of these tools are handy for epidemiologists and other public health types who study large, diverse groups of people. "In fact, the old charts may have been more useful for individuals, because they considered frame size," says Richard Cotton, a spokesman for the American Council on Exercise. The best gauge of what you should weigh, Cotton says, is in your closet. So stop sweating the charts, he advises. Exercise, eat right, and rely on that trusty pair of jeans to track your weight.

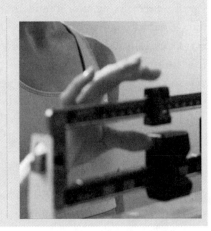

Belly Dance Your Way to a Better Body Image

Shimmying can loosen your hips—and your inhibitions.

BY DOROTHY FOLTZ-GRAY

Belly dancing never struck me as an athletic endeavor. But when, on separate occasions, two fitness buffs mentioned this Middle Eastern ritual as a boost to body and ego, I was suspicious—and curious. I found a class, and once assured belly baring was optional, I signed up.

The class met in a dance studio in Knoxville, Tennessee, with full-length mirrors across one wall. Instead of exotic-looking temptresses, the other 10 or so women in the group were reassuringly ordinary, in their 20s to 50s. Most were plump or out-of-shape office workers, doctors, even bartenders looking for a fun way to shake off stress. One 34-year-old beginner said, "If I don't start moving soon, I never will."

And move we did. Mere seconds after instructor Debbie Ashton, a dancer turned physical therapist, started the music, we were hoisting our rib cages and rotating our hips. The movements were simple and natural, our pelvises turning in circles and our torsos winding in figure eights. Halfway through the hour-long session, our brows were damp and our legs ached from dancing with slightly bent knees.

It's a workout all right, but for me, the class also could have counted as a one-hour massage. My normally tight back felt loose and limber. Gyrating my pelvis and rib cage actually eased my cramped back muscles—even the tiny ones between each vertebra that jogging or walking doesn't stretch.

We all felt more relaxed. As we faced the mirror, our hips and stomachs—some draped in colorful scarves jangling with decorative coins—turned provocative, curvy, and sexy. We began laughing, exaggerating the swivels. Our femininity had been set free. (Certainly our hips had.) The burden of skinny expectations shook loose as well. "What's affected me is seeing both overweight and thin women doing this and looking sexy," says Stacy Smith-Foley, 27, a radiology resident who has lost 30 pounds since taking up the pastime. "This shows me that, no matter what the scale says, I can be OK with my body."

"We spend so much time trying to get rid of these beautiful hips," says Karen Andes, a Middle Eastern dance teacher and author of *A Woman's Book of Power*. But belly dancing changes that, Andes says. "You accent that area, you decorate it, and so you start to have ownership of your hips, thighs, and buttocks as they are."

Barbara Enloe, a 5-foot-9-inch, 300-pound 40-year-old, agrees. "If you can walk, talk, and breathe, you have the skills to do this," she says. "Size doesn't matter, because there's such elegance and power to the movement. I see the way I'm moving, and it looks and feels wonderful."

As I watch Ashton, who has been teaching this art for 26 years, shimmy forward, lifting and lowering her seemingly double-jointed hips, I find that it's true—the dance's energy is celebratory, not critical. It doesn't induce the lose-weight-or-else grimace that stairstepping and kickboxing can. It has a kind of whimsy that lifts the spirits as well as the rib cage.

"Hip, hip, shimmy, drop," Ashton chants. "Now I see the music in your butt." ▪

Dorothy Foltz-Gray is a contributing editor.

259

Take These Steps to a Healthy Body

Use Pilates to get more from your walking workout.

BY DOROTHY FOLTZ-GRAY

A physical therapist once told me that he could almost always predict which runner would win a race just from observing his or her hip motion. "The more control you have over your hips," he said, "the better you perform."

I thought about that during a Pilates workshop devoted to improving my walking technique at Head-to-Toe Pilates Training, a studio near Huntsville, Alabama. I don't think much about how I walk, but as co-owner and workshop instructor Daniel Tripp would say, that's precisely the point. Everyone could be walking smarter, he asserts, whether they're lacing up for a daily turn around the park or schlepping from the sofa to the fridge.

Aside from looking less than graceful, a sloppy gait is a waste of energy and a sure way to injure yourself. By delegating some of the load to your abdominal and hip muscles, you can walk faster and more efficiently, reduce your risk of injury, and eliminate much of walking's joint-jarring impact. With fewer pains and strains, you might even walk farther. And that means you'll burn more calories.

Learning to rely on the deep stabilizer muscles in your trunk is the central tenet of Pilates, an exercise philosophy developed by Joseph Pilates in the 1920s that is one of the hottest fitness phenomena around.

Tripp's workshop is based on one offered by New York City's Physicalmind Institute, which trains Pilates instructors in Europe and North America. (For more info on workshops, call 800-505-1990 or visit www.the-method.com.)

Tripp starts his class by asking us to analyze our walking patterns. We dip our feet in finger paint, then walk across a long sheet of paper, revealing the individuality of our gaits. We become self-conscious, like teenagers in swimsuits, while Tripp points out the idiosyncrasies of our strides as we stroll around the studio. Some walk with freakishly still heads and hips, others move as if their shoulders and arms are welded in place. Some turn their feet and knees inward, splay their feet outward, or favor one leg. A few take short, constricted steps, squelching the flow of a longer, more natural walk.

Each of these posture and movement problems can hamper your ability to move fluidly. "In a perfect gait, you have muscle balance, or equal strength in the opposing muscles," says Christine Romani-Ruby, a physical therapist at PowerHouse Pilates Wellness and Rehabilitation near Pittsburgh. "But when you start using one muscle more than the others, it creates an imbalance that affects how you move and walk."

Correcting such imbalances reintroduces ease into your stride. For example, when Tripp asks me to roll each hip forward smoothly before I step, relax my shoulders, and hold in my stomach, I feel tension leave my lower back, where I often experience post-workout pain. "If your hips aren't rotating," Tripp tells me, "the force of hitting the ground ends at your hip joint instead of dissipating through the rest of your body." He points out that any change in gait will seem awkward at first. "But if you remain conscious of your movements, it won't take nearly the amount of time to do them right as it took to do them wrong," he says. "The mind will shape the body. Practice daily, and you'll see change within weeks."

For our next exercise, we sit on the floor with our legs extended in front of us. Tripp asks us to "walk" in this seated position, swiveling one hip forward, then the other, swinging our arms to help propel us. We scoot along on our behinds, arms pumping,

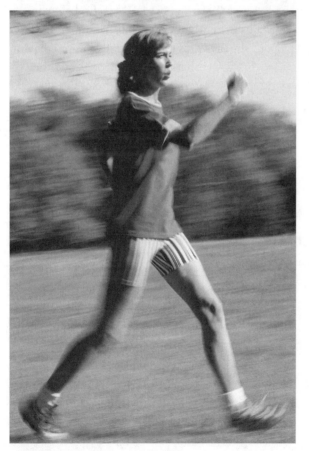

looking like Ls in locomotion. He wants us to sense how our arms move in opposition to our hips and how involved our pelvis and stomach muscles should be in moving us forward. Removing our legs from the equation convinces us how hard the muscles below the surface work—or could, if we let them.

So how do we let them? It starts and ends with awareness, Tripp says. If you think about how you walk and you know the correct way, you'll simply do it better. This walking-awareness checklist will get you started.

Pull your navel toward your spine. Your abdominal muscles will form a girdle of stability, and your movements will be more controlled (you'll have great abs, besides). As you walk, let your arms swing, but try not to swivel your torso—its job is to support movement.

Consciously engage your butt and thigh muscles. As you prepare to take a step, focus on your trailing leg, creating a crease where your butt and thigh meet by lifting your cheek and tightening your hamstring. Continue to use those muscles as you bring that leg forward. Notice how your inner thigh muscles keep your knee pointed forward and stabilize your leg.

Walk with your toes pointing forward. "Turning your toes out can stress the knees," Tripp says. When you walk, allow your heel to strike first, then push off from the big toe, flexing at the ankle.

Relax your shoulders. Hold them back and down, and resist the tendency to hunch or shrug.

Hold your head high. Loping forward headfirst stresses your neck and throws your gait off balance. To distribute the force of gravity over your body along the natural curves of your spine, walk as if you're suspended by a string attached to the top of your head. Or just recall that old charm-school drill of walking while balancing a book on your head.

Sure, it takes work to imagine—and place—your body into a perfect walking posture. But in the two months since I attended the workshop, I've been surprised at how aware I am of the way I move and stand. I haven't revolutionized my walk, but for now, it's nice to know I'm moving in a healthier way. ■

Going the Distance

Preparing for their first 5K, these women discovered resolve they never knew they had.

BY MICHELE J. MORRIS

Four years ago, the most exercise Jill Smedley could fit into her busy schedule was chasing after her two toddlers. Long gone were her high school days of running track and playing softball. She was burned-out and overweight.

Today, Smedley is 30 pounds lighter, and, at 38, a fast-moving mother of three children, ages 9, 6, and 2. At 5:30 each morning, she's off for a run, a practice she says has resurrected her spirit and the active person she used to be.

She found her outlet in the company of other women bent on reaching a common goal: to walk or run their first 5K race. They were part of First Strides, a 12-week class that has helped more than 400 women in the Allentown, Pennsylvania, area out of their ruts since its creation seven years ago by Jane Serues, a financial planner and long-time runner.

Newcomers in the female group are teamed with an experienced runner to train for the Allentown Women's 5K Classic, an annual fund-raiser for breast-cancer research and treatment. "The mental, emotional, and even spiritual rewards of running

> You find out you can walk farther than you used to, or run faster or longer. It's that measurable improvement that motivates people.
> —Jane Serues

have been incredible," Smedley says. "The mentors who coached me were great cheerleaders. They had mountains of faith in my abilities and encouraged me every step of the way."

First Strides does wonders for women's confidence levels, says 54-year-old Serues. "You find out you can walk farther than you used to, or run faster or longer," she says. "It's that measurable improvement that motivates people, and they tend to impress themselves."

Class participants pay $40 for weekly group training and support. To 54-year-old Ann Gastinger, that was a bargain. Running regularly with other women was what she needed to help her cope with her husband's death after his three-year struggle with Lou Gehrig's disease. "I really didn't care about anything. I was using food and school to fill the hours between work and sleep," says Gastinger, a chemist for a gas and chemical company in Trexlertown, Pennsylvania.

"I feel better about myself now," Gastinger says. "And even if I have a little setback, the class taught me that I can gradually do anything—if I have patience and a plan." ■

Need a Reason to Run?
Benefits of running—not just for younger set

Who says you need to run five or six miles at a time to reap health benefits? A recent Stanford University study says that running as few as six miles per week can provide men and women ages 55 and over with a bundle of body bonuses, including greater bone density, less pain, and—here's the kicker—the ability to stay active longer. Don't like to run? Study co-author and professor of medicine Jim Fries, M.D., says that any cardio activity of similar intensity—such as brisk walking, hiking, or hill climbing—can give you the same gains. As for the younger set, it's never too early to begin habits that will keep you going strong into your senior years.

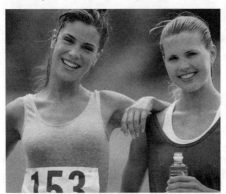

Lace Up Your Skates for a New Type of Marathon

While marathons for runners are nothing new, a small but growing number of women looking for a challenge have begun to lace up their inline skates to cover the 26.2-mile distance. And we're not just talking shiny-suited pros—a *Health* staffer recently skated her first marathon alongside a 59-year-old grandmother and a 40-something mom with her teenage son. Because skating a race requires less training time than hoofing it and is considerably gentler on joints, adding wheels to the mix opens the long-distance door to people who otherwise wouldn't be able to participate. Don't get us wrong: You still have to prepare, and 26.2 miles is no joke any way you cover it. Intrigued but looking for something a little less hard-core? Consider a half-marathon instead. Check out www.active.com to find an upcoming race.

Q + A

FITNESS BALL BUYING GUIDE

I'm shopping for an inflatable fitness ball to use at home. How do I know which size to get?

We're big ball fans, too (in fact, several of us use them instead of desk chairs). Generally, your knees and hips should be at the same height when you sit on the ball. Can't try before you buy? Use these guidelines: If you're less than 5 feet tall, opt for a 45-centimeter ball; if you're between 5 and 6 feet, try one that's 55 centimeters; and if you're over 6 feet, go with a 65-centimeter model. Don't skimp: Bigger balls may be harder to find and more expensive, but working out with one that's too small can overstress your back.

If you're a beginner, you may want to go a size or two larger than what's recommended for your height. The bigger the ball, the more support it offers, making exercise easier.

How to Choose
THE BEST BIKE
for Your Body

BY DIMITY McDOWELL

If you've ever found yourself stretching like Gumby to reach the handlebars of a bicycle and endured that torture in the name of fresh air and exercise—or given up on cycling altogether—listen up. Today's bikes are engineered to fit women's bodies better and reduce strain; plus, they're easier to find and more affordable than ever before. That's welcome news for women who want to take advantage of this low-impact, perfect-for-spring activity but haven't had very much luck with conventional frames, which are based on a man's body proportions.

If the last bicycle you owned had streamers and a banana seat, you could probably use some buying advice.

A woman who is 5 feet 6 inches or less will benefit most from choosing an anatomically correct bike. (Taller women may have an equally difficult time finding bikes that fit, but it's easier to adjust men's cycles to their physiques.) A female-friendly frame has a shortened top tube (it runs from the seat to the handlebars) and a lengthened head tube (on which the handlebars sit), helping position a woman's shorter upper body more comfortably. The handlebars, grips, and gears are all scaled down for a woman's narrower shoulders and smaller hands, and the saddle is designed to ease pressure on the genitals.

Women-specific bikes aren't exactly new. Terry started making them in the mid-1980s, but because of their limited distribution, the early models weren't easy to come by. Today, all the major bicycle manufacturers—including Specialized, Cannondale, Trek, and Giant—make tailored frames, fueled by the growth of women's cycling. According to a survey conducted by the National Bicycle Dealers Association, 5.8 million women rode at least 10 monthly miles during 2000.

Still, if the last bicycle you owned had streamers and a banana seat, you could probably use some buying advice. Try a hybrid or comfort bike; both are sturdy, with flat handlebars that allow you to sit in a more upright position than the typical road rig. Hybrids have skinnier wheels, which are better suited for roads and paved paths, while the wider tires of comfort models make negotiating dirt roads somewhat smoother (the knobby, superwide tires of mountain bikes offer the most comfortable off-road ride of all, though).

Expect to spend at least $300 for a quality cycle. The higher the price, the lighter the bike; you'll also get better gears and brakes. "The main difference you'll feel between a $300 bike and a $700 one is that you can climb hills easier and accelerate faster," says Kay Caunt, owner of Criterium Bicycles in Colorado Springs, Colorado. Regardless of your bike's weight, it can last as long as 10 years with annual tune-ups.

Because a specific model is tailored to the female form doesn't mean it's the right one for *your* form. Here's our expert's bike-shopping advice.

Play dumb. "When you go in, identify yourself as a beginner," Caunt says. "That way, somebody should take the time to measure and fit you, and explain things thoroughly."

Go for a test-drive. Ride long enough that you become familiar with how the bike works and feels. Are your back and shoulders comfortable? Stand up while pedaling to make sure your knees don't graze the handlebars. Take a couple of corners to see how the cycle handles turns.

Pick the gear shift you like best. Opting for a rapid-fire shifter, which lets you change gears with your index finger and thumb, or a grip shifter, which does the same thing with a turn of the grip (like the choke on a motorcycle), is merely personal preference.

Ride at least three different bikes. "If you can't feel a difference between them, you haven't ridden them long enough," Caunt advises. ▪

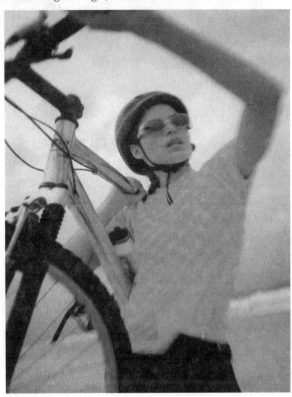

Warm Up to Work Out Longer

Your Spinning instructor may urge you to feel the burn, but you might be able to spurn the heat while working just as hard. A recent study published in the journal *Medicine & Science in Sports & Exercise* found that when stationary cyclists warmed up with some easy pedaling plus a few bursts of more strenuous work before going full speed, their muscles produced less lactate—that's the stuff responsible for the searing sensation that makes most folks want to give up and go lie on the sofa. The study looked only at cycling, but lead author Susan C. Gray, Ph.D., of Napier University in Scotland, suspects the results may apply to other intense sports as well.

Is Your Water Bottle Hibernating?

Staying hydrated during winter workouts is just as important as it is when you're exercising in the heat of summer, says Nancy Clark, R.D., director of nutrition services at the SportsMedicine Association in Brookline, Massachusetts. Your body's still heating up under those layers, and frigid air can be pretty dry. So be sure to tank up before and after your workout.

LATE BLOOMERS

Five women realize it's never too late to discover the athlete within.

BY DOROTHY FOLTZ-GRAY • PHOTOGRAPHY BY DANA EDMUNDS AND TOM RAYMOND

I was born to be an athlete. The trouble was, my body didn't know it. I was the fat kid always picked last for the team. I couldn't serve a volleyball or climb a rope. Still, I was spellbound by the Olympics. I yearned to be lean and sleek, capable of impossible feats.

Those longings resurfaced when, at age 25, I met the man I'd later marry and realized I wanted to live forever. So I took up swimming and jogging. Then my body awoke. I came to love the peace I felt after a good run and the silky slide of moving through water. I began participating in short races and signing up for classes at the YMCA. In short, I became an athlete.

Thousands of women, including the following five, tell a similar story. As children, they shied away from exercise because they felt clumsy, left out, or bored. But as adults, they took a chance and tried something new. Suddenly, they, too, unlocked a passion for sports and the feel-good, look-good dividends that come with it. Their stories have convinced me anew that it's never too late to set your inner athlete free.

MARTY BARRY
SWIMMING

Age: 70
Hometown: Novato, California
Profession: Retired caterer

As a child, Marty Barry loved swimming in the ocean, but her school didn't have a pool, and she knew of no girls' teams. She didn't want to get whacked on the knees playing field hockey and hated sweating when she ran. So she grew up sportless. At age 45, newly divorced and emotion-

ally devastated, she visited a holistic doctor who prescribed exercise to relieve her stress and depression. Swimming was the obvious activity of choice—a knee injury precluded other sports—so he put her in touch with

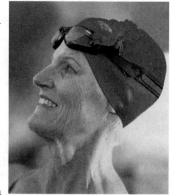

a masters team. At the first practice, she couldn't even swim a lap. "I thought I was going to die," she says. She persevered, though, and in three months she was swimming 18 laps at a time. Two years later, she started competing. She also remarried—a brief, unhappy union, this time to an alcoholic. To support her family, she started a catering business. "I discovered that swimming was holding my life together. Even when I'd only had two hours of sleep, if I could get up and swim, I knew I had a place on earth where my life was together."

Now retired and happily remarried, Barry swims at least 100 laps five times a week and goes to several regional meets a year. In 2002, she placed first in five events at one competition; she is also nationally ranked in several events among swimmers her age.

KIM MITCHELL
KARATE
Age: 30
Hometown: Horsham, Pennsylvania
Profession: Senior account executive at a public-relations firm

Kim Mitchell was an overweight, uncoordinated kid who found sports tough going. Still, she was fascinated by karate, an offshoot of her love for Bruce Lee movies. At age 6, she ventured into a martial-arts school to watch but fled, terrified, when someone threw a flying kick over her head. Twenty-two years later, a colleague told her he was offering a free karate class at a local church. She signed up and immediately fell in love with its mystique, its discipline, and the connection it offered to another culture. "There's an exotic nature, a formality to it that I respect," she says. Mitchell is astounded by her new skills, which include crunches, push-ups, snap round kicks, and backbends. "I wasn't one of those little girls who could do them," she says. "But now I can, and it's so cool." Today, she has her yellow belt (the third of seven

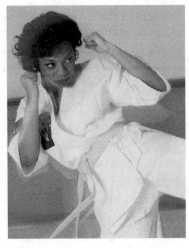

colors—she dreams of someday earning a black one) and attends a karate class four times a week. "At first, I'd see people doing things and think, 'I can't do that.' But now I think, 'If I can do this kick, then I can conquer X, Y, and Z as well.' " That confidence has carried over to the rest of her life. And she's delighted with her newfound athleticism and energy.

ELLEN MASSEY
SOCCER
Age: 39
Hometown: Knoxville, Tennessee
Profession: Human resources director for a regional orthopedic practice

Although she dabbled in basketball and softball as a child, Ellen Massey realized by middle school that it wasn't cool for girls to play sports—so she quit. But

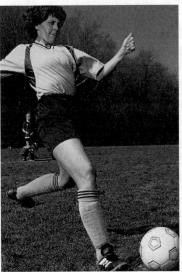

at age 29, after the birth of her second child, she was ready to get in shape. She hired a trainer, began lifting weights, and started running. Still, it took eight more years for Massey to discover her true athletic passion: soccer. When her three children took up the game, she and her husband signed on as coaches and took to kicking the ball around at home. The couple had been looking for a sport to play together, so they gathered a team of friends to play in an adult league. The first season, they didn't win a single game. They stuck together and found a coach to help them, and their tenacity paid off.

In 2002, the team lost only two games. During the final match, Massey fractured her shinbone and spent two months on crutches, but her enthusiasm hasn't wavered. "I love the sheer physicality of the game—the running, the sweating, the slide tackling," she says. "And I love the after-game bonding,

As children, many women shied away from exercise because they felt clumsy, left out, or bored. But as adults, women are taking chances and trying something new. By doing so, they are unlocking a passion for sports and the feel-good, look-good dividends that come with it.

hanging out and rehashing heroic plays." She also welcomes the outlet for her competitive spirit and relishes the knowledge that her aging body is still strong and capable of learning new things. She likes what it's done for her family life, too. "My kids see

me as a cool mom because I actually play soccer. And now that I'm my husband's teammate, he has more respect for me as an athlete."

RHONDA FRIEDMAN
PILATES

Age: 47
Hometown: Damariscotta, Maine
Profession: Potter

"I was the kind of kid who got hit in the head with the ball on the basketball court," Rhonda Friedman says. "I was completely unathletic." But nine years ago, she read something about the Pilates Method and became intrigued by its emphasis on building long, slender muscles and correcting body alignment. Friedman has slight scoliosis (curvature of the spine) and was looking to relieve the occasional pain in her left shoulder and her lower back. "Pottery involves a lot of heavy physical work," she says. "So my lower back would go out, and I'd be down for a week." But no one in the area taught Pilates until, several years later, a studio moved into the building in which Friedman owns

Q + A PUSHING EXERCISE TOO FAR

I lift weights three days a week, and I've just started taking yoga two other days. I'm surprised at how sore I am. Am I overdoing it?

You may want to cut back on one of your weight-room sessions. As your sore muscles are trying to tell you, you're already getting good resistance training with yoga, especially if you do Ashtanga or another power variation that strengthens your chest and triceps. Many yoga classes these days mix forms, so talk to your instructor if you aren't sure.

It's fine to alternate between weights and power yoga as long as you target different areas. On strength-training days, use your soreness as a guide: If your upper body aches, focus on your lower body and abs. Also, don't step up to heavier weights too quickly—you should increase the amount you lift by no more than 10 percent every week or two. Of course, if you're supersore, wait a day before heading back to the gym or yoga studio: Your muscles need some downtime to rebuild torn fibers and become stronger.

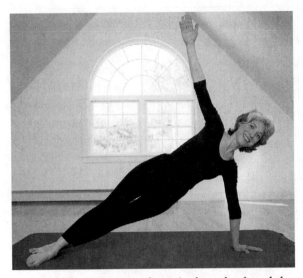

NAN WEINER
SALSA DANCING

Age: 51
Hometown: San Francisco
Profession: Magazine editor

Nan Wiener has always thought of herself as graceful, but she never liked team sports in high school. By her senior year, she was overweight. A college modern-dance class stirred something inside of her, and she found she enjoyed the exercise. But she was convinced that only people who had begun dancing as children could excel, so she never pursued it. Instead, she took up aerobics in graduate school. Five years ago, while loitering after a noontime class, she heard salsa music coming from a workout studio and was enthralled. "I couldn't tear myself away," she says. Wiener stayed for the Latin American dance class and has been enjoying salsa in classes and clubs at least once a week ever since. "Salsa isn't exercise, it's art. You're moving with a partner to beautiful music. And the dance pulls you in. It's like I'm hypnotized, moving to some sort of rhythm I can't control." Wiener also found that dance released her from the belief that

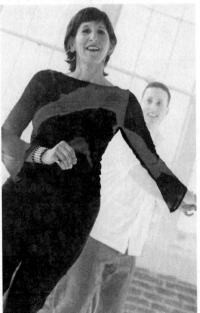

you're either born good at something or you aren't. "Now I have the opposite feeling. I'm willing to work at this, to spend months just learning how to do a complicated turn." ∎

a pottery shop. She signed up. At first, she found the method a bit confusing, but she soon realized that it was engaging her mind as well as her body, and then she was hooked. "The exercises require a focus that is very centering," she says. "And with practice, you gain a refined sense of movement." Now, after six years and countless lessons, Friedman takes Pilates instruction twice a week and practices four additional days on her own equipment. She loves the feeling of physical control it has given her, and her pain has vanished. "Pilates has changed the way I feel about my body," she says.

Q + A

A SECRET TO STRETCHING

How long should I hold a stretch?

Anywhere from 15 to 30 seconds is the ideal, explains Richard Cotton, chief exercise physiologist with the Web site MyExercisePlan.com. "Ten seconds is OK if you're in a hurry, but it's best to hold it a little longer," urges Cotton. As you stretch, note when the muscle "lets go" (you'll feel it relax) and be sure to hold through that point to get the most out of the stretch. But be careful not to force things. "If it hurts, something's wrong," Cotton cautions.

vital *stats*

88

Percentage of Americans who make NEW YEAR'S RESOLUTIONS each year

1

Rank of DIETING and WEIGHT LOSS among New Year's resolutions in 2001

10

Rank of DIETING and WEIGHT LOSS among New Year's resolutions in 2000

1, 2

Ranks of "ENJOY LIFE MORE" and "spend more time with friends and family" among resolutions

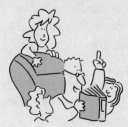

15

Number of minutes it takes to get a BOTOX injection

$500

Average COST of a Botox injection

2 to 4

Number of BOTOX INJECTIONS required yearly to maintain results

---

1 in 4

Chance that someone in your household gets MIGRAINE headaches

$13 BILLION

Amount lost each year by employers because of missed workdays and poor performance due to migraines

43

Percentage of migraine sufferers who have headaches at least five days every three months

55/47

Percentage of men vs. women who keep track of IMPORTANT DATES by memory

16/11

Percentage of men vs. women who keep track of dates by WRITING THEM ON THEIR HANDS

60/75

Percentage of men vs. women who were able to recall EMOTIONALLY CHARGED EXPERIENCES after three weeks

1

Rank of WINTER among most popular seasons to have LASER SURGERY, face-lifts, and chemical peels

---

$122

Average amount spent by a MAN on Valentine's gifts

$50

Average amount spent by a WOMAN

37-29-40

Measurements of an AVERAGE woman

38-18-28

Measurements of a Barbie doll adjusted to real-life scale

LESS THAN 1 IN 100,000

Chance that a real woman has Barbie's measurements

15

Percentage of people on antidepressants who experience SEXUAL DYSFUNCTION as a side effect, according to product labels

37

Percentage of users who actually report SEXUAL DYSFUNCTION as a side effect, according to a University of Virginia survey

---

80

Percentage of Americans who are "cyberchondriacs": NET USERS who research health info online

93

Percentage of those CYBERCHONDRIACS who believe the health-care information on the Internet is trustworthy

51

Percentage of those cyberchondriacs who would BUY PRESCRIPTION MEDICINE ONLINE without consulting a doctor

45

Percentage of clinical information on health Web sites that physicians found COMPLETELY accurate

33

Percentage of people who have taken more than the RECOMMENDED DOSE of an OTC medication

79

Percentage of medical professionals who believe this is a SERIOUS problem

Sources: GNC New Year's Resolution Survey, Harris Interactive Poll, *Journal of the American Medical Association*, Brown University Psychopharmacology Update, American Academy of Cosmetic Surgery, American Academy of Facial Plastic and Reconstructive Surgery, National Council on Patient Information and Education, Health Behavior News Service of the Center for the Advancement of Health, Museum of Science/The Changing Face of Women's Health, International Mass Retail Association—Reported by Laura Riccobono

chapter 6

healthy looks

**a busy woman's guide to
looking and feeling her best**

The *faces* of
HEALTH

The winners of our third annual contest share how they renew their spirits and let the beauty inside shine through.

BY LYNNE CUSACK • PHOTOGRAPHY BY JAYNE WEXLER

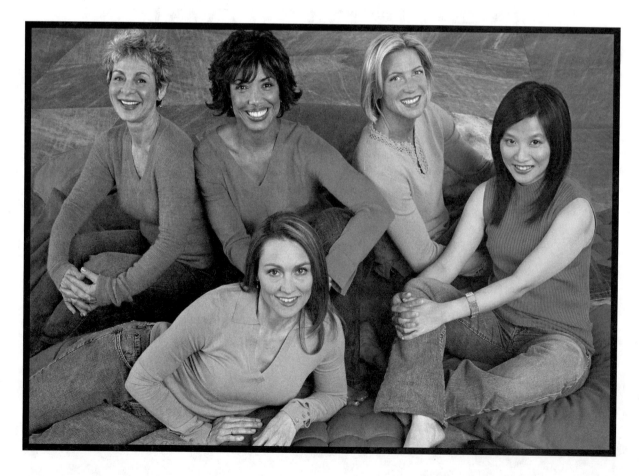

It all comes back to balance. Whether you're talking about the most nutritious diet, the best approach to fitness, or the essence of spiritual health and happiness, the center is the place to be. And these women, the winners of our 2003 Faces of Health contest, are right there. They manage to live big lives yet keep the details in perspective; to exude passion but embrace their limitations; to seek out challenges but know when they need to retreat and recharge. Each finalist has earned $1,000 from competition sponsor Dove—in addition to our undying admiration. We hope their stories inspire you to embrace your own true beauty.

MICHELE SPENCER

40, major, U.S. Army

"There is a seriousness about what I do: teaching army leadership skills to ROTC cadets. Eventually, my students—those who stay with the military, anyway—will be responsible for someone else's life. The importance of that has never been more clear than right now, because of where we are as a country with the war in Iraq. How I address my students is how I try to live my life, with purpose and passion. Being mindful of my purpose is how I avoid stress and create balance. I try not to set unrealistic goals. So many women reach for an idealized image of happiness and lose themselves along the way. I recognize that I am a work in progress, and that keeps me centered."

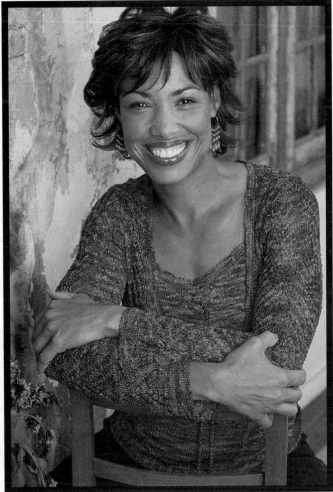

Michele's Balanced Beauty

- Michele's no-fuss approach to her looks clearly works. But she does have her challenges. "My hair is dry and porous," she says. "To keep it healthy and well-hydrated, I blend olive oil and a few drops of lavender and patchouli oils. I use the mixture as a moisturizer on my body as well."

- Although she keeps her makeup to a minimum because it suits her style on and off the job, Michele likes the natural glow she gets from Aveda's Cooling Calming Color, a cream blush stick. "There's no need for a brush. I simply blend it in with my fingers," Michele notes.

- For occasional breakouts, Michele likes to use Dermalogica's Medicated Clearing Gel and Multivitamin Power Recovery Masque because they leave her skin feeling and looking its best—and they also contain all-natural ingredients.

Michele's words of wisdom: I recognize that I am a work in progress, and that keeps me centered.

JUNE BISANTZ EVANS
55, artist and teacher

"In addition to creating my own art, I teach graphic design and digital art at Eastern Connecticut State University. My students are always pushing the envelope, always teaching me things. My last piece of digital art, called *It's a Balancing Act*, reflects on life's precariousness—and the give and take—that create balance. I believe you find true happiness when you make a commitment to do what gives you pleasure. For me, it's creative pursuits. For others, well, a little self-examination can open up a world of possibilities."

June's Balanced Beauty

- "I use a hydrating jasmine moisturizer made locally by Pam Brundage, a woman who started her own line of botanical skin-care products," June says. "It not only does a great job, but it smells heavenly."

- June doesn't spend a minute more than necessary on her signature no-frills hairstyle. "I keep it extremely simple—short and natural—even though I've received considerable pressure over time from stylists and others to color it."

- She rarely wears makeup but admits to a weakness for lipsticks in colors that look natural. Her favorite: Revlon's Super Lustrous Lipstick in Fleshtone.

- About once a month, June treats herself to a customized facial and deep-tissue massage—for the pure joy of it.

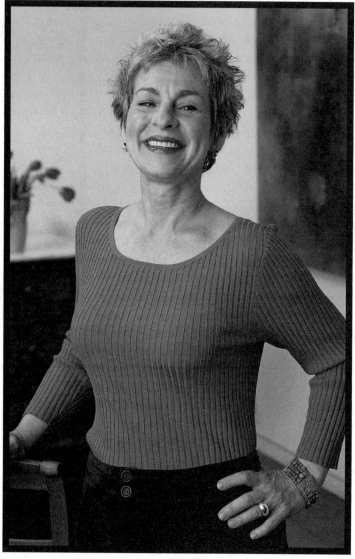

June's words of wisdom: You can find true happiness when you make a commitment to do what gives you pleasure. For me, it's creative pursuits.

Jean's words of wisdom: I believe balance is spiritual as well as physical ... I have to allow myself some breathing space and take time to refresh my outlook.

JEAN TAO
29, financial analyst

"Leading a healthy lifestyle is my passion. I eat well and have been practicing yoga for six years, because I believe balance is spiritual as well as physical. But it hasn't always been easy to think that way. The world in which I was raised is very work-focused. Many people in my culture feel it's wrong to have a life outside of your job. I work more effectively when I allow myself some breathing space, whether that involves making time for friends or traveling to refresh my outlook. I make my workout and my relaxation time priorities, because I've learned they're just as important as my career."

Jean's Balanced Beauty
- Jean mixes up her own facial mask (one egg yolk combined with 1 teaspoon honey and a few drops of lemon juice). "I use it weekly on my face for 10 minutes." She likes the way the egg and honey moisturize her skin; the lemon juice absorbs oil.
- She keeps her hair nourished and glossy by occasionally massaging in a little olive oil as a conditioner.
- "In the winter, I like to apply camellia oil to my face and hair," Jean says. "It comes from a tea tree found in southeastern Asia and has been popular in Japan as a moisturizer for centuries."
- Jean prefers the silky texture of glosses over the heavier feel of lipstick. "They provide a hint of color, and many of them are long-lasting." Her favorite? Neutrogena's Moistureshine Gloss.

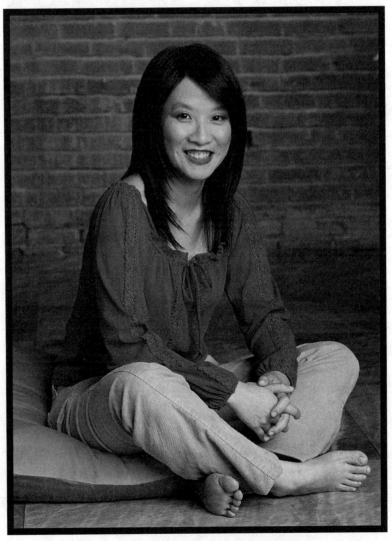

KRISTY ABBOT

43, homemaker and athlete

"I've always been athletic, but it was only after my mom died 10 years ago that I started spending a lot more time swimming, running, and biking. In fact, it was my athletic drive that saved my life. I was sore after lifting weights one morning, and as I massaged under my arm, I discovered a lump.

I was diagnosed with breast cancer on Mother's Day two years ago. Being an athlete kept me balanced in my quest to become cancer-free. My friend Gina accompanied me to my radiation sessions; we'd wear our workout clothes to the center, then jog around the beautiful lakes in Minneapolis. That made all the difference in the world."

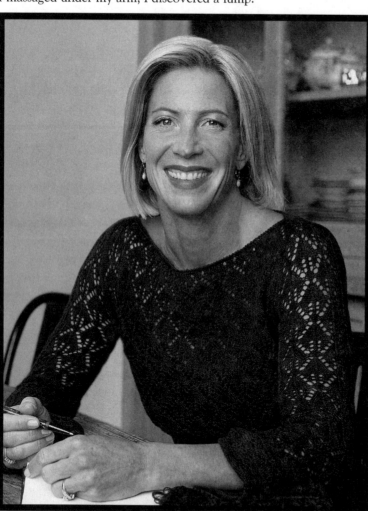

Kristy's Balanced Beauty

- When she's training for a triathlon, Kristy might work out as many as five hours a day. "I'm constantly battling dry skin," she says. Her secret? A superconvenient softening spray called Pevonia Botanica Dry Oil Body Moisturizer. "It's fantastic, and it smells like Hawaii!"
- Kristy's developed a couple of beauty tricks during her many years of swimming. "I never wash my face before I swim laps, because I think the natural oils give a little extra protection from chlorine." To banish all traces of chlorine after swimming, she uses a clarifying shampoo, Redken Hair Cleansing Creme.
- Regardless of where her training and family life take her, Kristy's makeup routine remains simple. "All I use is a tinted moisturizer and a clear mascara, so I don't have to worry about streaks when I sweat." (She likes CG Smoothers Natural Lash and Brow Mascara.)

Kristy's words of wisdom: Being an athlete kept me balanced in my quest to become cancer-free. It made all the difference in the world.

Judith's words of wisdom: I spend a lot of time outdoors.
I think of nature as a place to retreat and replenish.
It's helped me become more accepting of myself.

JUDITH O'KEEFE

47, fly-fishing-equipment sales rep
"It's the time I spend outdoors
hiking, exploring rivers, and
fly-fishing with my husband
that gives me a sense of balance.
When you're surrounded by trees
or walking along the shoreline,
where things are peaceful, with
no real-life interruptions, you
are able to put things into perspective. I think of nature as a
place to retreat and replenish.
The balance it offers has helped
me become more accepting of
myself. I don't believe any one
person or product is going to
unlock the secrets of eternal
youth—we would all do ourselves a favor if we accepted that
fact with grace. I intend to grow
old with a smile on my face,
laugh lines and all."

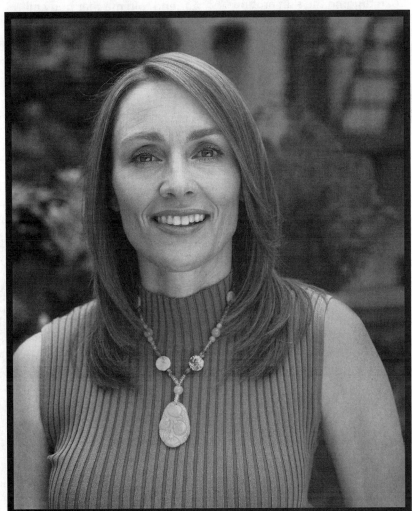

Judith's Balanced Beauty

• Rain or shine, Judith wears a
sunscreen on her face (Nivea
Visage Q10 Plus Wrinkle Control Lotion SPF 15).
When she fly-fishes, sun reflecting off the water
is as much a concern as rays from above, so she
uses water- and sweat-resistant Clinique Super City
Block SPF 25 and reapplies every couple of hours.

• "With an active lifestyle, a good haircut makes
all the difference," Judith says. "I need a low-
maintenance look with enough layering that

I can style it without having to use a lot of
products and appliances."

• "I'm the bath queen," Judith admits. "I have a
deep claw-foot tub, and I love being able to sink
into the water past my shoulders—it's such a
soothing sensation. Lavender-scented baths are
great. I even recently planted a quarter-acre
lavender crop."

Q + A

YOUR SKIN IS TOUGHER THAN YOU THINK

Can tugging the skin around your eyes while applying pencil liner cause wrinkles and sagging?

Luckily, you don't have to give up pretty eyes today to prevent wrinkles tomorrow. "Your skin is a fancy fabric, but it's also resilient and forgiving," explains cosmetic surgeon Jay Burns, M.D. "To cause wrinkles, you'd have to pull or rub your eyes excessively throughout the day for years. Applying makeup for a few minutes each morning is going to have minimal, if any, impact." Of course, a gentle touch is always best, so use just a little pressure and buy products that go on without a lot of effort. We like Bobbi Brown's Long-Wear Gel Eyeliner, which you apply with a brush. The pigment really sticks to the bristles, and the light gel glides on in one smooth stroke. Not up for using a brush? Try Madina Milano Eyeliner Classic. It combines the convenience of a pencil with the ease of a gel.

Q + A

No matter how much moisturizer I use, the skin on my arms and legs stays dry and flaky. A friend told me that body oil works better than lotions or creams. Is she right?

Your friend knows her stuff. "Most moisturizers are made with water, which tends to evaporate off the skin," explains Jeanine Downie, M.D., of Image Dermatology in Montclair, New Jersey. "Oils, on the other hand, form a film that seals water in and prevents moisture loss." Any pure oil—baby, massage, or essential—will get the job done. For best results, exfoliate once or twice a week to smooth your skin's top layer. When you get out of the bath or shower, rub in some oil, and pat dry. Then apply a moisturizer for extra softening. "Damp skin allows for better absorption and helps lock in moisture," Downie explains. We love Fresh's Rice Formula F21C Dry Oil, which has a calming fragrance and

WHEN DRY SKIN NEEDS MORE THAN LOTION

absorbs quickly—you can slip your clothes on right away, without worrying about stains. Another pick: Bath & Body Works' Aromatherapy Relax Blue Lavender Palmarosa Soothing Body Oil, which leaves your skin satiny and lightly scented.

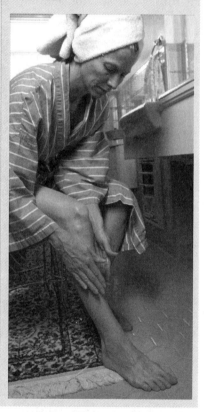

Pure oils are good for dry skin because they form a film that seals water in and prevents moisture loss.

Banish Your Skin Blotches

If you have brown blotches (aka melasma) on your face and neck, you know it's tough to fade them. Now, a cream approved by the U.S. Food and Drug Administration called Tri-Luma combines three previously separate treatments—a lightening agent, retinoid, and steroid—in one tube. The prescription-only cream is used nightly for eight weeks. In studies, 78 percent of patients showed some improvement, while 29 percent saw spots clear completely. A word of caution: Although melasma affects 70 percent of moms-to-be, you shouldn't use Tri-Luma during pregnancy or if you're nursing.

Get the Goods on Grains

Discover what's behind this new trend in skin products.

In ancient times, Japanese women with flawless skin were called *nuka-bijin,* or "bran beauties," because they supposedly rubbed their faces with rice bran. New skin products are borrowing from that ancient tradition by incorporating rice into powders and exfoliators.

"Rice is highly absorbent, so it will reduce oil and help makeup set," says Audrey Kunin, M.D., the dermatologist behind Derma doctor.com, a skin-care Web site. Powders containing rice starch are great for people who have oily skin, are acne-prone, or have rosacea. "Powder is less likely to block pores than liquid products,"

Kunin says. Try T. LeClerc's powders with rice starch—they're extremely light and not chalky.

Rice exfoliates by sloughing off dead skin cells mechanically, in the same way an apricot-seed scrub does. We love Prada's Exfoliating Mask/Face, which incorporates rice granules into a creamy cleanser (and comes in single-use, travel-friendly packaging). As this gentle product dries, its salicylic acid and clay provide even more polish.

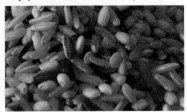

Q + A — SAY GOODBYE TO "FACE" DANDRUFF

I have red, scaly, itchy patches on my forehead and around my nose. None of my usual dry-skin solutions are helping. Any thoughts?

Apparently, you've been faked out by your flakes. If typical strategies, such as moisturizing and washing less frequently, haven't helped—or have even made matters worse—then you've probably got dandruff (yes, you can get it on your face, too). Known as seborrheic dermatitis, this common condition affects millions of women.

"Though your skin looks chapped or flaky, it's actually not dry at all," says Nancy Silverberg, M.D., associate clinical professor of dermatology at the University of California, Irvine. "The redness is caused by inflammation, and the scaly patches are due to a buildup of cells." Seborrheic dermatitis typically appears on your scalp, your forehead, in your eyebrows, around your nose, and on your chest; those areas have the highest concentration of oil-producing sebaceous glands. Experts are still unsure

what causes dandruff—yeast organisms are the offenders in some cases—but they do know that heredity plays a role; for now, there's no way to prevent or cure it. But you can treat it by washing your face once or twice daily with dandruff shampoo. Dermatologists like Nizoral, which was once prescription-only but is now available at drugstores for about $10. A mild over-the-counter cortisone cream can reduce redness. If things haven't cleared up in three to four weeks, see a doctor.

The 7 Biggest Beauty Breakthroughs

These advances could enhance your looks—and perhaps even your life.

BY CHRISTINE COBURN

The cosmetics industry is based on a slightly cynical principle: Hope in a bottle sells. That's why "new" and "improved" are the words most bandied about by marketers. Whether that describes a "groundbreaking" six-in-one moisturizer or a "miraculous" face-lifting procedure, the hype is so pervasive that it sometimes causes you to turn a blind eye to the true breakthroughs out there.

Well, listen up. We're going to fill you in on some truly remarkable beauty solutions. More than just bottled hope, the following seven innovations deliver results. Get ready to share this article with a friend.

THE SILENT BLOW-DRYER

This ear-friendly appliance is five times quieter. Industrial science has transformed the morning hairstyling routine. Revlon's Quiet Dry, introduced in 2002, boasts advanced engineering and 1,875 watts of power, yet emits a barely audible blast of air. "We basically rebuilt the blow-dryer motor from scratch," says Jeff Katz, director of marketing for Helen of Troy, a leading designer, developer, and worldwide marketer of brand-name personal-care

products. "We used a belt-driven motor in the handle of the appliance to minimize sound." As a result, the noise level is significantly lower than that of the typical dryer: 65 decibels versus 85 to 90. The difference could help prevent hearing loss, since research has proven that sounds above 75 decibels can damage ears. And, happily, a redesigned fan cuts suction that often catches long hair in the vent.

TRULY SAFE TANNING

For those who have trouble with their at-home technique, a new spray-on version guarantees nonstreak results.

The smart option for women (and men) who can't quite give up their quest for a little summer color: UV-free self-tanning, courtesy of two companies that are bringing patented spray-jet booths to a town near you. After disrobing, you step into a private cubicle where, for about 40 seconds, dozens of jets mist a light coating of self-tanning formula onto every inch of your body, including your face, if you like. (Before getting started, you cover your hair with a cap, coat your fingernails with moisturizer, and keep your eyes shut.) The result is a head-to-toe, streak-free tan that lasts about a week and dries almost immediately. After a quick buffing with a towel, you can dress and go, without worrying about staining your clothes.

This tanner uses the same active ingredient found in do-it-yourself products: dihydroxyacetone, a harmless protein that reacts with the melanin in your skin. Extremely light and nongreasy, the lotion is loaded with emollients that leave you feeling silky, not sticky. And with its UV-based competition bringing in 1 million customers a day (which translates to $4 billion a year), this sunless alternative may spare tanning aficionados from becoming skin-cancer statistics. Prices range from $15 to $25 an appointment, depending on the salon. To find a location near you, visit www.mystictan.com or www.mist-on.com.

ACNE-ERASING LASERS

Here's great news for those seeking lasting relief without side effects from breakouts.

According to recent studies at the Johns Hopkins University School of Medicine and the University of California, San Diego, the same new lasers being used to tone sagging skin can curb overactive oil-producing glands, preventing acne flare-ups. Two of these lasers, the Clearlight and the SmoothBeam, were approved by the U.S. Food and Drug Administration in late 2002 to treat acne. "They bypass the epidermis and shrink the specific glands that cause overproduction of oil, which leads to acne," says Harold Brody, M.D., clinical professor of dermatology at Emory University and communications director for the American Academy of Dermatology. "This is a real change from the old pulsed-light treatments that destroyed acne-causing bacteria but did nothing to control oil production." Because improved technology targets the deeper layers of skin, there is no oozing, redness, or recovery time, nor is there any of the dryness, itching, flaking, or increased light sensitivity associated

with most topical remedies (such as lotions and creams). Early research shows that a series of three to six sessions spaced over the course of a month or two typically keeps acne sufferers blemish-free for years (exactly how many years is yet to be determined, though). "But these treatments are being looked at as having the potential to be a permanent or nearly permanent solution to breakouts," Brody says.

FEATHERWEIGHT, FLAWLESS FOUNDATION

The secret that gives starlets their too-good-to-be-true natural look is coming to a spa, makeup counter, and home near you.

Originally conceived as a safe, effective method for applying cosmetics to the healing skin of post-op plastic surgery patients, airbrushing (the equipment is a scaled-down version of what pros use to give cars precision paint jobs) is now being made available to the masses. At about $40, the technique allows makeup artists to cover a variety of imperfections, including birthmarks, scars, and stretch marks. A handheld gun is used to apply an ultra-light spray of foundation to the client's skin, creating a finish so light and natural-looking, it's barely perceptible. Surprisingly, this faint hint of tint lasts much longer than traditional foundations—up to 12 hours without touch-ups. It benefits your skin,

A makeup marvel: Spray-on foundation leaves your skin feeling hydrated and healthy all day long.

too. "Since you apply the foundation with a spray jet, there is no risk of cross-contamination from a makeup brush," says Oakland, California-based dermatologist Katie Rodan, M.D. Most of the formulations also provide sun protection, avoiding another heavy layer on your face.

Limited availability at beauty salons, spas, and makeup counters used to make airbrushing an option primarily for special occasions. But that changed in 2002 with the introduction of Era Face, a home version. The 2.25-ounce aerosol foundation comes in 10 shades and contains enough product to last nearly 12 weeks, depending on use. You simply hold the metal can at arm's length and spray in a zigzag motion across your face for a few seconds. Era Face offers ingredients similar to those of its salon counterpart, including SPF 20; soothing botanicals, such as aloe vera and chamomile; and such antioxidants as vitamins C and E. You can find salons or spas offering airbrushed makeup at www.dinair.com. Era Face is available at department stores; call 866-372-3223 or visit www.classifiedcosmetics.com.

FAST, FEARLESS, (REVERSIBLE) HAIR COLOR
Salon services just got quicker, and no-risk shades are giving colorphobes the courage to try something new.

As any bottle blond, brunette, or redhead will tell you, coloring your hair is the epitome of beauty drudgery, even in a salon. Removing your natural pigment and replacing it with something new and lasting typically requires at least 40 minutes of malodorous applications—and that doesn't even include the wait at the sink, under the dryer, and in the sitting area while your stylist runs the standard 10 minutes late. Two new one-step formulas are drastically shortening the process, however. That's terrific news for the 55 percent of women in this country who color their hair regularly.

Clairol Professional's Violet Kaleidocolor lightens hair four levels (for example, from medium brown to light blond) in less than 10 minutes. The product also offsets brassiness with built-in toners. This used to require a separate, final step—and up to 30 additional minutes in the chair.

Similarly, Goldwell's first globally launched product, Elumen, comes in 20 permanent shades ranging from jet black to platinum, plus a clear shade to enhance shine; it also works quickly, in about 10 minutes. Unlike traditional permanent color, it eliminates the need for ammonia or

peroxide with negatively charged dyes that are drawn into the positively charged hair shaft like magnets ("great for people with dry or porous locks," says Pierre Goneau, Goldwell's national education manager). Even better, it's completely reversible. If you cringe when the dryer hood comes off, your colorist can apply what's known as a "return," which pulls out all the offending pigment. Or she can remove just a little to soften overly dramatic effects. If you're game, she can completely redo your color on the same visit, because the ammonia-free process won't damage hair. Prices for both the Clairol and Goldwell services range from $50 up to $300, depending on the salon and city. For details, log on to www.elumen-haircolor.com or contact your local professional beauty supplier.

PAINLESS VARICOSE AND SPIDER VEIN REMOVAL
Here's a quick way to improve the look of your legs. Treating varicose and spider veins, which afflict more than one-third of the women in this country, has never been pleasant. The top two procedures, surgical stripping and saline injections (which can cause burning, cramping, sores, or lightened skin patches), have enough downsides to deter most women from getting these often-uncomfortable conditions corrected.

One-shot wonder: Glycerin-foam injections guarantee legs free of varicose and spider veins—and pain—with a single trip to the dermatologist.

Prepare for some extraordinary news. "Glycerin-foam injections are a revolutionary solution to unwanted veins," says Mitchell Goldman, M.D., a clinical professor of dermatology/medicine at the University of California, San Diego, whose study on the treatment was recently published in a peer-reviewed medical journal. "The procedure is basically identical to the one used with saline injections, but is essentially free of side effects." Glycerin foam is injected directly into the affected veins, causing them to shrivel and disappear virtually overnight. The discomfort experienced with saline injections frequently requires doctors to limit the number of veins they can treat at one sitting, meaning that complete removal can take up to six sessions and several months. "Glycerin turns vein removal into a one-time appointment," Goldman says. More good news: Glycerin-foam injections typically cost no more—and often less—than saline (about $400 a leg).

A SURGERY-FREE FACE-LIFT

Multipurpose lasers firm while also reducing fine lines, age spots, and large pores.

Once upon a time, if you wanted to tighten loose skin, you had two effective choices: a face-lift or resurfacing with a carbon dioxide or erbium laser. Both of these options could require weeks of downtime; potential side effects included swelling, discoloration, and scarring. That changed in 2002, when the FDA approved a new category of lasers (sold under such brand names as Lira, Aura, CoolGlide, and CoolTouch II) for a procedure called facial toning. "These all-purpose skin-rejuvenating lasers bypass the epidermis completely and stimulate collagen production deep in the dermis to firm and tighten," dermatologist Brody says. Because they don't break the skin, they pose none of the risks associated with resurfacing lasers, making them feasible to use on such delicate spots as the neck, chest, and throat—areas that were difficult or impossible to treat before. Long-term results can require three to six appointments ranging from about $100 to $500 a pop over many weeks. And since this technology is so new, experts don't yet know if its benefits will last. To find a dermatologist or plastic surgeon who offers laser toning or lifting, visit www.aboutskinsurgery.com. ■

Q + A STRIVING FOR STRAIGHT HAIR

How do I know if I am a good candidate for the new hair-straightening technique?

Thermal reconditioning—aka Japanese hair straightening, ionic retexturizing, or thermal restructuring—is a hot topic in salons (expect to pay $200 to $900). But not everyone should try it. Because the process uses chemicals and a flatiron to permanently change hair's structure, you need to start with strong, healthy locks. The ideal prospect is someone who's never had her hair highlighted, lightened with a heavy-duty product, double-processed (e.g., colored and highlighted simultaneously), or relaxed with sodium hydroxide, says Sonya Byun, thermal-reconditioning specialist at the Frédéric Fekkai Salon in Beverly Hills. The treatment is also not advised for African-American women; to prevent breakage, they'd have to grow 4 inches of "virgin" hair before getting a touch-up. But anyone who's had a single-process coloring or a perm with no ill effects can still go for it.

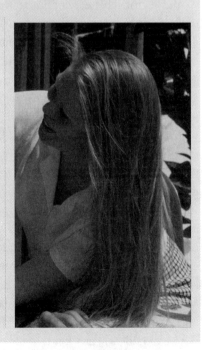

BEYOND BOTOX

Discover what you should know about the latest breed of antiaging injectables.

BY NANCY KALISH

It seems like a beauty fantasy come true: A few quick, almost painless needle pricks, and your crow's-feet, forehead furrows, and other wrinkles vanish for six months, sometimes more.

You've probably heard of Botox, a purified form of the toxin that causes botulism, an occasionally deadly type of food poisoning. You may even have been tempted to try it yourself. Millions of Americans have since it was approved by the U.S. Food and Drug Administration (FDA) for cosmetic use just over a year ago. You're probably less familiar with some of the other, newer wrinkle fixes, such as the fillers Restylane and Artefill. But chances are, they'll soon be just as popular with the baby boomers who have been jumping on the Botox bandwagon. In fact, to many women, receiving these fast, easy antiaging injections is no different from having their hair colored—they even attend parties where they can socialize while getting Botox shots. But this lax approach is a real concern, says Stanley Jacobs, M.D., director of the Center for Facial and Cosmetic Surgery in Santa Rosa, California. "The injection of Botox and fillers of any kind should be treated the

same way that you would a face-lift or even a heart transplant," he advises. When one of his patients requests Botox injections, Jacobs says, "I have consultations, informational sessions, and follow-ups. This is a medical procedure, and some people have started handing out Botox like candy."

The demand for wrinkle-free skin is so high that some doctors are willing to break the law in order to provide it. For instance, the filler Restylane—made from hyaluronic acid, a synthetic substitute for collagen, which is found naturally in human joints and skin—is not approved in the United States for use on humans. But that isn't stopping physicians and their clients from taking advantage of it. "I've been hearing that both doctors and patients are going out of the country to bring it back here for use, even though that's illegal," says plastic surgeon V. Leroy Young, M.D., co-chairman of the American Society of Aesthetic Plastic Surgery's Emerging Trends Task Force.

While there are considerable differences among Botox, Restylane, and the other injectables on the horizon, one thing is certain: The casual attitude toward these wrinkle erasers could yield unforeseen

284

consequences, both physical and psychological. Here's a look at the ways Botox has changed the complexion of the cosmetic-surgery scene, and what women need to know about the newest options for smoother skin.

THE LURE OF AN UNLINED FACE

Botox was first approved by the FDA in 1989 to treat crossed eyes and uncontrollable blinking. Doctors who administered it began to notice an interesting side effect: It also smoothed lines around patients' eyes by paralyzing the underlying muscles that cause wrinkling. Some physicians started using it off-label (without FDA approval) at low doses to zap crow's-feet, vertical forehead creases, and other lines. The drug, which takes effect after several days and lasts from two to six months, only works on wrinkles caused by muscle contractions beneath the surface, not those resulting from sun exposure, smoking, or normal aging. Much higher doses have also been used safely and successfully to treat migraines, excessive sweating, overactive bladder, back spasms, muscular problems following strokes, and other ailments.

But the big money lies in softening wrinkles. Not surprisingly, Allergan, the maker of Botox, applied for FDA approval in order to promote the drug as a legitimate wrinkle cure. It received the government's blessing in April 2002 for use on frown lines between brows; approvals for other parts of the face, such as the forehead and outer-eye area, should be coming soon. "Botox has had a long and excellent safety record, whether it's used for eye disorders or for eye-area wrinkles," Jacobs says.

Likewise, Restylane and Perlane (another filler made from hyaluronic acid) have been used safely in Canada and Europe for several years, explains Lisa Donofrio, M.D., assistant clinical professor of dermatology at Yale University. Unlike Botox, which paralyzes facial muscles, Restylane and Perlane fill wrinkles in the same way collagen does. "Restylane can be used to diminish the crease that might still appear even after Botox," says Donofrio,

who has used Restylane in her training schools in Switzerland for years. "The two treatments can easily be used in conjunction with each other."

All safety claims, though, assume that these materials are injected by skilled physicians. With Botox, that's increasingly less common, Jacobs says. "It's been getting into the wrong hands."

WHO'S CALLING THE SHOTS?

Although Botox used to be the province of plastic surgeons or dermatologists, who know exactly which of the 44 facial muscles to inject and how much to use, the surge in demand has prompted gynecologists, dentists, even veterinarians to start offering Botox treatments. The trouble is, inexperienced doctors can mistakenly target the wrong muscles or overparalyze them with too much of the toxin, increasing the risk of drooping eyelids or a frozen-looking face.

Once approved, Donofrio predicts, other wrinkle remedies will be offered by inadequately trained practitioners as well—and with similar risks. Doctors who use injectables need both anatomical knowledge and aesthetic artistry to produce good results. "You don't want someone who's just taken a weekend course practicing on you," Donofrio says. In addition to seeing a dermatologist or plastic surgeon, she recommends making sure the doctor handles the injections herself. "I could make a lot more money if I let my nurses do Botox," she says. "Only a highly trained physician should be giving these shots."

Even when administered by an experienced M.D., Botox doesn't always work as intended. "A doctor gave me shots around my brows, but it only worked on one side," reports Alice Scott, 42, of New York City. "For five weeks, I could only raise my right brow." Things went worse for Shelley Fichtel of Houston. She became alarmed when the doctor who had promised to get rid of her forehead furrows seemed to be injecting her brow rather haphazardly. "A week later, my eyelids were drooping down so far into my eyes that a co-worker asked me what was wrong with my face," says the 37-year-old.

Botox injections on the lower face can be riskier still. "When it's used around the mouth, even a small mistake can result in lopsided lips," explains Bahman Guyuron, M.D., clinical professor of plastic and reconstructive surgery at Case Western Reserve University School of Medicine in Cleveland. In one case, Donofrio notes, a soap-opera actress had to stop working temporarily when a misplaced shot rendered her unable to speak properly for three months.

Skill and training are perhaps even more important when injecting substances like Artefill—a collagen-and-synthetic filler that is made partly from the same chemicals as Plexiglas—because the results are permanent. Though an FDA panel recommended that Artefill be cleared in February 2003 (at press time, final approval was still pending), some U.S. doctors are wary of it. "We've seen Artefill migrate to other locations and lump up; it has also eroded through the skin," Young says.

BUT, I *AM* SMILING!

Botox's potential problems aren't just limited to the physical, though. Sure, those vertical frown lines that you thought made you look so old and angry have disappeared. Now, however, you can't look angry at all, even if you want to. A skilled practitioner strives to relax wrinkles while retaining expressiveness. But just a tad too much Botox can disable the very muscles that convey displeasure, puzzlement, happiness, and intelligence. (Wrinkle fillers, such as collagen, and its newer competitors, Restylane and Perlane, don't pose the same threat because they still allow facial muscles to move.) In fact, directors, such as Martin Scorsese and Baz Luhrmann, have complained that some actresses are so heavily Botoxed, they can no longer emote convincingly on camera.

"A lot of communication is nonverbal," explains Richard Friedman, M.D., a New York City psychiatrist and director of the Psychopharmacology Clinic at New York Weill Cornell Medical Center. "So one bad Botox shot can have a profound effect on the way you interact with others for months." What happens when a patient can't smile around the eyes when her boss gives her a plum assignment or frown at her husband during an argument (a truly ironic situation, considering that women have complained for years that men can't read their emotions)? "Women put a premium on being understood," Friedman says, "yet they don't realize that Botox can make it harder. One woman came to me because her boyfriend kept accusing her of being unsympathetic. This was really distressing to her, and it was no surprise why. Her face didn't look distressed at all, and that was the problem. Too much Botox had made her look weirdly blank."

New moms in particular might want to think twice about being treated with Botox. One of the first ways an infant learns about emotion is by observing its mother's facial cues. Artificially stifling that communication can adversely affect the fledgling parent-child relationship. "Babies use their parents as a model of expressiveness and rely on that nonverbal communication way before they use language," Friedman says. "Any diminished facial expression on the part of the mother could come across as cold and emotionally distant, and disrupt the bonding process. Parents are willing to spend tons of money on stimulating toys and accessories for their babies, yet they have no problem dulling their own expressions."

The over-Botoxed face is such a new phenomenon that no studies yet exist regarding exactly how it affects other people's perceptions, although some research is in the works. Scientists have, however, examined victims of Parkinson's disease, a degenerative neurological disorder. These people often suffer from facial masking, a condition that flattens expression and looks eerily similar to the effects of a Botox overdose. "Many people with Parkinson's can smile with their mouths, but they can't activate the muscles around their eyes that allow those crinkles of pleasure," explains Linda Tickle-Degnen, Ph.D., an occupational therapist and social psychologist at Boston University's Sargent College of Health and Rehabilitation Sciences. "Without that, their smiles just don't seem genuine. Our research has shown that people perceive them as negative or emotionless."

Like smiles, brow furrows are an important component of facial communication. "While they can make you look angry, they also indicate that you're engaged and interested," Tickle-Degnen says. "When you're unable to furrow, you come across as apathetic. I'm baffled that some people would voluntarily choose to change their faces that way." Other observers, though, are hardly surprised that a woman would gladly trade the outward manifestation of her personality for temporary youth. "Many women are more than willing to give up some expressiveness to turn back the clock," says Nancy Etcoff, Ph.D., a professor of psychology at Harvard Medical School and author of *Survival of the Prettiest: The Science of Beauty*. "As a culture, we've pretty much given up on authenticity."

A SOCIETY OF FROZEN FACES?

Despite the possible drawbacks, experts worry that some women may be unable to resist the appeal of a wrinkle-free face. "Botox is not physically addicting, and most patients are realistic and know when to stop," Guyuron says. "But others become emotionally addicted."

That dependency translates to lots of repeat customers, especially as more quick wrinkle fixes become available. "And what will happen then?" asks Deborah Sullivan, Ph.D., associate professor of sociology at Arizona State University and author of *Cosmetic Surgery: The Cutting Edge of Commercial Medicine in America*. "Will we become a society of frozen faces?" This idea isn't so far-fetched to anyone who's studied American culture. "We love a fad, and we have a history of embracing anything that will make us look younger and more beautiful, without much regard for the consequences," Sullivan says. "With too much Botox, our faces could become so hard to read that it interferes with communication on a societal level. Humans are good at compensating, but finding a whole new way to read each other's emotions is asking a lot." ∎

Nancy Kalish is a freelance writer in New York City.

What's Next?

These new wrinkle cures are coming soon to a dermatologist (or social gathering) near you.

RESTYLANE AND PERLANE These are two brand names for hyaluronic acid, an injectable wrinkle filler that could be approved by the Federal Drug Administration (FDA) in the near future. Restylane works on fine lines, the thicker Perlane on deeper creases. Both offer advantages over collagen, since hyaluronic acid causes no allergic reactions and lasts twice as long (six to nine months) as its natural counterpart.

ARTEFILL Used in Europe since 1994, Artefill is a combination of polymeric microspheres (an artificial material) and collagen. It works by encouraging the growth of your own collagen around the microspheres, which stay in place forever. That may sound good, says plastic surgeon Stanley Jacobs, M.D., but "if there is any sort of adverse reaction, you cannot remove it without cutting part of the face."

CYMETRA Skin harvested from human cadavers is treated with chemicals and ground into small particles to form this gel, recently approved by the FDA for filling lines and augmenting lips. Like hyaluronic acid, Cymetra poses little risk of allergic reaction. Effects last six to eight months.

RADIANCE Also derived from a human source—teeth and bones in this case—the drug, first approved to treat vocal-cord paralysis and urinary incontinence, is now being used off-label to minimize wrinkles. Results reportedly last two to five years. Reactions are rare, but, like Artefill, Radiance can potentially migrate to other areas.

Smooth Out Wrinkles
fast

A new cream may give Retin-A a run for its money.

BY MICHELE BENDER

Move over, prescription wrinkle treatments: There's a new kid in town. Tazarotene (aka Tazorac), a vitamin-A derivative in the same chemical family as Retin-A, has been used to fight acne and psoriasis for years. But new research suggests it may reduce signs of aging even better than some of its relatives.

In a recent study conducted by several universities to determine Tazorac's safety and effectiveness as an antiager, dermatologists graded the severity of fine wrinkles, sun spots, and discolorations on the faces of 563 participants (mostly women), then divided them into two groups. One group applied a 0.1-percent tazarotene cream, the other placebos. After 24 weeks, 22 percent more of the people who used tazarotene, compared with those given placebos, saw their fine wrinkles improve, while 45 percent found their spots and discolorations had faded. As a result, the cream was approved by the U.S. Food and Drug Administration in 2002 to treat aging skin and is now available under the trade name Avage.

So how does it stand up to other vitamin-A treatments? Studies comparing tazarotene cream and Renova (which contains tretinoin, the same active ingredient in Retin-A) found that the former worked faster and yielded better results. "Though its exact mechanism is unclear, tazarotene is unique because of the special binding properties that make it adhere to the skin," explains Nicholas Lowe, M.D., lead author of the study and clinical professor of dermatology at the University of California, Los Angeles. Although both products can produce the same side effects, including peeling, redness, and dryness, tazarotene may be a better choice for people with sensitive skin. "Because of its ability to bind to skin, you can wash it off 5 to 10 minutes after

> Tazarotene is different from other vitamin-A treatments because of its special binding properties, which may make it a better choice for people with sensitive skin.

applying it and still absorb enough to get the benefits," Lowe says; this reduces the chance of irritation. (Most patients, though, can keep the cream on overnight.) Plus, Avage's light consistency makes it less likely to cause acne than thicker formulations. Just keep in mind that you need to protect your skin from the sun and that you should avoid using Avage if you're pregnant or nursing. ∎

New Alternative to Face-lift

A cosmetic breakthrough can help you look youthful without the pain and recovery time required by a typical face-lift, according to a study published in *Plastic and Reconstructive Surgery*. A surgeon passes Gore-Tex fibers (the same material used in outerwear) through two tiny incisions in the creases between the nostrils and lips, then threads them through fat tissue to another incision above each ear. There, the sutures are attached to a Gore-Tex anchor patch beneath the skin. The procedure repositions fat, tightening the area just above the jaw. "It's best for someone who doesn't have too much sagging skin, but whose smile lines have gotten more prominent and who has noticed some fullness above them," says Gordon H. Sasaki, M.D., creator of the technique and clinical associate professor of plastic surgery at Loma Linda University in Pasadena, California. The surgery, which costs about $4,000 and takes approximately an hour, can be performed at a hospital or doctor's office. Bandages are unnecessary, and there's no recovery time. After four years, 85 percent of patients still see positive results, but Sasaki says more studies are required to determine whether the benefits will last.

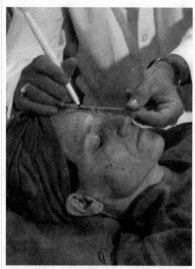

A new surgical procedure may lessen the demand for face-lifts.

The Truth About Cellulite Creams

Cosmetics companies know that women—up to 90 percent, say dermatologists—are trying to get rid of cellulite. (We'd like to meet the other 10 percent.) Perhaps that's why stores are filled with products that claim to smooth things out. The newest contain substances, including caffeine, creatine, soy protein, and ginseng, that manufacturers say can reduce the appearance of cellulite. "These ingredients may work temporarily," says dermatologist Mitchel Goldman, M.D. "But if they work at all, they only do so when they are used continually." Whether they do any good is still unclear, as no controlled studies have determined the effectiveness of a cellulite cream's individual components.

One theory holds that slow circulation causes cellulite; such chemicals as caffeine, then, may stimulate blood and lymphatic flow. Other ingredients supposedly break down fat cells.

So how do you know which—if any—of the remedies will *really* help reduce your dimples? Goldman suggests using a cream on one leg for a few months and then comparing it to the untreated one. Here are two of the newest cellulite fighters: Shiseido Body Creator and Avon Cellu-Sculpt Anti-Cellulite Slimming Treatment.

Test your cellulite cream by only using it on one leg for a few months and compare it to the untreated leg.

10 Quick Tips for a Flawless
FAKE TAN

These step-by-step instructions will give you a fabulous faux glow.

You've heard it a hundred times: The only safe tan comes from a bottle. But getting one without telltale streaks or splotches isn't always easy. Ann Marie Cilmi, director of training at Bliss Spa in New York City, teaches aestheticians how to apply a natural-looking tan. Who better to give us streak-free secrets?

1. Exfoliate first to help tanner go on evenly and ensure long wear (DHA, the active ingredient in most formulas, clings best to freshly buffed skin). Avoid creamy oil-based exfoliators; their residue will keep your skin from absorbing the tanner. Give extra attention to knees, elbows, wrists, ankles, hands, and feet.

2. To get your skin even smoother, shave, rinse thoroughly, and dry well.

3. Apply moisturizer to your ankles, heels, tops of toes, kneecaps, and elbows. The moisturizer keeps them from soaking up excess tanner and turning unnaturally dark.

4. Pour tanner in your hands, then rub them together so the product evenly coats each palm.

5. Start applying with long, full strokes, then rub in a circular motion. "By spreading in all directions, you'll blend it better and avoid streaks," Cilmi says.

6. Work from your lower body up, covering the area between each ankle and knee first. Apply the tanner that remains on your hands to ankles, knees, and the tops of your feet, which don't need

as thick a coat. Do the same with your arms, using leftover tanner on your elbows and the backs of your hands.

7. If you're flexible, you may be able to reach your shoulders and back yourself. To be sure you don't miss a spot, though, ask a friend to help.

8. To lessen the likelihood of clogged pores and breakouts, use a product made specifically for your face, which contains less oil than a tanner made for your body. Facial formulas also tend to be lighter in color and, therefore, more natural looking. Apply to spots the sun naturally highlights: nose, cheeks, and midpoints of the chin and forehead. Then blend into your hairline using light strokes.

Top 3 Self-Tanning Mistakes

1. Applying tanner when you're in a rush. You're bound to miss a spot, and it won't have enough time to dry.

2. Exercising within eight hours of application or putting on makeup within three. Both can decrease absorption and increase streaking.

3. Using too much. "It's like seasoning chili: You can always add more spice, but you can't take it out once it's in," says aesthetician Ann Marie Cilmi.

9. Most self-tanners contain ingredients that dry your skin so moisturize diligently to maintain results (wait about eight hours after applying tanner).

10. You may have to sample several products before finding one that works. To narrow your search, here are two we've tried and loved:

• Lancôme Flash Bronzer Self Tanning Moisturizing Mousse, with its weightless colored foam, gives you tawny skin immediately, helping you see any missed spots.

• Shiseido Self-Tanning Protective Face Cream SPF 8 is a breeze to apply. Enriched with plant extracts and vitamin E, it leaves skin feeling soft. And the sunscreen lets you show off your golden glow outdoors, while protecting you from UV damage. ■

Another Strike Against Tanning
The government adds UV light to its hit list.

You've heard dermatologists and health experts warn that ultraviolet light (UV) can cause skin cancer, the most common form of the disease in the United States. To make that message even louder and clearer, the federal Department of Health and Human Services recently added UV radiation from the sun and from artificial sources to its comprehensive list of known carcinogens. This biennial report is mandated by Congress to make the public aware of substances and circumstances that may cause cancer.

Of course, this addition isn't without controversy. Some in the indoor-tanning industry say that research has only found beds and sunlamps to be probable causes of cancer, not known ones. Skin-cancer doctors disagree. "Numerous studies have shown time and time again that overexposure to ultraviolet radiation can lead to skin cancer," explains Fred F. Castrow II, M.D., president of the American Academy of Dermatology. In fact, according to one study published in the academy's journal, tanning at a salon can create molecular changes that potentially lead to skin cancer.

The report's critics also point out that UV light helps the body make vitamin D, which is crucial for calcium absorption and may reduce the risks of other diseases, such as breast and colon cancer. Those who support the listing counter that foods (such as eggs and milk), vitamin supplements, and incidental exposure to the sun are safer ways to get your D than baking outdoors or in a tanning booth.

Our advice: Whether UV rays are on the list or not, skin cancer is a disease we'd like to avoid. So we'll say it again: Stay in the shade.

Coming Your Way:
Total Sun Protection

Despite improvements in sunscreen formulations over the last 20 years, the only way to completely safeguard your skin against the sun is to stay out of it. That may be about to change: Researchers at L'Oréal have developed a new ingredient called mexoryl that experts are calling the next big thing. "This agent will provide much more protection from UVA rays than any currently on the market," explains Vincent A. DeLeo, M.D., associate professor of clinical dermatology at Columbia University. Recent studies show that screening out UVA rays—which penetrate deeper into the base layer of the skin than UVB rays and can weaken the body's immune system—is crucial for preventing skin cancer. Until now, no ingredient has shut out UVA completely. Though L'Oréal has been hush-hush about details, experts predict products containing mexoryl will be available in a year or two.

You can prevent most problems with sunglasses by remembering to always handle your eyewear with care.

Q + A
SAVE YOUR SUNGLASSES

My favorite pair of sunglasses is stretched out—they're sliding right off my face. Is there a way to fix them, or should I just buy new ones?

Stretched frames, which often result from wearing your glasses on top of your head or from banging them around when they're not in their case, can typically be repaired at your local optical shop. "There, an expert can either heat plastic frames to mold them back into alignment or use special tools to do the same to metal frames," says Cindy Elkin, a spokeswoman for the Vision Council of America. Many shops will perform this quick procedure free (especially if you bought your pair there) or for a nominal charge of $5 to $10. Some stores, such as LensCrafters or Sunglass Hut, extend this service for the life of your glasses.

Loose or missing screws may also present problems, as they can cause earpieces or lenses to fall out. A professional can tighten or replace them. Or you can do it yourself with a repair kit, available at drugstores and optical shops. If you've lost an earpiece or lens, you can find replacements at the store where you bought your glasses or from the company that made them (if the brand is well-known).

To prevent problems in the first place, handle eyewear with care: Store your shades in a case, preferably a hard one, when you're not wearing them; don't place the lenses facedown; don't leave sunglasses in a hot spot (like a dashboard) where frames can warp; and clean lenses with a soft cotton cloth (tissue can scratch).

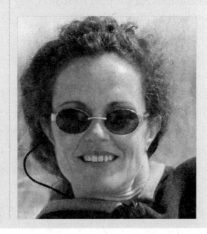

Q + A
SAFE SUNBATHING

I hear so much about the sun being bad for me. Do I have to avoid it completely?

Despite the real threat of skin cancer, you don't have to sit inside all summer with the curtains shut tight. You need some sun to make and store vitamin D. Recent research suggests that UV-phobes and workaholics may not get enough of the "sunshine vitamin" (which is actually a hormone). Adequate levels may help keep bones strong, lower blood pressure, and reduce the risk of diabetes. Some studies have found that vitamin D may also lower your risks of colon, breast, prostate, and ovarian cancer. To get your dose without chancing skin damage, spend time outdoors at least three times a week, but no longer than a quarter of the time it normally takes for you to start burning. For instance, if that usually happens after an hour, limit your time to 15 minutes; if it takes only 10 minutes, come in after two. Don't slather on sunscreen until after your time is up; products with SPF 15 or higher reduce your ability to make vitamin D by 98 percent. To learn more, pick up *The UV Advantage*, by Michael F. Holick, M.D., Ph.D., and Mark Jenkins, currently in bookstores.

Caffeine: The Latest in Skin-Cancer Prevention

Topically applied caffeine may protect against sun-induced skin cancer, according to preliminary research. Rutgers University scientists exposed mice to ultraviolet light twice a week for five months to make their risk of tumors similar to that of humans who got too much sun early in life. Then one of three solutions—one formulated with caffeine, one made with a chemical in green tea called EGCG, and one containing no active ingredient—was applied to the skin of different mice five days a week. After 20 weeks, caffeine had reduced benign tumors by 44 percent and malignant ones by 72 percent, while EGCG reduced them by 55 percent and 66 percent, respectively.

Though both showed positive results, the effects of caffeine opened researchers' eyes. "Both ingredients may have increased the body's ability to destroy cells that contain damaged DNA," says study co-author Allan Conney, Ph.D. "But caffeine is a more stable compound than EGCG, so it may last longer, both on the shelf and on your skin."

Although early data is promising, the days of rubbing coffee on your body to erase sun damage are still far off. Beauty products made with caffeine or green tea won't do the trick,

either. In order to work, such preparations would have to contain those ingredients in certain amounts and in specific forms; further research is needed. In the meantime, use a broad-spectrum sunscreen every day while researchers take their next step: studying the effectiveness of these compounds on humans who are at high skin-cancer risk.

Early data is promising, but more research is needed before you can start rubbing coffee on your body to erase sun damage.

Soy: The New Skin-Saver

The benefits of soy have been touted for years—it may reduce the risks of some cancers, lower cholesterol, and keep your heart healthy. Now there may be another advantage, one that was discovered quite accidentally. In animal studies, Australian researchers set out to observe the way a compound called NV-07a affected inflammation. Although this substance, a synthetic derivative of one of the major isoflavones (phytochemicals that are abundant in soy), did prove to be a weak anti-inflammatory, the scientists stumbled across an additional effect: NV-07a protected skin from ultraviolet (UV) light damage, which can lead to cancer. Human clinical trials suggest that applying the compound after sun exposure reduces harm to both skin's DNA and its immune response. It may even ward off UV-induced wrinkles. Further tests are being conducted, but Novogen, the company that makes NV-07a, hopes to market it for use in after-sun products or cosmetics, such as moisturizers and foundations. You won't find these on drugstore shelves for several years, and researchers say they don't know whether topical lotions that already contain soy would have similar effects. For now, our usual advice applies: Wear a wide-brimmed hat and slather on a broad-spectrum sunscreen. Our favorites are Clinique City Block Sheer Tint SPF 15 and Origins Sunshine State SPF 20 Sunscreen.

The Dirty Side of Pedicures

Don't set foot in a salon before you read this.

BY MICHELE BENDER

You've finally found some of the "me" time that self-help gurus tout, and you're happily soaking your soles in a tub of sudsy water during a pedicure. But watch out. You could be walking away with a contagious disease from the tools and foot spas in salons. According to the American Academy of Dermatology, these health risks include such viral conditions as warts or hepatitis B and C; bacterial illnesses, such as staph or strep; and fungal infections, like athlete's foot and nail fungus. Several news stories confirm this: A California salon with contaminated foot baths passed on a bacterial disease called furunculosis to more than 100 women, and a recent inspection of New York City salons found that 1,700 out of 2,000 had violated local health regulations.

All told, these are serious consequences for a treatment that's supposed to leave you de-stressed. But this doesn't mean you can never indulge. Simply heed the following advice to make sure the only thing you leave your salon with is nice-looking toes.

- Don't shave calves or ankles before your pedicure. You may think you're saving the technician from rubbing stubble, but "shaving can cause cuts or subtle abrasions that you don't even notice," says Kevin Winthrop, M.D., a medical epidemiologist with the federal Centers for Disease Control and Prevention. "These provide a porthole of entry for bacteria."

- Make sure both the salon and the technician have state licenses. They should be posted—if they're not, ask to see them.
- Check and see if the pedicurist washes her hands between customers. If you don't know whether she has, ask her to do so.
- Ask if whirlpool footbaths are routinely drained and washed with detergent and disinfectant between customers. Their filters should be removed and cleaned daily—it was bacteria in a buildup of hair and skin debris behind these screens that caused the California outbreak. You really have no way of knowing if these steps have been taken unless you ask.
- Don't let the technician cut your cuticles. "When this protective barrier gets cut or removed, it's easy for bacteria and fungus to enter," says Shelley Sekula-Gibbs, M.D., clinical assistant professor of dermatology at Baylor College of Medicine.
- Watch how the salon disinfects its instruments. Steam sterilization under pressure for a minimum of 15 minutes is ideal, but if a chemical disinfectant is used, look for the phrase "with tuberculocidal activity" on the label. Instruments should soak for at least 10 minutes between customers.
- Bring your own set of tools, such as nail buffers and cuticle pushers. These cannot be sterilized, and it's not always likely, even in the most pristine salon, that they are replaced with each customer.

Be Sweet to Your Feet

Try this cocoa soak—it's guaranteed to have you begging for seconds!

You've sworn chocolate will never touch your tongue, but what about your toes? Give them their just desserts with this tantalizing recipe created by Tara Oolie, co-owner of New York City's Just Calm Down, A Jewel of a Spa. "The lactic acid in the milk softens dry skin," Oolie says, "while the scents of cinnamon, vanilla, and peppermint have an uplifting, rejuvenating effect." And the calories won't go to your hips (the smell is a good test of your willpower, however).

For the soak:

8 tablespoons cocoa powder
6 tablespoons powdered milk
4 drops cinnamon essential oil (available at most health-food stores)
4 drops peppermint essential oil
1 teaspoon vanilla extract or vanilla oil
8 large marshmallows
20 chocolate kisses (plus extra ones for snacking)

For the scrub:

1 cup sugar
½ cup extra-virgin olive oil

1. Fill a basin with warm water to cover ankles. Add the first 6 ingredients (through marshmallows); stir well. Unwrap the kisses and keep them nearby.
2. In a small bowl, mix the sugar and olive oil, and set aside.
3. Soak your feet in the cocoa concoction for about 4 minutes. Next, drop the kisses into the basin (most will land pointy side up) and rub the soles of your feet over them for a ticklish massage. Once the kisses have melted, push your sweet-smelling feet into the soft-as-clouds mess of chocolate.
4. While one foot soaks, take the other one out; using very light circular motions, massage your foot and calf with the sugar-oil mixture. Switch feet and repeat.
5. Rinse both feet with water, pat dry (use an old towel, since it will turn chocolate-brown) and then slather on your favorite moisturizer.

Q + A   SHAVING WITHOUT IRRITATION

My husband's dermatologist suggested that he use an electric shaver to fight irritation. Can I try it, too?

Yes, this tool can be a savior if you have sensitive skin—from armpits to legs to such delicate areas as the bikini line. "A traditional blade is in direct contact with the skin, so it not only shaves the hair but also the skin," says David Green, M.D., clinical assistant professor of dermatology at Howard University Hospital in Washington, D.C. "The cutting edge on an electric shaver makes contact with the hairs through a screen that acts as an interface between the shaver and the skin." The only downsides: You typically don't get as close a shave, and you sometimes have to go over the same spot more than once.

An electric shaver that's made for women will probably give you better results than a men's model, since the head is especially designed to fit the angles of your body. The wet/dry shavers are the most convenient—you can use them either in the shower with shaving cream or at the sink when you need just a quick touch-up, say, under your arms. Even better, many of these female fuzz busters, such as the wet/dry Conair Satiny Smooth Lady Pro, have women-specific features, such as a pop-up bikini trimmer to groom longer hairs.

Unclutter Your Cosmetics

These five tips are sure to help you get your makeup in order.

BY MICHELE BENDER

It's 8:15 a.m., and the search is on. You dig through your purse, but your lipstick is missing. You fish around in your coat pocket, only to find a roll of LifeSavers. As a last resort, you dump the contents of your makeup bag onto the bed. Having found the tube at last, you smear the deep-red color across your lips. Wait, you wanted pink.

If this sounds like a scene from your life, it's time to clean up your beauty clutter—and not just for cosmetic reasons. "Having products at your fingertips not only enables you to leave the house on time, but also sets a pleasant tone for the rest of the day," says Julie Morgenstern, author of *Organizing from the Inside Out*. Here, Morgenstern helps clear things up.

Get back to basics. Toss any beauty product you bought six months ago but still haven't touched. In the end, you should be left with just one item per purpose: a single foundation, powder, mascara, and eyeliner, plus a lipstick or two. "We always hang on to too many of those extra lipsticks 'just in case,' but then never actually use them," Morgenstern says.

Hold everything. If your storage spot is visible—such as a countertop, shelf, or back of the toilet—try to organize your products in baskets or containers. Round or oval ones work best for lipsticks, compacts, and foundations; tall, upright ones are better for pencils and brushes. Try Bobbi Brown's Brush Holder, a chic-looking black-leather container with two sections for your supplies. The holder's weighted bottom ensures it won't tip over no matter how full it is. If you have drawer space, invest in some organizers to keep things from rolling around and out of your children's reach. Bed Bath & Beyond's Expandable Cutlery Tray has sections in a variety of sizes to accommodate items of different shapes, and it can expand from 9 to 16 inches to fit most drawers.

Clear medicine out of the medicine chest. "That prime space should be reserved for the things you use daily, not the cold medicine or first-aid items you only need once in a while," Morgenstern says. (Those can go on a high shelf in a linen closet or in a locked cabinet underneath the sink if you have kids.)

Don't neglect makeup brushes. Get a case with individual compartments for each brush. This makes them easy to find and keeps bristles in shape. We like Laura Mercier's Brush Sets (available in three sizes: mini, travel, and large), which fold up virtually flat and feature an extra zippered compartment.

Choose your bag wisely. Put as much thought into selecting a makeup carrier as you do an evening bag. It should be small enough to tote easily but have an opening wide enough to let you find your mascara without everything else spilling out. Choose such materials as cotton or plastic, which are washable and can withstand being tossed around in your purse. (Silk and satin are luxurious but delicate and can easily get stained or torn.) Also look for a plastic or vinyl lining that can be wiped clean when needed (once a month or so). We love the Cindy Make-Up Bag from Buzz by Jane Fox. It zips up to a slim silhouette but opens to a wide, roomy square, so it's easy to dip your hand in and out. It comes in such patterns as polka dots, florals, and green bamboo.

Q + A
EYE-POPPING LASHES

I'd love to try colored mascara but don't want to look like I'm going to the prom. Any tips?

We agree that one stroke can cross the line from classy to clownish. "However, applied with the right technique, colored mascara is a simple way to make eyes pop," says makeup artist Carol Shaw. Here's how: Coat your top lashes with black mascara, then brush a more vibrant hue on the tips. When you want to ditch black altogether, try rich but understated shades of plum, wine, navy, and olive. Here are some examples: Shiseido's The Makeup Distinguish Mascara in Deep Bordeaux, ideal for the color-shy because it's just one notch lighter than black; Aveda's Mosscara in Jade Vine, an army green that highlights gray, green, or light brown eyes; and Agnès B.'s Curling and Thickening Mascara in Navy Blue, which brightens blue or blue-green eyes.

Q + A
PRODUCTS FOR LONGER LOCKS

Recently, I've seen products formulated espcially for long hair. I have always used regular shampoo and conditioner on mine, but I'm wondering if I should switch.

Women with long hair do have needs different from those of their shorter shorn friends. "The ends of long hair are old and tend to be dry and fragile," says dermatologist Jeanine Downie, M.D. "You need products that really moisturize and condition. If the long-hair products you choose do that, then great. But others not labeled 'long hair' can do the trick just as well."

How do you know what to buy? Look for ingredients that hydrate and protect, such as fatty alcohols (like cetyl alcohol and oleic acid) or silicones (like dimethicone). Our picks: Redken's So Long Shampoo and Conditioner and L'anza's Be Long Long Hair Formula Cleanse and Condition. To give long locks some extra TLC, apply conditioner to the ends of your hair before you lather to avoid overcleansing, Downie says.

Q + A
LONGER LASTING LASHES

I've heard about a mascara that lasts three days. It seems great for my hectic lifestyle, but is it safe?

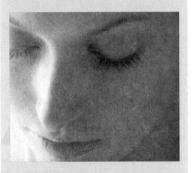

Marathon mascaras, like Revlon ColorStay Overtime Lash Tint, should be "perfectly safe," according to Seth Matarasso, M.D., associate clinical professor of dermatology at the University of California School of Medicine. You're just dyeing the outer layers of the hairs, he says; that's not a problem as long as you don't get the mascara in your eyes. To be extra-cautious, put on a light test coat. "People do have allergic reactions, but it's from the makeup itself, not from leaving it on too long," Matarasso says.

We were surprised by how natural the Revlon product looked (and that we didn't wake up with raccoon eyes). The color fades in three days; you can remove it sooner with an oil-based remover.

One Size Doesn't Always Fit All

New technology promises to make finding the right fit a lot easier.

BY MICHELE BENDER

Though fashion changes faster than you can hand over your credit card, the sizing standards for clothing haven't budged since the 1940s. Back then, the U.S. Department of Commerce measured various body points on 10,000 American military women and assigned each a size between 2 and 20. Today, manufacturers still follow these guidelines, even though the average woman has gone from 5 feet 2 inches and 129 pounds in the '40s to 5 feet 4 inches and 142 pounds today. "We've gotten taller and wider, but most clothes aren't cut to reflect that," says Karen Davis, a spokeswoman for Textile/Clothing Technology Corp. [(T2)2]. As a result, more than 50 percent of consumers are unsatisfied with the fit of off-the-rack items.

Some companies try to soothe women's bruised egos with clothes in so-called vanity sizes—that is, a size or two smaller than the pieces really are. "If I can wear a size 8 in one brand instead of a 10 in another, I'll go back to that line because I'd rather be an 8," Davis says. In fact, our own size-4 tester tried on skirts from three different stores and found she was a size 6 at Ann Taylor, a 4 at Banana Republic, and a 2 at J.Crew.

To address this often frustrating inconsistency, [(T2)2] has kicked off a National Sizing Survey funded by manufacturers,

retailers, and the Department of Commerce. The organization is traveling the country, using a light-based scanner to take dozens of measurements from tens of thousands of people. [(T2)2] plans to complete the survey by June 2003 and pass its findings on to stores and apparel firms, who hopefully will use the information to make clothes with measurements closer to real life.

In the meantime, consider custom clothing for a personalized fit. LandsEnd.com and Levi's offer jeans and khakis made to your specifications. In fact, although they're $20 to $35 pricier than off-the-rack items, 40 percent of all chinos and jeans bought at LandsEnd.com are customized. ∎

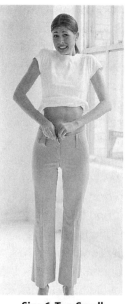

Size 6: Too Small
Hennes by H&M

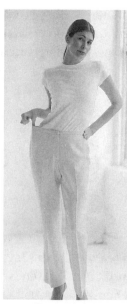

Size 6: Too Big
Jones New York

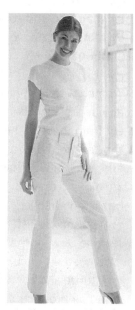

Size 6: Just Right
Banana Republic

What's Your Style?

In order for us to get inside your heads—or at least your closets—*Health* conducted a Web poll to find out how fashion fits into your world. Almost 700 of you responded; here's what you had to say.

<u>You like the latest.</u> Sixty-one percent of participants described their style as "somewhat trendy;" only 1 percent said it was "totally trendy." Almost 20 percent called their look "classic."

<u>Forever in blue jeans.</u> Almost half said that jeans are their most-worn wardrobe staple.

<u>Husbands, listen up.</u> Forty-three percent of those surveyed said jewelry was the key to dressing up an outfit, followed by almost 36 percent who said that shoes did the trick.

<u>Your credit cards are warm.</u> Forty-three percent of respondents said they shop for clothes once a month, while almost 38 percent said they hit the mall once every other month.

<u>No fashion slaves here.</u> Seventy-one percent polled said comfort was more important than style when deciding what to wear.

How Smaller Thighs Are Leading to Bigger Breasts

A study presented at the American Academy of Dermatology's annual Derm Update found that women who had undergone power-assisted liposuction on their abs, hips, and thighs got a bonus: bigger breasts (by an average one cup size) two to six months post-op. "One thought is that the abs, hips, and thighs are areas where fat cells metabolize testosterone. By removing those fat cells, you increase the amount of estrogen in the body," says study co-author Bruce Katz, M.D. "Since breast tissue is sensitive to changes in estrogen, it swells." A second possibility: Liposuction changes the way your body distributes fat. "If women gain weight post-op, the fat may have gone to their breasts," says Naomi Lawrence, M.D., a spokeswoman representing the American Society for Dermatologic Surgery.

Q + A

GET THE SKINNY ON YOUR SKIVVIES

I've heard that thong underwear can cause health problems. True?

You don't have to give in to panty lines; just choose your skivvies wisely. "The constant friction of a thong's thin strip of material can result in cuts, fissures, and skin irritations on and around your vagina, your rectum, and the area between them, the perineum," says David Soper, M.D. "It may also transport bacteria from the rectal area, leading to bladder or vaginal bacterial infections." (Not all doctors agree on this, though, as the evidence is anecdotal, rather than scientific.) To avoid these below-the-belt maladies, choose a thong with a wide back panel. The extra material reduces movement so that bacteria won't spread; it also keeps the panty from getting wedged in too far, ensuring that it doesn't cut into delicate tissue. As you should with all underwear, look for cotton or mesh fabric and a cotton crotch, both of which breathe and wick away moisture. Finally, if you're tempted to wear a thong while you exercise, don't. You'll just add more friction.

Which styles passed our test for comfort and met our experts' criteria? Calvin Klein's Seamless Thong, for one. It's made of superfine cotton, and its generous back panel stays put. If you wear low-rise pants and don't want your undies peeking out, try Cosabella's Soiré Lowrider mesh thong.

Will you age like your MOTHER?

You may have inherited your mom's brown eyes or your dad's Roman nose, but according to the latest research, aging gracefully is largely up to you.

BY PATRICIA J. O'CONNOR • PHOTOGRAPHY BY JENNY ACHESON

During a family dinner not long after my now husband and I started dating, the conversation turned to the royal family of Monaco. We were debating whether or not Grace Kelly's daughters looked like the legendary beauty icon. My future husband argued that they did, noting, "The apple doesn't fall far from the tree." He then looked over to my mother.

What is he staring at? I asked myself. I considered my mother's beauty—blemishes and all—part of the extraordinary package that made her who she was. But how did I know whether the wrinkles around her mouth owed to 30 years of smoking True Blues? Or if her move to a warmer climate more than two decades before was the precursor to her age spots? Her gray hairs were easy: After a month of living with me, my husband knew exactly where they came from.

Whether genetics or lifestyle plays the greater role in aging has been fiercely debated for years. Science, it seems, can now provide us with answers. The particular package you inherited from your parents does determine in part whether your hair will go gray and, to some extent, where your wrinkles will form. However, lifestyle factors, such as sun exposure and stress, seem to be stronger determinants. Experts now believe that 80 percent or more of premature skin aging is sun-induced and that smoking is equally, if not more, damaging to the skin. Darrick Antell, M.D., a New York City plastic surgeon whose research focuses on identical twins, says that a twin who smokes looks, on average, 6 to 10 years older than her nonsmoking sibling. And though the correlation is harder to prove, studies have linked high stress levels to everything from increased wrinkling to hair loss.

Curious about how this could affect you? We invited Debra Jaliman, M.D., clinical instructor of dermatology at Mount Sinai School of Medicine in New York City, to take a look at four sets of mothers and daughters. Each woman revealed her one main beauty gripe, whether she perceived it to be inherited or not. We wanted to see what steps our subjects could take to safeguard future good looks. Jaliman's prognosis was positive: With a few smart lifestyle changes, along with help from some high-tech products and dermatological procedures, it seems there's a lot these women—and you—can do to prevent and even reverse signs of aging.

Not too long ago, I asked my husband if he was looking at my mother in order to gauge how I might age. A bit embarrassed, he answered, "Yes." Then he added, "But I've always thought of freckles as sexy."

BEAUTY LEGACY: WRINKLES
Kay, LuAnne, and Martha

Daughters' Stories: Kay clearly remembers an unfortunate sun experience. "I used a tanning lamp in college and burned my face so severely that I had to go to the infirmary for ointment." Now, as editor of *Coastal Living* magazine, Kay is constantly traveling to beach locations. "I'm careful about wearing sunscreen every day, especially since my mom was diagnosed with skin cancer," she says. Like her mother and sister, she now has lines around her eyes that bother her.

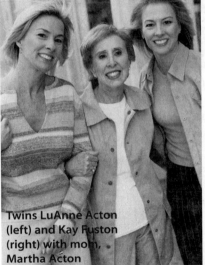

Twins LuAnne Acton (left) and Kay Fuston (right) with mom, Martha Acton

LuAnne also recalls a few bad sunburns in her teens on family beach vacations. Since her 30s, she's been more conscientious about wearing sun protection. "I now live in Florida and still love spending time outside, but I always make sure to wear sunscreen," she says. Since she started seeing fine lines at the corners of her eyes and between her brows, she's been using an over-the-counter retinol cream at night and a vitamin C cream with SPF during the day.

Mom's Story: Although she's fair-skinned, Martha never gave sun protection much thought. "I used baby oil and iodine at the beach, and I ended up with some pretty bad burns," she admits. Besides

having significant wrinkles around her eyes and mouth, Martha underwent surgery to remove a squamous cell skin cancer from her nose a few years ago. Since then, she makes a point of always wearing a hat and a broad-spectrum sunscreen with SPF 30 whenever she goes outdoors.

The Diagnosis: Martha's cancer puts her and her daughters at increased risk for sun-related skin conditions. Luckily, there's a lot they can do to avoid potential problems. The effectiveness of topical antioxidants is still controversial, Jaliman says, but new research from Duke University shows that using sunscreen with L-ascorbic acid (the only form of vitamin C the skin can absorb) and 1-percent alpha tocopherol (vitamin E) minimizes the DNA damage that can lead to skin cancer (try Primacy C+E by SkinCeuticals, the only product of its kind containing both these nutrients in their pure forms). Preliminary studies also suggest that eating a diet rich in omega-3 fats, such as those in fish and nuts, can lower your risk of the disease.

"All three women could use Renova or Retin-A, both vitamin-A derived prescription creams that improve the appearance of fine lines and rough texture," Jaliman says. If that doesn't smooth out Kay's and LuAnne's skin, monthly glycolic acid peels ($75 to $250) can help. Derived from sugar cane, these treatments exfoliate the top layer of dead skin, revealing smoother skin below. "For Martha's deeper and more pronounced wrinkles, I'd suggest a peel with a nonablative laser. The laser stimulates new collagen and creates better hydration in the outer layers of the skin," Jaliman explains. It can also be used close to the eyes and requires no recovery time. Patients typically require five sessions spaced one month apart (each runs from $400 to $1,000, depending on location).

BEAUTY LEGACY: PREMATURELY GRAY HAIR

Amy and Nattari

Daughter's Story: What did Amy Hale get for her 25th birthday? A few strands of gray. "Great present!" she laughs. "They're especially noticeable because my hair is dark." Amy inherited her thick, straight mane from her Thai mother, and it has always been her favorite feature. "But the gray really bothers me because it is a different texture than the rest of my hair, more coarse and brittle," she says. So far, she hasn't seen enough gray to warrant covering it, but she knows a trip to the colorist is just around the corner.

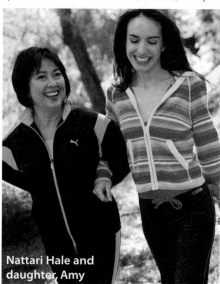

Nattari Hale and daughter, Amy

My long, dark hair is my favorite beauty feature. Seeing gray in my early 20s really took me by surprise.
—Amy Hale, 27

Mom's Story: "Amy worries about her grays. I, too, saw them in my 20s, but they never bothered me," Nattari says. (According to an ancient Thai legend, pulling out one gray hair will offend three ancestors, leaving three more in its place.) Nattari waited until she was 50 before she colored her hair. She now uses an ammonia-free, semipermanent home product to avoid the harsh chemicals sometimes included in permanent color. But she'd prefer something that didn't wash out every six weeks.

The Diagnosis: Studies suggest that certain stress-related hair-loss conditions may cause premature grayness. But according to Jaliman, the pigment-making cells in your hair follicles are more or less genetically programmed to produce color for a fixed length of time. "Typically, the darker your hair, the faster you'll go gray. We think this is because it takes more pigment to make dark brown and black

hair," Jaliman explains. "I compare it to the ink in a printer—the darker the type, the faster the ink will be used up."

Although the link between graying and stress isn't definitive, Amy and Nattari may benefit by incorporating some relaxation time into their lives, especially since Amy describes her mom as a "self-proclaimed worrier." Because Amy is seeing only a few gray hairs, she can simply pluck them or use a cover-up stick (such as 'Tween-Time Temporary Haircolor Touch-Up Sticks). If her hair stays less than half-gray, highlights (such as L'Oréal's Féria Colour Strands) will provide coverage for up to three months. But when hair becomes more than 50 percent gray, as in Nattari's case, only permanent color camouflages completely. Clairol's Nice 'n Easy Multi-Tone Permanent Color Formula would be a good choice for her. It uses a new technology that enables extra dye molecules and conditioners to penetrate hair, making it softer and more natural-looking without strong chemicals.

BEAUTY LEGACY: SUN SPOTS

Anne Marie and Patricia

Daughter's Story: Although 100-percent Italian, both Anne Marie and her mother have fair skin and light eyes. "In my teens and 20s, I spent a lot of time at the beach," Anne Marie says. "And like most of my friends, I did the baby-oil thing. I also went to tanning salons. It wasn't until my mid-20s that I even started to wear sunscreen." Anne Marie's face and chest freckles bother her, so for the last two years she's worn a daily moisturizer with SPF.

Mom's Story: Like her daughter, Patricia was a tanning enthusiast during her younger years. "I remember Anne Marie getting sunburns, but back then we just thought burning was part of the process, something you had to go through to get a nice tan," she says. Patricia has noticed sun spots on her arms, legs, and face; she also has wrinkles around her eyes and mouth. She now doubles up for safety—her foundation and moisturizer both contain sunscreen.

The Diagnosis: Everyone, no matter what their skin tone, is born with melanocytes, cells that produce melanin, the pigment that gives skin its natural color. When melanocytes are exposed to UV light, they can turn into freckles. "And just like a tan or sunburn, freckles should fade after sun exposure," Jaliman says. "If they don't, as in Patricia's case, they're referred to as sun spots." Technically known as lentigos, these spots are the products of cumulative, longstanding sun exposure. "Freckles look like healthy normal skin under a microscope, whereas sun spots show signs of underlying skin damage," she notes.

Both freckles and sun spots can be bleached with Tri-Luma, a new prescription cream combining tretinoin (aka Retin-A) and hydroquinone. Anne Marie and Patricia will see some lightening in two to four weeks and additional improvement in six to eight weeks.

> We just thought burning was part of the process, something you had to go through to get a nice tan. —Patricia Sancilio, 58

Anne Marie and mom, Patricia

The most effective way to remove spots, however, is the Versapulse laser, which can be used all over the body. In one visit to a dermatologist (about $300), the blotches are zapped, after which scabs form (they fall off in one to two weeks). To maintain clear skin, though, mother and daughter need to use a sunscreen that contains UVA/UVB protection and an SPF of 15 or higher every day. Also, as light-eyed and light-skinned women are at higher risk for skin cancer than their darker counterparts, they both should have their spots checked annually.

BEAUTY LEGACY: UNDER-EYE CIRCLES
Rachel and Beverly

Daughter's Story: "I'm generally pretty happy with my skin, but my dark circles have always bothered me. They make me look tired even after a good night's sleep," Rachel says. She suspects she has a genetic tendency toward them, because her grandmother, her mother, and even her 9-year-old daughter, Bianca, have them. Concealers provide some coverage, but Rachel has yet to find one that makes her circles completely disappear. She grew up on the Jersey Shore but only got serious about sun protection in her 20s. She now uses sunscreen when gardening or spending time at the pool.

Mom's Story: People have asked Beverly if she and her daughter are twins, which, of course, gives her endless pleasure, but Beverly is also frustrated by under-eye circles. "I've tried different eye creams, but nothing seems to work," she says. Because Beverly lives on the coast, she's outside a lot. "But like Rachel, I've become more focused on sun care. I now wear a daily moisturizer with sunscreen for extra protection," she notes.

The Diagnosis: Jaliman first asked whether Rachel, Beverly, and Bianca suffer from seasonal allergies. The answer was yes. "Allergies cause inflammation around the eyes, and women of African-American heritage have a tendency toward hyperpigmentation, or skin discoloration, once the puffiness subsides," Jaliman explains. The time that they have spent in the sun has added to their circles, as the delicate skin under the eyes is vulnerable to ultraviolet damage and darkening.

In addition to wearing sunscreen around their eyes (nonirritating products containing zinc oxide, such as DDF Protective Eye Cream SPF 15, work well), Rachel, Beverly, and Bianca should wear sunglasses that extend just above the brows and block 100 percent of UV rays,

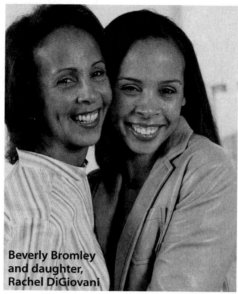

Beverly Bromley
and daughter,
Rachel DiGiovani

> Despite eight hours of sleep and the latest in antiaging creams, I still have dark, puffy under-eye circles.
> —Beverly Bromley, 53

Jaliman advises. For allergies, Rachel and Beverly can use a prescription anti-inflammatory cream, such as Eladil, daily to prevent darkening. To lighten circles, Jaliman recommends a prescription combination of Renova .02 percent and Solaquin Forte cream, which contains the bleaching agent hydroquinone. "While you won't get rid of the discoloration completely, you'll see a significant lightening after a few months, so dark circles are easier to cover with makeup." (Experts suggest a cream-based, yellow-toned concealer one to two shades lighter than Beverly's and Rachel's foundation. Our pick: Black Opal, Flawless Perfecting Concealer.)

Patricia J. O'Connor is a freelance writer who specializes in beauty and health.

Q + A

THE JUICE BEHIND FRUITY BEAUTY PRODUCTS

A lot of beauty products supposedly contain fruits. Are these claims for real?

Technically, yes. But no one's been squeezing fresh mango juice into your favorite shampoo. If that were the case, you'd have to store your cosmetics in the refrigerator. The label may tout the words *papaya* or *orange,* but "most of the time,

'fruit' means extract—material taken from the skin or pulp that has had some of the phytochemicals removed from it," says Rebecca James Gadberry, an instructor of cosmetic sciences at the University of California, Los Angeles. Look at the ingredients, and you'll see that such words as *acid, extract, oil,* or *enzyme* follow the name of the fruit. The higher this

component is on the list, the more potent the concentration.

Why choose these products? They smell delicious. Try Jaqua Girls' Facial Kit, tiny tubes of cleanser, scrub, mask, and moisturizer in such flavors as cherry and papaya, and Clairol's Herbal Essences Fruit Fusions Revitalizing Shampoo, which leaves hair smelling like an exotic fruit salad.

Revitalize Summer Faces with This Homemade Cleanser

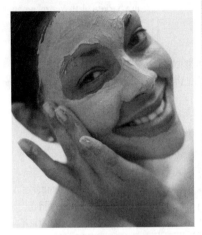

Unless you spend the summer at the movies, your skin is bound to suffer. Sun, sweat, and wind can leave your face irritated, greasy, and parched. To the rescue: this yogurt-honey cleanser created by Linda Collins of Salon Blue in Carle Place, New York. "The lactic acid in yogurt softens and soothes the skin, while the honey cleanses and moisturizes it," says dermatologist Audrey Kunin, M.D.

WHAT YOU DO

1. In a bowl, mix together 1 cup plain yogurt and 2½ tablespoons unflavored honey. Because people who are allergic to pollen may also be allergic to honey, Kunin says, you might want to patch-test the mixture first behind one ear. Wait one hour, watching for any irritation.

2. With clean hands or cotton pads, apply the mask liberally to your freshly washed face and neck (even your décolletage) and leave on for five minutes.

3. Rinse well with warm water, lightly pat dry, and follow with your favorite moisturizer. Repeat one or two times a week.

ADD A SPRITZ

If you have oily skin, you can try adding ½ teaspoon lemon juice in Step 1 in order to control shine.

Q + A

My chest seems to be aging faster than my face. Is there anything I can do about my freckles and wrinkles?

Your chest is giving away your age—or even adding a few years—because you've probably been neglecting it. "Most people put sunscreen on their faces but forget about their chests," says Linda K. Franks, M.D., assistant clinical professor of dermatology at New York University Medical School. Plus, as you walk to work or go for a run in the park, your chest catches some incidental rays. With chronic sun exposure, skin wrinkles and pigment darkens, causing brown spots.

An over-the-counter retinol product, used for three to five months, can help diminish some of the damage; so can nonprescription treatments containing 2-percent hydroquinone, such as Rodan &

DON'T LET YOUR CHEST AGE YOU

Fields Radiant Skin Lightening Lotion. Neither works as quickly as a doctor-prescribed remedy, however. For faster results, ask your dermatologist for Retin-A or Renova, which will each help get rid of wrinkles and blotches. "After several months, have any remaining spots evaluated by a dermatologist, who can treat them with a chemical peel or laser surgery," Franks says. A doctor can also determine if the discolorations are harmless.

To prevent further damage, protect your chest daily. "When you apply your morning SPF facial moisturizer or sunscreen, put a bigger glob than you need in the palm of your hand," Franks suggests. "When you're through with your face, use what's left over on your neck, chest, and the backs of your hands." Then give your chest the same respect as your face by covering up when you go outside.

vital *stats*

5
Percentage of people who have purchased DRUGS from another country to save money

40
Percentage who WOULD consider it

62
Percentage who don't know whether it's ILLEGAL (it is)

3.56
Number of serious actions (revocations of licenses, suspensions, probations) by STATE MEDICAL BOARDS per 1,000 doctors in 2002

11.87
Number of serious actions per 1,000 doctors in Wyoming

1.07
Number in Hawaii

1
Number of ounces in a suggested SERVING SIZE of cereal

1.6
Number of ounces most WOMEN consider one serving

2
Number of ounces MEN consider a serving

55
Percentage of women who believe they regularly consume the RDA for IRON (18 milligrams)

10
Percentage who actually do

51
Percentage of people planning to take a SUMMER VACATION

54
Percentage of people who say they return from vacation FEELING TIRED

46
Percentage of vacationers who pack the DAY BEFORE their trip

10
Percentage who pack the DAY OF their trip

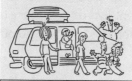

8
Average number of BIRTHDAY CARDS most people get

1
Rank of August among months with the MOST birthdays

45
Percentage of Americans who have thought about QUITTING or have quit their jobs in the last year

44
Percentage who say their jobs are more STRESSFUL now than they were a year ago

83
Percentage of people who believe their households don't contain MOLD

88
Percentage of WINDOW SILLS that contain mold

36 MILLION
Number of Americans who are potentially ALLERGIC to mold

51
Percentage of women who just "HOLD IT" when there's a long line at a public rest room

27
Percentage who use the MEN'S ROOM instead

17
Percentage of women taking CONTRACEPTIVES who don't use backup birth control when on antibiotics

28
Percentage who have been prescribed ANTIBIOTICS without their doctors' asking if they take the Pill

21
Recommended number of days a Pill user should use BACKUP BIRTH CONTROL if she takes antibiotics

67
Percentage of FLOWERS purchased by women

34
Percentage of flowers people purchase for themselves

94
Percentage of homes with SMOKE DETECTORS

20
Percentage of those homes in which the smoke detectors DON'T WORK

Sources: Cigna Behavioral Health, Cambridge Consumer Credit Index, Avelox, Sanofi-Synthelabo Inc., University of Arizona, Asthma and Allergy Foundation of America, Society of American Florists, Hallmark, Cream of Wheat, U.S. Consumer Product Safety Commission, *Wall Street Journal*/Harris Interactive, U.S. Food and Drug Administration, Uristat, Public Citizen Health Research Group—Reported by Laura Riccobano

relationships

**the secrets to happiness for
work, love, and play**

The 7 Friends Every Woman Should Have

BY LIZ WELCH

You might say Leyla Sharabi has a friend for every occasion. Kimberlee, for example, is a fellow photographer who helped her land a job for *Time* magazine and always gives great lighting tips. Vicky, a wife and mother of one, gives the recently married Sharabi advice on relationships. For matters of the soul, the half-Palestinian 34-year-old reaches out to Zeina, who lives in Beirut, Lebanon. "My friends enrich my life in so many ways," Sharabi says. "They keep me balanced and in touch with who I am."

Sharabi has realized that she needs different types of companions to tap into various parts of her personality—and not just to fill her social calendar. As Bruce Rabin, M.D., medical director of the Healthy Lifestyle Program at the University of Pittsburgh Medical Center, says, "The more varied behavior you engage in with different types of friends, the better your health will be."

Strong friendships are primarily a woman-to-woman phenomenon, experts say. "Even though men and women form adult partnerships, women continue to confide in female friends, and have more close friends than men do over their lifetimes," says psychologist Shelley E. Taylor, Ph.D., author of *The Tending Instinct*.

In fact, the very definition of friendship embraced by some psychologists rules out platonic male-female relationships altogether. "Women need same-sex friends for those bonding experiences that you don't have to explain," says Jan Yager, Ph.D., a sociologist and author of *When Friendship Hurts*.

Here, we identify the seven types of friends a woman needs to live her healthiest, happiest life.

THE **BEST** FRIEND

Technically, by definition, you can have only one best friend, Yager says, but a woman often has different kinds: one in her community, one from school, one from a former job. Whether it's one person or more, your best friend is the first person you call after your husband and family members to share news, good or bad. "She's the one person in your life you can say anything to, and you know she'll understand and love you no matter what," explains Margaret Gibbs, Ph.D., a professor of psychology at Fairleigh Dickinson University. She knows your darkest secrets, most embarrassing moments, and painful insecurities. "A best friend is important because she affirms and reaffirms you," Yager explains. "She grounds you, helps you through self-doubt, and never judges you."

For Liz Subin, a stay-at-home mom in Vermont, Nancy Benerofe has played that role for her since the ninth grade. During their years together, they've

> **Women continue to confide in female friends and have more close friends than men do over their lifetimes.**
> —Shelley E. Taylor, Ph.D

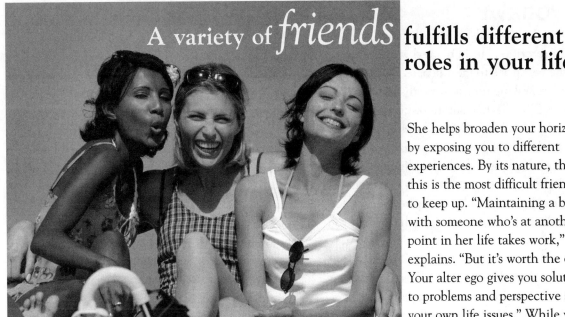

A variety of *friends* fulfills different roles in your life.

She helps broaden your horizons by exposing you to different experiences. By its nature, though, this is the most difficult friendship to keep up. "Maintaining a bond with someone who's at another point in her life takes work," Sills explains. "But it's worth the effort. Your alter ego gives you solutions to problems and perspective about your own life issues." While you may seem like you're poles apart, Tamara Traeder, co-author of the national bestseller *Girlfriends: Invisible Bonds, Enduring Ties*, believes that friendships like these serve an important purpose. "When you hang out with your opposite," she explains, "it's usually because she represents a part of yourself that's not being recognized."

been to Grateful Dead concerts, endured obnoxious boyfriends, backpacked in South America, and even gone through pregnancy together. "Nancy has witnessed every major event in my life," Subin, 35, explains. "When I went into labor with my first child, she drove from southern Vermont to upstate Maine to be by my side. My contractions were two to three minutes apart, and I was telling my husband we needed to wait for Nancy!" Benerofe pulled into the driveway just as Subin was leaving for the hospital.

Benerofe, 35, has also helped Subin through some of life's low points. She was there for her friend when she miscarried a year and a half later, not only talking her through the heartbreaking experience but also taking care of Otis, Subin's son, while Subin went to the doctor. "Nancy is a compassionate, nonjudgmental, and loving soul," Subin explains. "I know she will always be there for me."

THE **ALTER EGO**

You not only need a friend who is your closest confidante, but also one whose life is just the opposite of yours. You're married with children and living in the suburbs; she's single and renting an apartment in the city. You're an adventurer; she's a homebody.

For Shira Miller, a 36-year-old divorcée who runs her own publicity and marketing firm in Atlanta, that would be Christy Dennis, a 29-year-old stay-at-home mother in Knoxville, Tennessee, who used to work for her. Miller lives in a hip urban neighborhood, while Dennis lives in a quiet suburb with her husband and 2-year-old son. Miller, a vivacious redhead, flaunts formfitting clothes and knee-high boots; Dennis, a wholesome brunette, prefers the ease of blue jeans and sneakers. "I've encouraged her to dress up more," Miller says, laughing. It's those differences that fuel their friendship. Miller could never imagine giving up her job to raise a child, but she finds comfort and stability in Dennis. "I'm in awe that she can make her son the center of her universe and not miss having a career," Miller explains. "I tend to go in a million different directions, and she's always calm and supportive. She is serenity personified."

THE WORK PAL

Back in college, friends were easily found in classrooms or sororities, but in the real world, work is often the best place to meet people. "Most people spend more waking time at work than anywhere else," says BJ Gallagher, author of *Everything I Need to Know I Learned from Other Women*. "Whether you're celebrating a promotion or commiserating about a terrible boss, a strong bonding takes place." Beyond making it through each day together, work friends also help each other navigate their careers. They really listen, give advice, pitch in when you need help, and often make you better at your job because they want you to succeed. Danielle Flagg, a 36-year-old art director at an advertising agency, learned the importance of a work pal firsthand through Jennifer Smieja, the colleague who produced Flagg's first TV commercial. "I had just moved to Portland for my job and didn't know anybody," Flagg explains. "I felt like I had no idea what I was doing, and Jennifer, who had a ton of experience, rescued me without belittling my lack of knowledge. The day of the commercial shoot, she gave me confidence that I have carried with me and built on ever since." That was the beginning of a six-year friendship that has grown far

> The work friend listens, gives advice, pitches in when you need help, and makes you better at your job because she wants you to succeed.

beyond the office. The women carpool to work, where they have spent many late nights—and shared a few tense moments. Occasionally, they've also shared a few after-hours margaritas. "Jen's insight and support have helped me become a better art director," Flagg explains. "I can bounce an idea off her, and she will push it in six directions. She reminds me not to take things so seriously, while I inspire her to stand up for herself in the office and be more proactive. We're a great balance for one another."

THE GO-TO GIRL

When Jennifer Bates, a Los Angeles attorney, was too busy to think of a Halloween costume, she called her college friend Sandi Yi. "At work, I'm always under such intense pressure to make important decisions that I often leave little time for fun personal choices," Bates, 30, explains. Within minutes, Yi, 29, came up with a long list of great possibilities, including Mae West, a Girl Scout, and an '80s prom queen. "She even met me at the costume store and helped pick things off the rack for me. Bates also turns to Yi for her house-hunting tips, dinner-party recipes, and etiquette questions. She even helped Bates choose her wedding dress. It's not only Yi's wealth of knowledge that keeps Bates coming back for more, but also her nonjudgmental attitude, an important quality all go-to girls have in common. "She never makes me feel bad, no matter how ridiculous my requests may be," Bates says. "And, unlike some of my other friends, she always calls me back immediately!"

The go-to girl makes your life easier and enjoys doing so. According to Emily Miles Terry, co-author of *It's a Chick Thing: Celebrating the Wild Side of Women's Friendship*, she's also irreplaceable. "Today, women are often required to be multitaskers," Terry explains. "The go-to girl takes off the pressure by being a treasured friend and an essential resource." She is a problem-solver who eliminates unnecessary stress from your life. "She is crucial, because women are expected to do so much," Terry says. "We need to work, parent, entertain, and buy gaskets at Home Depot. She helps us with constructive shortcuts, saves us time, and keeps us sane." But as much as you need her in your life, you probably play that role in another friend's life, maybe without even knowing it. "People need to share their knowledge," Yager insists. "Too often, people think, 'Who are my friends?' without considering who they are as friends."

My Magnificent Seven

Marion Winik, National Public Radio commentator and author of Telling, *pays tribute to the friends she can't live without.*

Best Friend: Sandye

Sandye has been my best friend since I was 9 and her family moved to my street in New Jersey. Our friendship has weathered girlhood hurts, high school wildness, and over-crowded postcollegiate living situations, though for decades now we have lived far apart. One time, I asked her, "If my car broke down in Buffalo and you were in Arizona, would you come get me?" It turns out she would.

Alter Ego: Emma

It's my stepdaughter, my 15-year-old, purple-haired, high school art student/performance artist/punkette/vegetarian, Emma. Being around her makes me feel young. Sometimes, when we're alone together, I have an insane urge to find a rave and dance all night. She also makes me feel old, as she tosses shoes and socks and magazines around with an abandon once my own, and I pick them up with a grim compulsiveness I once thought only my mother's.

Work Pal: Judy

Judy and I met at a software company while working on a project that went on for months. By the time we finished, we were friends for life. Good thing, because that's when the big waves started to roll in:

Judy's marriage fell apart, then my husband became ill, and inappropriate office relationships loomed. Then corporate disasters, layoffs, and buyouts finished things up tsunami-style. Today, we live quite far apart, but we are still one another's first choice for airing long stories of frustration that might bore others.

Go-To Girl: Ellen

First, a bow to my mother, who knows everything (almost), and who is present somehow in every decision I make. Second, my sweet friend Ellen, who took care of me when I was a single mom. Ellen helped me reorganize my house (she had a decorating business), shop for clothes (she worked in a dress shop), and plan vacations (she took us to her parents' place in the country and on ski trips). I miss her every day.

Cerebral Match: Jim

They say you would marry your cerebral match if she were a man. Well mine is a man, and I can't marry him because he's the husband of another beloved friend. But I'd make Jim an honorary woman if I could, because he's a stay-at-home dad, and he likes to talk on the phone. Jim and I are both writers, control freaks, and gossips. We love to read, cook, eat, drink, and dance; we are both crazy about our families but not easy

to live with. We disagree about practically everything, yet somehow the love always wins.

Childhood Friend: Nancy

My sister Nancy and I are joined in our hearts and our brains. We grew up fighting over Devil Dogs and Barbies, and, later, boys and drugs. But long after we thought our paths would have diverged, our lives continued to run parallel: Each of us was widowed by AIDS while still young; each was left with two sons to raise. We both remarried and, in our 40s, had baby girls. When we laugh together, it is the helpless, unstoppable laughter of children.

Mirror Image: Theresa

Four years ago, I moved to rural Pennsylvania, where I knew no one but my soon-to-be second husband. Then I met Theresa at a local 5K. In her, I found a running partner, an unpaid therapist, and a name to put on my kids' school-emergency cards—all in one package. As both our children and our elderly parents start dating, as our hormones drive us mad, the hours we spend trotting the trail keep me going in body and spirit.

Wait a minute. I didn't list Margaret, Liz, Naomi, or Jessica, and each of them is as stuck with me as those I mentioned. Can we add a few categories to the list?

311

THE **CEREBRAL** MATCH

All the friend types mentioned here feed various parts of oneself, but the cerebral match is perhaps the most satisfying. This is the friend who challenges you intellectually, who pushes you to see things in a new light, who doesn't let you off the hook, and who leads you to important life epiphanies.

Cathy Cohen met Patty Davis at a cocktail party five years ago in the Hamptons, where each has a summer home. They clicked instantly, despite their different lives. Both are married stay-at-home mothers—Davis, 56, has an 8-year-old adopted daughter; Cohen, 46, has six children, two of whom are still living at home. "We have similar views on what's important and what's not," Cohen says. "With other acquaintances, often I find myself talking about what everyone else is wearing, because there's nothing else to say. Patty and I transcend that. We discuss our relationships with our spouses, our kids, our emotional lives, even our dark sides. We can talk about world issues and how they affect us." During the school year, Cohen and Davis chat every 10 days and see each other only once a month, but they easily pick up where they left off. "A lot of women want to talk several times a week," Cohen says. "Patty isn't needy at all. I can tell her half the story, and she gets it."

THE **CHILDHOOD** FRIEND

A childhood friend isn't necessarily your oldest one as much as she is a witness to your many reincarnations. "We're so many people over the course of a lifetime," explains Judith Sills, Ph.D., a clinical psychologist and the author of *Excess Baggage*. "If people meet you when you are a very productive, hardworking young mother, they're oblivious to the fact that you once were a rebellious partier. But a childhood friend keeps that part of you alive." She's vital, because she knows who you are at your core and where you're from, and she reminds you what you were like when you were young, Sills explains.

Jane Buckingham, a 34-year-old mother and owner of a market-research company in Los Angeles, grew up with Clare Ostermeyer, who lived in the same Manhattan apartment building. "We played 'Charlie's Angels' after school," Buckingham remembers. "I was Kelly, and she was Sabrina." Ostermeyer, 34, knew Buckingham when she had braces and a bad perm, but their friendship runs deeper than memories of eighth-grade dances.

> A childhood friend knows who you are at your core and where you're from, and she reminds you what you were like when you were still young.

"My mother died when I was 21," Buckingham says. "That Clare knew her is a constant gift. She remembers what my mother had in her handbag or an outfit she would wear. Sometimes, Clare will say something that reminds me what my mom was really like—not just what I remember over the years."

Best of all, Ostermeyer acts as Buckingham's barometer. "She doesn't buy any of my crap!" Buckingham laughs. "If I whine about my work or life, she'll remind me of silly things we wanted as children and how lucky we are now."

THE **MIRROR** IMAGE

When Susanne Sanchez, a 33-year-old marketing executive in Miami, discovered she was pregnant with triplets, she immediately searched for other mothers in her situation. "They all said, 'If we did it, so can you,'" Sanchez remembers. "It was so reassuring." From them, she learned that only a Chevy Suburban will accommodate three baby boys and their gear, and that hiring a night nurse is a must for the first three months.

Sanchez has grown closest to Amy Tamara of Hollywood, Florida, who was also pregnant with triplet boys when they met through a mutual acquaintance. The two have spent hours on the phone but have yet to meet face-to-face. Tamara, who is in her early 30s, had her boys in November 2002, the same month that Sanchez was put on mandatory bed rest (she delivered on December 24). Still, they continue to compare notes and speculate about what their future lives will be like when their sons hit puberty.

Whether you're a working parent, a divorcée in your 40s, or the future mother of triplets, you need to share your experiences with someone who is going through the same things. In fact, Yager's research found that women who fail to make new friends after major life changes are more prone to isolation than those with support. "Yet so many women feel guilty about developing new friendships," she says. They think, 'Is it that important to have someone to wheel my toddlers around the mall with?' The answer is yes!"

You're probably wondering, "Can my best friend also be my go-to girl?" or "I think my mirror image and my childhood friend are the same." You'll have some overlap, but experts agree that having a variety of friends to fulfill different roles in your life is what's important. "Women dare to be vulnerable with each other, and vulnerability is accompanied by intimacy," says Joel Block, Ph.D., a psychologist and the author of *Naked Intimacy*. "People who experience true intimacy live longer and better lives." ▪

Is It Time to Dump Her?

Sad to say, not all friendships last forever. In a recent survey of 180 people, 68 percent said that a "casual, close, or best friend" had betrayed them, says Jan Yager, Ph.D., author of *When Friendship Hurts*. Even if that isn't the case, sometimes you still have to say good-bye for your own sanity. Take our true/false quiz to see whether that time is now.

1. You always screen her calls. Sometimes you're just not up for another one of her sob stories. ❏ T ❏ F

2. Speaking of calls, the two of you seem to talk less and less. You can't remember the last time you got together for a movie or lunch. ❏ T ❏ F

3. You tiptoe around her feelings. In fact, she's still mad about the time you signed up for that cooking class without her. ❏ T ❏ F

4. When you throw a party, you feel like you have to invite her or else. ❏ T ❏ F

5. You cheer her up, but she seldom returns the favor. ❏ T ❏ F

6. You told her something in strict confidence, and she spilled the beans—again. ❏ T ❏ F

7. She looks bored whenever you mention your marriage/ children/career/house/pet/ vacation plans. ❏ T ❏ F

8. You two would get along fine if only she'd stop criticizing your new man. ❏ T ❏ F

9. When you argue with each other, it's hard for either of you to see the other's side. ❏ T ❏ F

10. Being around her just isn't as much fun as it used to be. ❏ T ❏ F

Answers: "True" to four or more questions could mean you need to call it quits, especially if there's a pattern of pal problems. For women today, time is precious, says Lauren Solotar, Ph.D., chief of psychology at the May Institute in Boston and a specialist in women's issues. "You have to think about your time like money: How do you want to spend it? Then make some decisions."

To say good-bye, you've got two choices: Stop reciprocating phone calls and dinner invitations, thus letting the friendship fade away, or confront her. "Raise the issues," Solotar suggests. "Say, 'This is too hard for me. I can't be friends with someone who isn't kind to my spouse.' Confrontation isn't easy, but it can help. Even if she never changes, you may change—and both of you might change for the better."

Giving Circles:
The New Clubs with a Cause

A growing number of women are turning "girls' night out" into a charitable event.

BY MAUREEN KENNEDY

Ten years ago, when Pamela Rosin received a substantial inheritance from her grandparents, she knew she was fortunate. But the money did raise a question for the now-31-year-old Boston artist and performer. For years, Rosin had written random checks, however small, to various charities. But now she felt overwhelmed by this large sum: How much should she give? And to whom?

To make her giving more focused, Rosin joined the Kitchen Table, a band of eight young women from disparate economic backgrounds who pool their money to aid worthy causes. Her group is one of a growing number of "giving circles," in which the desire to help and the bonds among members are more important than the size of the donation.

Sondra Shaw-Hardy, co-founder of the Women's Philanthropy Institute in Rochester, Michigan, and author of *Creating a Women's Giving Circle*, says that in the past seven years, nearly 2,000 women have joined or organized giving circles and that together they donate about $2 million to nonprofits each year. Just as investment clubs were a reflection of the moneymaking '90s, giving circles appeal to this decade's simpler values of community connection. Many are modest efforts, with members who do not necessarily have a lot to donate; others are made up of women with deeper pockets. What all these groups share is a mix of education, friendship, and action.

> **Some groups are modest efforts, with members who do not have a lot to donate; others are made up of women with deeper pockets. What all these groups share is a mix of education, friendship, and action.**
> —Pamela Rosin

"Spiritually, it's really powerful for me," Rosin says. "We've taken a journey together by talking about our personal ideologies and looking at ourselves and how we want to make an impact in the world."

While that may sound like a pretty lofty sentiment, it's only part of what's driving the trend. According to Stacy Palmer, editor of the *Chronicle* of *Philanthropy*, there is another dynamic at work here. Rosin and others like her are among a new generation of donors who are taking a hands-on approach to giving. "Younger people want to get more involved, to see that their money is being put to good use," Palmer says. Most giving circles, for example, spend nearly a year deciding which nonprofit to donate to. They invite guest speakers to their meetings, visit different service organizations in the community, and pore over annual reports. The Kitchen Table spent nine months learning about a variety of nonprofits before eventually donating $12,000 to two groups benefiting low-income youth. "We wanted to be sure we made the right decision," Rosin says.

Another reason behind the trend is that women have more to contribute than ever before. "Women earn more of their own wealth now, which makes them feel much more powerful in the world of philanthropy," Palmer says. And that increased spending power is only going to grow: Women stand to inherit much of the $10 trillion to $136 trillion that is expected to change hands over the next 50 years.

Sure, it's easier to simply mail a check in to a charity. But women who join giving circles get more out of their philanthropy than the satisfaction of knowing their donation is helping others. Boston resident Susan Priem, 57, who started a circle with nine friends nearly three years ago, has watched her group balloon to 44 members. The participants are busy with work and children, but Priem says the women have stayed in the club because of the relationships they've formed there. "It's been great to watch us mesh together and bond," she says.

In the end, that's the real power of giving circles: a chance for busy women to enjoy each other's company while doing good. "It's a way for women to get together and to work together," Palmer says. "Many of us don't have lots of opportunities to do that." ■

Maureen Kennedy is a freelance writer in San Francisco. Her work has appeared in Ladies' Home Journal *and other publications.*

How to Start a Giving Circle

You're sold on the idea of a charitable group. Now what? Here are the basics.

Set the ground rules.
Get as specific as possible: What will the group be named? How often will you meet, and where? How much will members contribute? Will there be a limit to how many people can join?

Write a mission statement.
Describe who you are and what issues the group will be focusing on.

Divvy up responsibilities.
Assign the logistical work to group members. You may want one person to schedule meetings, another to take notes, and another to contact nonprofits, for example.

Decide how to handle your finances.
You can open a joint checking account, partner with a nonprofit that acts as your financial administrator, or write individual checks to your chosen charity.

Do your homework.
Research and visit the nonprofits that are involved in your circle's area of interest, and invite guest speakers to your meetings. An organization worth supporting should be able to clearly communicate its short- and long-term goals and demonstrate proven results. Ask to see the charity's annual reports and consult the Better Business Bureau's Wise Giving Alliance (www.give.org) to get additional information about specific groups.

315

The New Matchmakers

Here's a look at the latest dating gimmicks from women who have tried them.

BY EVA MARER

The newest ways of finding a date make the Internet matchmaking craze seem dated. If you're divorced or tired of singing solo, you might be tempted to get back in the groove with one of these methods. "Each has its pluses and minuses, but ultimately it comes down to how you feel when you meet the person face-to-face," says Kate Wachs, Ph.D., a psychologist in private practice in Chicago and author of *Relationships for Dummies*. We asked Wachs to evaluate these dating trends, then got the scoop from women who have tested them.

THE TREND:
SPEED DATING

The moves: In this romantic version of musical chairs, you'll sit across from a new suitor every few minutes and move on when the bell rings. Held at bars, benefits, and even gyms, you'll see and rate up to 30 "dates" in a session. You'll only get phone numbers for the guys who gave you the thumbs-up, too. The original version—based on the philosophy that first-person first impressions are more telling than the inklings gleaned from your computer screen—was created by a rabbi for a Jewish social club, but it has spawned plenty of imitators.

Expert opinion: "Speed dating allows you to get straight to the point and ask important questions, which appeals to goal-oriented women," Wachs says. "Keep in mind, though, that this method tends to favor men who are smooth talkers, charming, and good at making first impressions."

She tried it: *Jennifer Hust, 29, technical recruiter, Atlanta*

"It's great because you just check yes or no, and you never have to see them again, which means no rejection dramas. Granted, three minutes is not much time to get to know someone. You should decide in advance what questions to ask so you can weed out the players. My strategy was to ask about their exes. If they said anything immature or hateful, then I just marked 'no' right away.

"Brian was the last person I saw. We met on a Wednesday, he called on Thursday, and we went to a tapas bar on Friday. Five months later, we were engaged. We're getting married in June."

Do it yourself: Visit such sites as www.hurrydate.com, www.speeddating.com (for Jewish singles), or www.crunch.com (for the athletic-minded). To nail down your speed strategy, pick up a copy of *Speed-Dating: A Timesaving Guide to Finding Your Lifelong Love,* by Yaacov and Sue Deyo, before you give this method a try.

THE TREND:
REUNIONS

The moves: Hunt down an old high school flame on Internet reunion sites, directories, and search engines. "Lost-love reunions often occur when 'first loves'—those who met before age 17—are 30-something, but this happens at all ages, from 18 to 89," says Nancy Kalish, Ph.D., who researches and writes on the subject of love and is a professor of psychology at California State University, Sacramento. "These couples also tend to have a higher success rate than other marriages," she says.

Expert opinion: "You need to be ready and willing to take whatever you get—the person may be married or changed in a way you don't like," Wachs says. "Meet for lunch in a public place and be willing to edit your knowledge of that person from the past, because everybody grows up."

She tried it: *Galen Malicoat, 39, full-time mom, North Truro, Massachusetts*

"Five years ago, my sister got to talking about how much she hated kindergarten. I said, 'The thing I remember most about kindergarten was kissing Beau Valtz under a table.' Every so often over the years, I would wonder what he was up to, but I couldn't find him. When the Internet came along, I plugged his name into a White Pages search, and it came up in 30 seconds. I was pleased when he said that he thought about me, too!

"Beau was heading East for a wedding that June, so he decided to come a little early—and I ended up going to the wedding with him. There was this really huge sense of connection, of already knowing each other. Yet at the same time, we had to ask each other these very practical questions, like 'Do you eat meat?' and 'Do you believe in God?'

"He moved East, and we were married the following June; a first marriage for both of us. We had our first baby, Clementine, in August 2002."

Do it yourself: Still thinking about your high school crush? He may have posted his name on such Web sites as www.classmates.com or www.reunion.com.

If you know what state he currently lives in, you can try tracking him down by using an Internet phone book, such as www.bigfoot.com or www.whitepages.com. For more tips on how to reconnect with a long-lost love, visit Kalish's Web site, www.lostlovers.com.

THE TREND:
TV REALITY SHOWS

The moves: Let the producers of one of the television dating programs set you up on a date. You won't have much say, if any, in choosing who he is, and you'll have to go through with it even if you're ready to split immediately after he says "hello." Plus, there could be some acting involved: With the cameras rolling, you might have to do more than one take.

Expert opinion: "If you're really serious about hooking up, you need a pool of prospects, so this seems kind of limited—but fun," Wachs says.

She tried it: *Shana Vitoff, 31, owner, Society Hill Dance Academy, Philadelphia*

"A friend heard that The Learning Channel's *A Dating Story* was looking for people in the area, and on a lark I decided to do it. My date was a nice guy, a jewelry designer. We went to a restaurant and then Latin dancing. The thing is, you can hardly call this a date—it's a TV show! We had never met before, but everything was planned, even though it seems impromptu to the viewer. We had a camera crew all over us, so it was hard to be intimate. On the plus side, though, I would say that you really do get to see how the other person reacts under pressure. We were thrown together into the same boat and forced to get along. So we did bond over that. In fact, we agreed that we would like to see each other again. I was pretty surprised that he never called me afterward."

Do it yourself: To find out how you can sign up, visit *A Dating Story* at tlc.discovery.com. Or look up the hit WB's show *Blind Date* at www.blinddatetv.com. ▪

BEDROOM
myth-busters

These women share what they didn't know about sex—and were delighted to learn.

BY JENNIFER MATLACK

Given today's sex-soaked culture, you'd think people would be experts on the subject. Yet, all those movie clichés aside, nobody really gets sex right the first time (or the second, third, or fourth, for that matter). It takes years before most women finally figure out what makes them scream with pleasure—and what simply makes them want to scream. Still, they wonder, "Am I normal?" The following three women discuss their sexual learning curves and reveal the insights they've gained.

MYTH: *There is only one correct way to have sex.*
REALITY: "When I was 30, I dated an older man who encouraged me to touch myself during intercourse, which I'd never considered doing in the past. Throughout my 20s, I had boyfriends who expected me to reach orgasm through penetration alone. Because I couldn't, I thought that something was wrong with me. Once I became comfortable with touching myself in front of a partner, I discovered other ways to make sex more pleasurable. Now when I begin a relationship, I take the lead and show my partner what it takes to make me happy in bed." —*Mary, 33*

THE TAKE-AWAY: Don't be afraid to stray from the script when you aren't satisfied. Experiment with moves that make having sex fun for you and make sure you share what works with your partner.

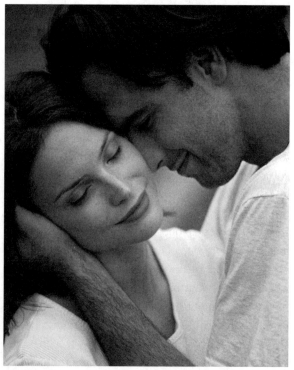

MYTH: *My partner is as critical of my body as I am.*
REALITY: "Five years ago, I was lying naked with my husband, who was then my boyfriend. I had always felt self-conscious about my thighs—they were too wide, too dimply, too soft—and I always kept them covered. That day, we were lying on top of the sheets, and my whole body was in full view. When my boyfriend's eyes reached my thighs, I cringed. With a look full of love, he told me I was the most beautiful woman he had ever seen. It was an incredibly poignant moment for both of us, and one that allowed me to relax enough to really enjoy sex." —*Michelle, 38*
THE TAKE-AWAY: Trust and confidence go a long way in the bedroom. It's hard to receive pleasure, or give it, when your focus is on whether you measure up to some mythical ideal. Believe your partner when he tells you that you're beautiful. Remember: There's nothing sexier than a woman who feels sexy.

MYTH: *Men always want sex more than women do.*
REALITY: "Before I met my husband 27 years ago, I'd just assumed that guys were always in the mood. While my husband and I both enjoy sex very much, the truth is I'm often the initiator. I'd like to make love at least three times a week. I wouldn't mind having sex every day, but my husband travels a lot, and sometimes he's too tired for sex. I accept that. There have been times in our marriage, such as after we had children and I was breast-feeding, that I wasn't into sex. Now I want it, and I'm not afraid to let him know it." —*Pat, 49*
THE TAKE-AWAY: It's perfectly OK to be the aggressor between the sheets. Allow the sexual roles of you and your partner to change with time and life events, and know that those changes are normal. Talk about your needs, and above all, don't let old stereotypes stand in the way of your pleasure. ▪

Shopping Versus Sex: *Which Would You Choose?*

Hard to believe, but a recent British poll found that most European smokers would rather give up sex for a month than cigarettes. That got us wondering what *Health*'s non-nicotine-addicted, mostly female readers prize even more than sex. The answers, according to our own Health.com survey: a full night's sleep, shopping, and exercise. We can understand how sleep got the top vote—we know that American women are tired. But shopping and workouts? Come on.

Yet at least one expert believes your responses make perfect sense. Sandra Leiblum, Ph.D., director of the Center for Sexual and Marital Health at Robert Wood Johnson Medical School and co-author of *Getting the Sex You Want,* says many women feel they can count on having more fun at the mall than in bed. "Every time you go shopping, there's a different adventure," Leiblum says. "For a lot of women, sex has become boring and predictable." Point taken—but jogging? "Exercise produces a rush of endorphins, and afterward women feel good about their bodies," Leiblum explains. "With sex, they may feel more self-conscious."

Overall, Leiblum says your answers reflect many women's attitudes toward sex. "There's a notion that people are having a ton of sex, and they feel deprived if they don't have it." In reality, she says, "giving sex up might be a relief for some women." (A recent survey by the Kinsey Institute found that 24 percent of the women surveyed felt "worried" or "distressed" about sex.) Luckily, you don't have to go quite that far. If medical concerns aren't causing your bedroom boredom, the old advice still holds true: Take stock of your needs and start talking to your partner. Hopefully, you'll end up like *Health* reader Maureen, who wrote, "There's nothing I'd give up sex for."

Save Your Marriage NOW

Has your relationship suffered from an "attachment injury"? Find out what it is and how to repair the damage.

BY AVIVA PATZ

Marcy Wendell (not her real name) was three months pregnant when she began bleeding heavily. Realizing that she was having a miscarriage, she tried to remain calm. "I thought that when my husband got there, everything would be OK," remembers the 39-year-old real estate agent in Kingston, Ontario. But it wasn't. "Rob seemed cold, like he wasn't upset," she says. "As he drove me to the hospital, I thought, 'He must not love me.' " At that moment, five years ago, the couple's marriage began to fall apart.

What Wendell experienced is called an "attachment injury"—a devastating blow that occurs when one partner fails to provide support and comfort when the other partner needs them most. "It could happen with something as obviously distressing as an affair, but it could be more subtle, such as a comment about someone else being attractive just when you've been dieting like mad," says University of Ottawa psychology professor Susan Johnson, Ed.D., director of the Ottawa Couple and Family Institute.

Whether a trivial aside or act of betrayal, the effect can be profound. Johnson is one of a growing number of experts who believe that an unresolved

attachment injury is the hidden reason many couples fail to get past their problems, contributing to a divorce rate that is more than 50 percent. Johnson describes the phenomenon in an article published recently in the *Journal of Marital and Family Therapy*. She had noticed in her practice that clients would often bring up the same incidents over and over as reasons not to trust their partners again. "Whether it happened six months or six years earlier, the event caused a fundamental loss of intimacy and trust," she says.

Is your marriage doomed if this happens to you? Not necessarily. Attachment injuries can be healed with a little-known counseling approach called Emotionally Focused Therapy (EFT), which Johnson helped originate 20 years ago. Studies conducted by Johnson and several colleagues show that about 73 percent of couples in troubled relationships report being happy with each other again after EFT, compared with only 35 percent of those who undergo conventional therapy. More than 90 percent of couples experience significant improvement.

"Attachment injuries are common in distressed relationships, but traditional marriage counseling often skips right over them," says Scott R. Woolley,

Ph.D., director of the graduate programs in marital and family therapy at Alliant International University in California. "Traditional counseling tends to focus on improving communication, encouraging people to do nice things for each other, and changing their views of one another. It doesn't deal with emotions, which are the reason people get together in the first place and the reason they get distressed."

But emotions are front and center in EFT. The idea is to restore the spousal bond by identifying and working through the event that first jeopardized it. "If you don't heal the attachment injury," Woolley says, "the wounds will fester for years."

Indeed, Marcy Wendell would bring up Rob's mistreatment of her every time the two of them argued. And the initial damage was compounded: When Wendell had a second miscarriage and later when she learned of her father's heart attack, Rob didn't comfort her, and her feelings of betrayal returned and intensified. Eventually, she was getting angry at Rob all the time; he would react by becoming silent and tuning out, which only made her angrier.

The cycle had brought them to the brink of divorce by the time they saw EFT therapist Judy Makinen. She asked the Wendells to go back to the beginning of their downward spiral. "First, I had to get Marcy to talk about the emotional impact it had on her when Rob was not responsive," says Makinen, a Ph.D. candidate in clinical psychology at the University of Ottawa. "And I needed him to listen to her without withdrawing. Once he was tuned in, he was able to explain his own perspective on what happened that day."

Rob said that he'd been afraid to comfort his wife; he felt that if he had shown any emotion, she would have fallen apart—and then so would he. Holding back was his way of protecting himself.

"Once he explained that, Marcy understood that Rob did care for her. Her relief had all the emotional power of the original event," Makinen says. "Marcy began to cry, and Rob was able to reach out to her and give her the comfort and care that were absent originally. It was like correcting history." Makinen suggested that the Wendells repeat this role-play at home. "You back up the videotape of life so you can replay it with a healthier ending," she says.

It worked for the Wendells. "Rob put both arms around me and just kept saying, 'It's OK,'" Wendell recalls. "Then it was done. It's amazing how that changed my view of my husband—and my marriage."

Start Healing Today
Is an attachment injury hurting your relationship? These steps may start the reconciliation process.

1. Identify the injury. Think about a time you felt vulnerable and were disappointed by your partner's response. Notice the timing, which can turn an otherwise-mundane slight into a major hurt.
2. Talk about it. Hard as it is, tell your partner how you felt. But try to frame your feelings in positive terms, says Susan Johnson, director of the Ottawa Couple and Family Institute. Saying "I'm still hurting because you're so important to me, and you weren't there when I really needed you" will get him listening more effectively than "You bum, you ran off."
3. Let your emotions show. Allow your partner to see how upset you were. Don't be afraid to ask now for what you didn't get then. You might say, "Right now, I just want you to hug me."
4. Express your needs. To make sure the injury doesn't repeat itself, tell your partner what you'll need from him in the future. It might be comfort when you're upset, more support for a project, or greater awareness of your feelings. Work to incorporate any changes in your daily lives that would help bring you closer together.
Caution: If, however, you've been feeling alienated for several months, Johnson encourages you to see a therapist. For some couples, though, it may be too late. EFT is not designed for couples who have tried unsuccessfully to connect for so long that they've already grieved for the lost relationship and become completely detached. It's also inappropriate for abusive relationships.

Is Your Man Too Vain?

To love another person, you've got to love yourself first. But a little self-esteem goes a long way. Researchers say that while a narcissist—someone with an all-me, all-the-time type of personality—may seem like Prince Charming, underneath he's all frog. "Narcissists often have good social skills," says W. Keith Campbell, Ph.D., assistant professor of psychology at the University of Georgia. "But they don't mind hurting people and moving on." In particular, Campbell and his colleagues found that narcissists are better than most people at playing relationship games, such as keeping partners guessing about how committed they are and having flings on the side.

Love may be blind, but you shouldn't be. If the statements below seem painfully familiar, it's probably time to dump him. (Chances are, he won't even notice).

You know he's a narcissist when …

1. You've been seeing him for months, and he still can't remember your middle name.
2. He gives you gift certificates for stores he likes.
3. At parties, he leaves you by the coatrack while he heads for the bar.
4. You say you're feeling down, and he replies, "Huh?"
5. He complains that your friends and family bore him to tears.
6. He cuts you off midsentence to talk about his cool new gym bag.
7. He says your pants make your butt look big—and then says that he was only joking.
8. Your best friends can't understand why you put up with him.
9. He brags that you'll never find anyone better than him.
10. He cheated on old girlfriends, but he says he'd never do that to you.

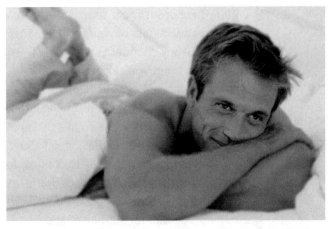

re•frig•er•a•tor rights *n.* **1:** A term coined by author Will Miller, Ed.D., to describe the privilege of nosing around in someone else's fridge: "As her boyfriend, Mike, searched for the mayo and mustard, Jill realized that their relationship had turned a corner; he had gained refrigerator rights."

Surprise! Study Shows That Men Are *More* Sympathetic Than Women

Your guy starts sputtering about why he forgot to pick up the dry cleaning. If you're like most women, his lame excuses just won't wash. (He was too tired after work? *Puh-leeze.*) A new study from Indiana University shows that women are far less likely than men to tolerate other people's flimsy reasons for failure. Regardless of whether the excuse comes from a man or woman, guys tend to be more sympathetic: "Of course you were too busy to research the company before the interview. Better luck next time, buddy." But women—perhaps because they value hard work so highly—are more prone to think, "Oh, get off your lazy butt and do it."

Hotheads May Be in for Heart Trouble

Unless you're like Red and Kitty Forman from *That '70s Show,* you and your spouse probably don't enjoy arguing with each other. That's a good thing: A new study shows that frequent fights can be hard on the heart—especially women's hearts. University of Washington researchers recently ran EKGs on 54 couples as they discussed such hot-button topics as money and in-laws. Some subjects (male and female) had trouble calming down afterward, but while men just felt riled up, the effects for women were both emotional and physical. Their parasympathetic nervous systems (PNS)—the body's antidote to an adrenaline buzz—weren't kicking in, says study author Sybil Carrère, Ph.D. That meant their heart rates weren't falling. "It's as if they'd stepped on the gas and couldn't find the brake," Carrère says. Earlier studies show that this can increase heart disease risk, she adds. Fortunately, you can help out your PNS. If spats with your spouse tend to escalate, get your temper—and your pulse—in check. "Say, 'I know this is important and we need to come back to it, but right now I just need a break,'" Carrère suggests. "Then take some deep breaths, meditate, or go for a walk." A long one.

Do You Kiss the *Right* Way?

Twice as many people tilt their heads to the right as to the left when puckering up for a kiss, say German researchers. The lifelong habit develops before birth; babies show a preference for turning their heads one way or the other while still in the womb.

Size Doesn't (Always) Matter

MYTH: A man's shoe size is a clue to what he's packing in his pants.
REALITY: Stop staring at his feet. Two urologists in Britain recently measured the stretched penises of 104 men, compared the lengths to their loafers, and found no correlation.

Wanted: A Man Who Does Chores

Sure, he'll marry you—but will he take out the trash? You may want him to move in first and see. Researchers at the University of California, Irvine, found that couples who live together before marriage do a better job of divvying up the housework.

Surveying 17,849 people in 22 countries, the study focused on chores typically performed by women: grocery shopping, doing laundry, cooking, and cleaning up after meals. Experts guess that couples who put off marriage are more likely to ignore traditional gender roles, thus making an important discovery: A toilet brush *does* fit a man's hand.

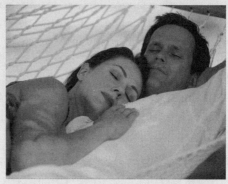

He loves to snuggle, but don't ask him to do the dishes.

re•la•tion•al dis•or•der n. 1: A newly proposed class of psychiatric problems defined by doctors as "persistent and painful feelings, behavior, and perceptions involving two or more partners in an important personal relationship," as in "after months of arguing over who would take out the trash, Warren and Amanda decided to seek professional help for their relational disorder." 2: A term we think could potentially send every couple in America into therapy.

Surviving Marriage Milestones

Discover how you can keep those troublesome times from throwing your relationship off course.

BY AVIVA PATZ

If only the journey through married life came with road signs like "Slow Down: Men Working (Late Again)" and "Danger: Infidelity Ahead." Maybe then so many relationships wouldn't hit dead ends. A 2002 Centers for Disease Control and Prevention report shows how marriages in America degrade over time: After five years, nearly a fifth have ended; after 10 years, divorce has claimed a third.

Still, many couples stay together in spite of demanding jobs, big mortgages, and parental pressures. How? "While all partners face inevitable soars and slumps

America's high divorce rate is alarming, yet many couples still stay together in spite of demanding jobs, big mortgages, and parental pressures. The question is: How?

at various points in their relationships, those who survive learn how to navigate them successfully," explains University of Denver professor of psychology Howard J. Markman, Ph.D., author of *Fighting for Your Marriage: Positive Steps for Preventing Divorce and Preserving a Lasting Love*.

We asked five couples to share how they have overcome some of the most common obstacles to wedded bliss. Their experiences, as well as advice from relationship experts, can help you and your mate travel more smoothly along that sometimes bumpy road.

THE FIRST BIG FIGHT

Larissa, 30, marketing manager • Robert, 32, international sales executive • Married one year

The issue: "We fought a lot, mostly over trivial things, and it was starting to erode our quality of life," Larissa says.

The turning point: "My husband has this chair that he always moves forward to watch TV. When he's not there, I move it back. We did this for months until one day he came home in a bad mood and said, 'Why are you constantly moving this chair? It's *my* chair.' I had dinner on a tray table, and he said, 'What if I decided to move your tray?' He took hold of the table, and my water accidentally flew off; in my anger, I flung what was

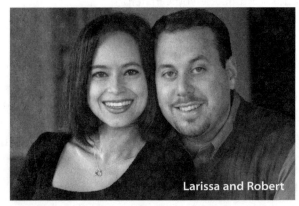

Larissa and Robert

left on him. We didn't talk the rest of the night or the next day."

The resolution: Larissa and Robert realized that their fight wasn't about the chair at all. The underlying problem was that they were both stubborn and easily angered. They committed to compromising more often and to controlling their tempers. "Now if I start to get mad, I walk away," Larissa says. "When he gets angry, he puts the discussion on pause. We're both trying," she adds. "We still move the chair back and forth, but now we can laugh about it."

Expert advice: "Larissa and Robert realized that their fighting was destructive, and they decided to work as a team to counteract it," Markman says. "What they still need to do on a regular basis is sit down when they're both feeling calm and discuss what annoys them. Having a safe place to talk about disagreements will decrease the chance of small events erupting into bigger conflicts."

THE BABY BOOM

Marguerite, 36, freelance writer • John, 34, lawyer • Married five years

The issue: "John was angry at our baby for disrupting our life and relationship," Marguerite explains. "He was clearly mourning the loss of his more carefree, childless days. And I was miserable because I had left a job that I loved, moved to a new city, and now had to keep this colicky baby quiet so my husband could study for the bar exam. I was disappointed because I thought John would be an excellent father; instead, he seemed to resent the role."

The turning point: "One night when John and I went out for dinner, he admitted that he still didn't feel bonded with Jake, who was already 9 months old. I told him that if it didn't happen soon, he would need to seek counseling. I explained that since my dad hadn't been around for me, it was especially important for John to be a good parent to Jake, and that if he didn't try, it would be a big problem for us."

The resolution: Afterward, John tried to be more patient when the baby cried at night, and in turn, Marguerite was more patient with John, allowing him to bond with Jake in his own time. They also invested in their own relationship by establishing a weekly date night and taking an 11-day vacation to Alaska by themselves.

Expert advice: "Marguerite clearly told John what she was unhappy about, what she needed, and that something had to change," says Bill Doherty, Ph.D., University of Minnesota professor of family social science and author of *Take Back Your Marriage*. "She also did it early in the problem and said it without threatening divorce. John took her message as a

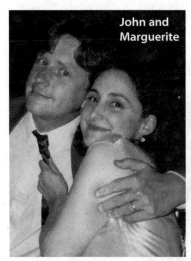

John and Marguerite

wake-up call and acted on it. He recognized that it was more than just becoming an involved father; he knew they had to work on their closeness as a couple as well. Going on weekly dates and taking a trip alone was a great way to do that."

NO MORE FIREWORKS

Mary, 44, special education teacher • Bill, 44, furniture-plant manager • Married 20 years

The issue: "We fell out of love," Mary says. "Over the years, it became harder to find time for the two of us—we were busy with the kids, church, our work. We stopped communicating. We grew apart. When we separated for nine months last year, I thought it was over."

The turning point: "During Christmas, I booked a trip to the beach with the kids, and for their sake, I invited Bill. After much hesitation, he agreed to come, and although we stayed in separate rooms, we ended up having a really great time. When we came home, we started going to counseling together, which ultimately helped us get back on track."

The resolution: The counselor had Mary and Bill fill out personality profiles, which highlighted exactly how they were different and why they found certain things so hurtful. They started changing the offending behaviors and spending more time together. Now they go out to dinner once a week, and they have become stricter with their children's sleep schedules. They have some time alone to talk before bed—and to enjoy each other *in* bed. Mary says, "We're back in love."

Expert advice: "Mary and Bill rediscovered the things that first attracted them to one another," says Baltimore psychologist Shirley Glass, Ph.D.,

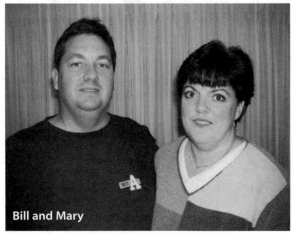

Bill and Mary

author of *Not "Just Friends": Protect Your Relationship from Infidelity and Heal the Trauma of Betrayal.* "When they gave themselves a chance to have fun and be together, they remembered why they got married. Couples need time alone so they can touch base and connect, to say 'How did your meeting go?' or 'A funny thing happened today.' Particularly in dual-career marriages, parents often feel guilty that they don't spend enough time with their kids, so when they have a spare minute, they spend it with family. The fact that Mary and Bill built time for each other into their daily schedule ensures it will actually happen."

FINANCIAL CRISIS

Pam, 42, owner of a credit-management outsourcing company • Bryan, 44, temporary vice president of sales for his wife's company • Married 15 years

The issue: "When Bryan got laid off from his technology company nearly a year and a half ago, he felt angry, numb, and ashamed," Pam says. "I was too busy worrying that we'd lose everything to realize he might need time to process those emotions. Instead, I pushed him to try harder to find a new

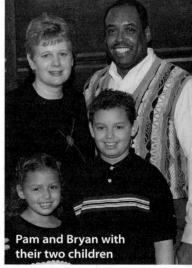

Pam and Bryan with their two children

job. I put a lot of pressure on him, and it caused a great deal of tension between us."

The turning point: "When Bryan joined a support group for job-seekers, I learned that some members had been out of work six months or more. That helped me see that Bryan might not get another job right away, and we had to solve the problem together."

The resolution: Pam and Bryan identified core needs and downsized everything else. Once they learned how to get by on half of what they had before, Pam was able to relax a little. Remembering how Bryan had supported her while she had children and built her business helped her let go of her resentment.

Expert advice: "Pam realized that getting laid off wasn't Bryan's fault, and it wasn't something he could just fix," Doherty says. "This attitude adjustment enabled them to work together to figure out how to cope with the financial downturn. Before that, it was only his problem—and his job to find the solution. In these situations, Doherty adds, "it's helpful for the unemployed person to contribute to the household in other ways, maybe by cooking or taking over some of his partner's chores. Any way he can make his wife's life easier and be a good companion will help."

THE AFFAIR

Mary, 48, homemaker • Rob, 51, government contractor • Married 30 years

The issue: "I had been seeing someone I met over the Internet," Rob says. "I was emotionally involved and seriously thinking of leaving Mary to start a new life with this woman. When I told Mary about the affair, she was devastated, and she threatened to commit suicide. Part of me wanted to run to this other woman, and another part of me felt obligated to stay because of the children."

The turning point: While doing an online search for "marriage help," Mary discovered the Retrouvaille Program, a Christian peer-support group. She signed herself and Rob up for a weekend session. "I didn't think it would help," Mary admits. "At first I went because I wanted to tell my kids I did everything possible to save the marriage. But in that one weekend, we went from complete despair to a glimmer of hope."

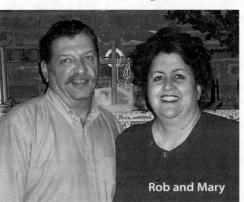

Rob and Mary

The resolution: The other group members inspired Rob and Mary to adopt the philosophy that "love is a decision more than a feeling," and the two of them pledged to make their marriage work. Through a series of follow-up sessions, they learned how to communicate better and to forgive and trust each other more. Mary says that she could not have done it all without her strong religious faith.

Expert advice: "Staying for the children's sake is a good place to start, but Mary and Rob took the next step and committed to recreating a loving relationship," Glass says. "It's important that they forgave each other, because Mary shares responsibility for what went wrong. After all, Rob had an emotional involvement with another woman because he had a need to share deep feelings and have another person accept him. Working on communication skills helped Mary answer those needs." ■

Hidden Attractions

Sure, you say you're "just friends." But according to an unpublished study at the University of Indianapolis, most men and women—both singles and those in romantic relationships—are secretly attracted to their opposite-sex friends. In a survey of 87 undergrads, 72 percent admitted that they found their friends physically attractive. Singles went even further: More than half said they wanted to kiss their pals, and about a third said they'd like to become bed buddies.

But that survey was limited to college kids. To see how our readers compared, we posted our own poll at Health.com. Nearly 90 percent of our respondents said that they found their opposite-sex friends attractive. While most people in the original survey said that, all fantasies aside, they wouldn't want the friendship to move on to romance, 66 percent of *Health* readers said, "Why not?"

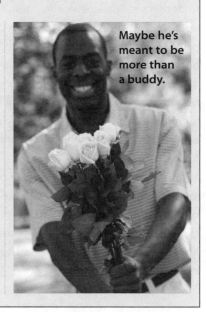

Maybe he's meant to be more than a buddy.

Real Life, Real Answers

Ali Domar, Ph. D., our relationships guru, weighs in on the issues that affect women most in their personal and professional lives.

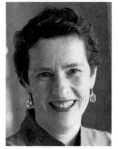

MISSING: MY **BACK-TO-WORK** BLUES

My maternity leave just ended, and I'm back to work full-time. I had expected I'd have separation anxiety, but I don't. I love being with my baby when I get home at night, but I relish my time at work because I feel like it belongs to me. Is it wrong for me to be so comfortable away from my newborn?

No, it's perfectly normal. In fact, I think you're probably more honest than some women. For every mother who is miserable being separated from her child, there's probably one who is totally OK with it.

I remember talking to a woman I work with in front of a male colleague who doesn't have children; we were discussing how easy work is compared to being at home. He was astonished; he sees every day how crazy our jobs can be. But we explained the difference to him. At work, we have adult conversations and complete projects. We can enjoy a sense of accomplishment. At home, you do the same things over and over, such as changing diapers, picking up toys, and doing laundry.

The fact is, you are meeting some of your needs at work and others at home. And the best way to have a happy child is to be a happy parent. Kudos to you for embracing a truth many women don't want to acknowledge: They have lives outside of being moms.

HOW TO KNOW WHEN A **FRIEND'S MAN** IS NO GOOD

Since my best friend got engaged, she's lost weight even though she was already thin. She now wears skimpier clothes, and she even checks with her fiancé first before going out with me. I'm concerned that there may be some abuse in their relationship. Should I say something?

Your suspicions may be valid. Women who are being abused will sometimes change their looks or ask permission to go out with girlfriends, but this can also be the case of someone who's simply trying to please her man.

You need to know for sure that your friend is in an abusive relationship before you act. I wouldn't say anything yet—she might tell her fiancé, who will probably get angry and might convince your friend to stay away from you. Then you really wouldn't be able to help her.

Instead, you should let her know she can trust you and be on the lookout for clues that she's asking for help. (For instance, she may start talking about a hypothetical friend in trouble.) Keep suggesting lunches, movies, and other things the two of you enjoy. It also wouldn't hurt to look into potential escape routes for her, including phone numbers of shelters for battered women. If she ever does need you, you'll be ready.

HIS PLACE OR YOURS?

I'm moving in with my boyfriend next month. He owns the house and has lived there a long time. It feels like a bachelor pad—how can I make it feel like my place, too?

Well, you could throw out his ratty chair and bowling trophies, but I'm afraid this situation calls for compromise. As much as you want the house to have your touches, remember that he may be feeling territorial, not to mention defensive about his taste (or lack thereof). If you can afford it—and if you can convince him to—go shopping together and buy a few pieces that you both like. This way, he probably won't feel so threatened. If you have the space, try designating a room for each of you. He can hang his prize trout on the wall, and you can have an area for your folk art. But if he indicates that you're invading his turf, go slowly.

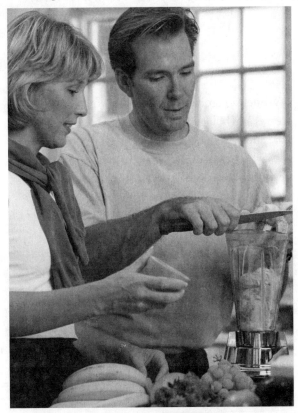

You need to feel at home if you choose to move in with your man.

ALONE FOR THE HOLIDAYS

As a single person who is between relationships, I'm worried about New Year's Eve and Valentine's Day. When I'm not involved with someone, these holidays always depress me. Any tips?

No doubt about it—the holidays, with all their hype, can be painful. But they don't have to be. Surround yourself with other singles. Throw a party for your closest buddies and ask each of them to bring another single friend. You'll end up with a roomful of people, and you could have a great time. Staying busy is another great remedy for the blues. Volunteer at a shelter or hospital, or do something you've always wanted to but have never had the time for. Just don't think that being in a relationship guarantees a great holiday.

DEALING WITH A
FAT-FOCUSED FRIENDSHIP

My size-6 friend has a habit of making rude comments when we see large women on the street, many of whom are the same size as me. I'm usually comfortable with my body, but around her I feel self-conscious. How do I confront her without seeming defensive?

Your friend obviously has an issue with weight. When she talks about a stranger's figure in front of you, her insecurity is showing. Before you confront her, think about what you want to accomplish. If you simply want her to stop, say something like, "It makes me uncomfortable when you say things like that. You don't know what other people are going through." Or you could go further and say, "Do you realize how that makes me feel?" If you're not worried about ticking her off, you could be even more direct and ask her why other people's sizes bother her so much. If you do that, be prepared to lose a friend. In this case, it might not be such a bad thing. ■

329

When You Don't Want to Be
Manager Material

Ambition may be nudging you up the corporate ladder, but staying on the lower rungs could be your key to happiness.

BY LAUREN PICKER

Ask a roomful of elementary school children what they want to be when they grow up, and invariably a handful will respond, "The president." With all due respect to Mr. Cheney, it's unlikely that even one of the kids would say, "The vice president."

The urge to be number one is a defining American characteristic, one that influences behavior from the school yard to, arguably, geopolitics. It's clearly at play in the workplace, where colleagues jockey for position, vying for the top spot and the perks that often go with it. "We tend to glorify leaders. We associate career success with leadership positions," explains Susan Battley, Psy.D., a leadership psychologist and clinical associate professor in the School of Health Technology and Management at Stony Brook University in New York.

If you aren't tailor-made to lead, you may still land the position, but you will pay a heavy price.

While you probably entered the workforce with big dreams and bold ambitions, you may conclude, with time and experience, that you're not cut out to be the boss, whether that's chairman of the board or several steps down as a division head or departmental manager. The discovery may hit you like a bolt out of the blue or dawn on you gradually. However it arrives, the decision to lower your sights and turn your back on what is practically a cultural imperative isn't necessarily easy. And it's especially tough for women, who experts say are more likely than their male counterparts to feel caught between professional aspirations and personal satisfaction. Knowing whether or not you've got the goods—or the drive—to take on a supervisory role doesn't simply affect your career. It can have a profound impact on your physical and mental health.

330

CLIMBING DOWN THE LADDER

Not everyone is a Barry Diller or a Donna Karan. But more and more people are admitting they don't want to be. In fact, a growing number of MBA students express no interest in the topmost rung of the corporate ladder, says Richard Boyatzis, Ph.D., professor of organizational behavior at Case Western Reserve University in Cleveland and co-author of the bestselling *Primal Leadership: Realizing the Power of Emotional Intelligence*. Twenty-five years ago, Boyatzis says, if you had asked a lecture hall full of business students who among them eventually wanted to be a CEO, you'd have looked out into a sea of raised hands; today, he estimates, maybe one hand in five would shoot up.

Boyatzis attributes this change to a shift in values. Where once the dollar reigned supreme, people now consider love, spirituality, and community more important. That's especially true in the aftermath of 9/11, which prompted many Americans to reorder

> **People say, "You must make good money," but who knows? You're so busy you don't have time to enjoy it.** —Richard Boyatzis

their priorities. "A lot of people are saying that being the CEO is not worth the costs," Boyatzis notes. He should know. Before becoming an academic, he was the chief executive officer of a prominent consulting company. "In 11 years, I took one two-week vacation," he says. As for the perks, he notes, "People say, 'You must make good money,' but who knows? You're so busy you don't have time to enjoy it."

Why are some people happy being number two, or for that matter, number 22? The preference may be a conscious choice, driven by any number of reasons. Maybe the top job doesn't play to your strengths or your interests. You could be happiest as what psychologists call an "individual contributor," meaning you'd rather design the costumes than run the show. Alternately, perhaps you want to spend more time with your family, or you simply like the idea of leaving your job behind at the end of the day.

BEST SUPPORTING ROLE

Consider Suzan Colon. Four years ago, this longtime writer and editor was given the chance to become editor in chief of a national women's magazine. "At first it was really flattering," remembers Colon, now age 39. "It's nice for someone to think you're good enough to be in charge." But the more real the job prospect became, the more Colon

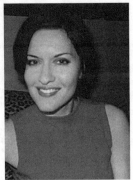

Suzan Colon 39, New York City
Freelance editor

began to wonder if it would be right for her. Family, friends, and co-workers told her she would be great in the role, but would she be happy doing it?

Colon's question is important. Forget the fancy title and the stock options; ultimately, the best measure of professional success is personal happiness. To achieve that on the job, leadership experts and psychologists stress the importance of "job fit," a term that means very much what it implies. Think of the physical parallels: If you like your size-8 body, why would you starve yourself into a skimpy size 4? Or bulk up to a size 16? "If you're going to be happy, you have to fit the job and the job has to fit you," says Beverly Kaye, Ed.D., author of *Up Is Not the Only Way* and chief executive officer of Career Systems International, a talent-management consulting company based in Scranton, Pennsylvania.

After weeks of deliberating, Colon knew the job wasn't for her. At the time, she says, "I thought to myself, 'I will run this magazine into the ground, not because I can't do it, but because it's not me.' I like to be part of the team. I'm the one who yells, 'Yeah!'—not the one who yells 'Charge!' "

Colon made a smart decision, but others rarely reject an opportunity to be in command. "Few people think, 'I like what I'm doing, I'm good at it, I want to keep doing this, and I don't need to do anything more or at a higher level,' " explains Douglas Soat, Ph.D., an organizational psychologist and president of Soat Consulting Psychology Inc., in Janesville, Wisconsin. "It is ingrained in our culture that you're supposed to want more."

To be certain that you're pursuing a job because it truly makes you happy, not because it's expected, you need to assess what you value most, both on and off the job. People who make better supporting players than superiors get their satisfaction from being, say, the detail person, the gatekeeper, or, like Colon, the creative type, Battley says. For these workers, managerial responsibilities aren't ego-boosting or exciting, just stressful. Those who are most content in secondary roles also may have made lifestyle choices that demand the kind of time that is unavailable to someone in a leadership position.

Colon had to make some sacrifices to follow her path. As a freelance editor, she has neither a 401(k) plan nor health benefits (she currently pays $600 a month for her own insurance). What she does have is harder to quantify: time to be with friends, to write books, and, most recently, to fulfill a decade-long dream of becoming a yoga instructor. Any regrets? "Not even for a second," she says.

THE BUCK STOPS OVER THERE

To find out if the job fits, you sometimes have to try it on. In that respect, Keri Kotz's former post was an illuminating dress rehearsal. Because the insurance company she worked for was undergoing a restructuring, Kotz, now 33, went through six managers in two years; for a while, the St. Paul,

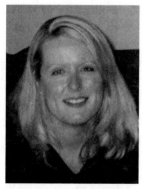

Keri Kotz 33, St. Paul, Minnesota
Marketing Manager

Minnesota, resident headed her department. An ambitious woman, Kotz was surprised to discover that she hated the responsibility. "It was excruciating," she recalls. "I didn't feel like I got anything done. There were all these hiring decisions and administrative details that needed

to be attended to. I was so relieved when I could get back to doing what I enjoyed."

If you aren't tailor-made to lead, you may still land the position, but you'll pay a heavy price. "You'll have to put in 100 times more effort to do the job," Kaye notes. For Kotz, the burden showed in the nearly 20 pounds she shed during her time at the helm. "I looked like a greyhound, and I ran around like one, too," she says, remembering the 12- to 13-hour days that left her feeling completely depleted. "I want to lose weight as much as the next person, but not like that."

Kotz managed to hang on to her good health, but the stress of a bad job fit could end up exacting a serious physical toll. A 2001 study in the *Journal of Applied Psychology* found that people who have high levels of control over their careers yet lack confidence in their abilities and blame themselves for negative outcomes are more vulnerable to such infectious diseases as bronchitis, colds, and flu. In fact, working at an occupation you hate can be a killer. A 1998 study in Stress Medicine found that in people who dislike their jobs, levels of the stress hormone cortisol rise within half an hour after awakening. Over time, high cortisol can raise blood pressure, heart rate, and blood sugar, all of which can increase heart-attack risk.

Even if your body holds up, your mental health may suffer. Feeling perpetually out of your depth can contribute to depression. A 2002 study in the *Annals of Internal Medicine* found that 76 percent of 115 medical residents surveyed experienced emotional exhaustion and a sense of low personal accomplishment; half of this group was also depressed. Conversely, enjoying your work can give you a mental lift. "When you're doing what gives you satisfaction, you'll have a lot of positive carryover effects—you'll be less irritable and more energetic in your broader life," Battley says. Odds are you'll also feel more motivated to take better care of yourself by eating right, exercising, even flossing your teeth.

Kotz, now a marketing manager who has no desire to do her boss's job, agrees. "I feel like a better employee now—more creative and more in control—since I left the insane workload behind," she says. "I also feel like a better person. At home, I'm more relaxed and content." It's no coincidence that she loves her current position, which is free of the paperwork, sticky personnel situations, and strategizing sessions she so disliked as a manager. "That's not appealing to me," Kotz notes. "I prefer to roll my sleeves up and actually do."

Her preference for producing the work instead of overseeing it, along with a lack of interest in office politics, is a hallmark of the individual contributor. It's a role that many women find inherently more satisfying than calling the shots. "Because of the way women are socialized, we tend to be more motivated by the desire to make a contribution—to make a difference in people's lives—and to build relationships," explains Tracey Manning, Ph.D., senior scholar at the University of Maryland's Academy of Leadership. "It doesn't mean we don't want high achievement," she says, but, rather, that most women want to forge strong relationships in the workplace and at home in addition to having a positive impact on the wider world. That's not true of all women, Manning adds, and certainly not of most who are at the pinnacle of their fields. "The higher women move in an organization, the more similar they are to men in the motivations, values, and interests they have at work," she says.

A DIFFERENT KIND OF STRESS

In 1986, Hikari Hathaway was about to sign a lease on a small store where she would sell her own clothing designs. After years of working long hours and traveling often, first as an executive trainee at a large department store, then as a vice president at a manufacturing corporation, she was on the verge of realizing a long-held desire to run her own business. When she was about to sign the lease, the landlord informed her that she'd rented the place to someone else. "I was devastated," recalls the New York City mother, now 47. Unwilling to find another location, Hathaway decided that, instead of starting her own company, the time was right for her and her partner to start their family. Her professional life hasn't been the same since.

The Makings of a Great Boss

Are you coveting the keys to the executive washroom?

According to leadership experts, you'll need ambition, dedication, vision, and energy. That doesn't discount the technical skills necessary to do the job; after all, a manager has to have a firm grasp of details, while also being able to think globally. Perhaps the most important job requirement, though, is your ability to work and play well with others.

Research suggests that the typical boss invests more energy in the job than in human connections. But the difference between an adequate leader and a great one, according to some experts, is being smart about emotions. "You cannot be a leader without followers. People want to work with leaders to whom they are drawn," says Richard Boyatzis, Ph.D., professor of organizational behavior at Case Western Reserve University in Cleveland. And what's good for the staff is good for the company as a whole. "Leaders' emotional states and actions affect how the people they manage will feel and, therefore, perform. How well leaders manage their moods, then, becomes not just a private matter but a factor in how well a business will do," he explains.

When it comes to emotional intelligence, Boyatzis says, women have an edge over men. "Women have—and use—a lot more self- and social awareness," he says. But it remains harder for women to reconcile the demands of a high-powered job with those of family life because they are typically less willing to sacrifice everything to pursue a single goal. "The characteristics and values that make someone a great leader are the very same qualities that might convince them to step off the ladder," Boyatzis notes. "It's a conundrum."

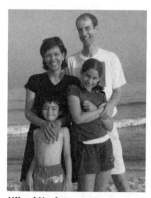

Hikari Hathaway 47, New York City • *Real-estate saleswoman*

If being at the top (or staying on the fast track to get there) requires you to surrender your life, the job poses particular problems, because professional women typically take on more responsibilities at home than men. "Women think more about the pressures of family," Kaye says. They are more likely to maintain social connections, foster familial ties, and, yes, ensure that everyone has clean socks. Children complicate things even further, and not simply because a mother's obligations multiply exponentially. For working parents, the old double standard is alive and well. "If a man isn't around a lot, he can still be perceived as a good father. But it's harder for people to consider a woman who isn't around very much a good mother," Soat notes.

That doesn't mean that motherhood and success in the workplace are mutually exclusive. But you do have to be creative. Because working moms typically find themselves juggling more tasks than their spouses, their professional decisions are complex and multifaceted. "You have to ask yourself how you want to design your life in terms of a career and family," Battley says. "You have to make those decisions with your eyes wide open." You may take time off when the kids are young, or work part-time and then get back to business when they reach school age. "It can work when it's thought out," Battley adds. "It's most successful when there's a plan in place."

Eight years and three children later, Hathaway did resume working, but in a very different capacity. Today, she is a licensed real estate saleswoman at a family-friendly agency. "I have a lot of freedom and flexibility. I'm managing my own time," she says.

Hathaway's fringe benefits go beyond picking her children up from school, joining their classes on field trips, and even taking off the entire month of August to be with her family. "I used to get the flu and colds. Now, I'm much healthier, physically and mentally. I don't feel there are the same stresses in my life that I had then," she says. "Right now, picking up my teenage daughter from a party at 1:30 a.m. is the only kind of stress I want to have," she adds, laughing.

WHAT WOMEN UNDERSTAND

Hathaway's career ambitions shifted when she became a mother. Lynda Rothman had her "Eureka!" moment shortly after she graduated from business school with a double master's in business administration and accounting. After landing a job at a top firm, the newly minted CPA looked around and was discomfited by what she saw. "There were very few women in high places, and none of them seemed to have lives outside the office," says Rothman, 35. At first, she attributed her observation to sexism, but in time she came to see it as a reality of the business world.

If she couldn't have it all, Rothman knew what she was willing to give up. After two years at the company, she got married and moved to Los Angeles, where she

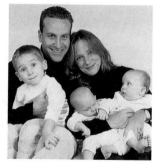

Lynda Rothman 35 (with husband, Mark, and sons [L-R] Max, Davis, and Grant), Los Angeles *Financial consultant*

interviewed for two different positions at an investment-banking firm. She took the slightly less demanding job that offered more flexible hours. "I wanted to have a balanced life," she says.

Rothman's less rigorous schedule (she went part-time after the birth of her first child; more recently, she switched to consulting) has given her time to travel, be with family and friends, and get involved in charity work. There have been trade-offs; though her job is lucrative, Rothman says, she is not making as much money as some of her business-school friends. Winning her colleagues' respect also took some time. Still, she says, "I showed I could contribute to the bottom line. That gave me credibility and value. You don't always have to be that top person to contribute to the group."

More importantly, you don't have to be in that slot to have a rewarding career and a fulfilling life. Women may intuitively understand this in a way that their male co-workers don't. "I think that status is more important to men," Kaye says. In fact, having a life outside of work can increase your happiness. A 2002 study in the *Academy of Management Journal* found that people with well-rounded lives have greater self-esteem and life satisfaction.

CHARTING YOUR COURSE

To ensure that your job fits your life and not the other way around, you need to navigate your own unique course. Battley suggests doing an annual "life audit," in which you take stock of your goals and how your career choices fit in with them. Revisiting the issue every year lets you take into account the natural ebb and flow of your life. You may have the right stuff to be a corporate leader, but the timing may be all wrong. "Someone who is devoting time to family may say that, at this point, being number two is consistent with her priorities," Battley says. Those can change, however, and professional direction along with them.

Society is more tolerant of different vocational paths than ever before. Thanks to modern technology, people are creating jobs that work for them, rather than vice versa. Case in point: Nearly half of all new small businesses are started by women. "Now, there are many more routes to being number one than in the old corporate model," Battley says.

Office Cliques: Harmful or Helpful?

You see them at the office all the time—the gang that works together, lunches together, and goes out for after-hours margaritas together. To see how office cliques affect *Health* readers, we took our own survey at Health.com. Sure enough, more than 85 percent of poll participants have observed these types of coteries where they work. Most view them negatively: 66 percent have sometimes felt excluded by the in-crowd, and more than half said that cliques at the office are "not helpful." Some of the top reasons: Such groups spread gossip, lower morale, and set up only a select few for success.

Most experts agree with our readers. "Many cliques are toxic," says Erika Karres, Ed.D., assistant professor of education at the University of North Carolina at Chapel Hill and author of *Mean Chicks,* which discusses cliques among girls and women. "Their only purpose is to be anti-productive and antisupportive."

But others disagree. "The term 'cliques' is an unfortunate one—it sounds like grade school," says Deborah Kolb, Ph.D., professor of management at the Simmons School of Management in Boston and author of several books on the workplace. Kolb encourages women to think of cliques as networks. "They can be the basis for proactive groups to take charge," she says. One such group, after discovering that they had all received the same warning from their superiors about being too assertive, formed a regular leadership breakfast to initiate change. Banding together helped the women uncover a systematic problem and find ways to solve it, Kolb says.

Make the most of your office posse. First set boundaries, says BZ Riger-Hull, an executive coach in Martha's Vineyard, Massachusetts. "No gossip, no complaining," she says. "Agree that if you're going to talk about a problem, you have to come up with at least two solutions."

Office Rage

Sure, work can make you cranky.
But has it ever caused you to go to extremes?

BY LAURIE HERR

A recent survey revealed that 51 percent of women—compared with 39 percent of men—said they've come close to striking a fellow employee. Top reasons: computer glitches, overwork, and annoying colleagues. Experts aren't surprised at these findings. Scott Geller, Ph.D., professor of psychology at Virginia Polytechnic Institute and State University, says that even though women have the same career demands as men, "they probably have more home responsibilities than the typical male. That causes frustration." While the original survey was conducted in England, office rage appears to be an international phenomenon, as these anecdotes illustrate.

When a co-worker blew up at me for no reason at all, I locked myself in my office for four hours. I cried, worked, and listened to music. I wouldn't leave or take calls. Staying inside was the only thing I could to do to keep myself and the other guy safe. —*Ellen, 38, computer programmer*

One day, when my boss was being totally unhelpful with a problem I was having, I stormed out of his office and slammed his door so hard that a picture fell and broke. He was so dumbfounded that he never said anything about it. I'm not proud of my reaction, and I know I should have been fired on the spot. —*Caroline, 58, food-service worker*

I once threw a chair in my cubicle. It received quite a bit of attention. —*Leah, 26, account executive*

I once got so furious at my boss that I threw a pencil at him, with the pointy end aimed right at his eyes. He thought it was funny, but I thought he deserved a lobotomy. —*Barbara, 39, business owner*

> ## Ease the Anger *Before you take it out on a co-worker, try these soothing strategies.*
>
> **Give your head a vacation.** It may be a cliché, but it works. Picture yourself in a calm locale and whisk yourself there mentally. If you can't manage it sitting at your desk, step outside or get a drink of water to transport your mind to another place.
>
> **Create a comfort zone.** If your office is a gray box that looks like it's from a Dilbert comic, no wonder you feel angry. Photos of family and friends will help remind you that you have a life outside of work.
>
> **Empathize.** "It's a word women know better than men," says psychologist Scott Geller, who researches workplace health and safety. Try to put yourself in the other person's shoes and give him or her the benefit of the doubt.
>
> **Write it down.** "You can't scream at someone while you write," Geller says. Getting your thoughts on paper may help you see the situation more clearly. Don't use E-mail, though—it could easily get into the wrong hands.
>
> **Talk it out—later.** "If you harbor your anger inside, it will only get worse," Geller notes. Wait until you're calm, then talk to the person involved (or someone in human resources). Ask questions: What happened? How can we prevent it from happening again? Show that you want solutions, not revenge.

Once I was so angry that I ended up in the ER. I thought I was having a heart attack, but the problem turned out to be anxiety. I quit the job. —*Diana, 40, former executive assistant* ∎

How to Ask for a Raise—and Get It

Times are tough, and you could really use more money. But in today's shaky economy, most companies are cutting costs more than ever. Still, many experts say that shouldn't stop you from asking for a raise, as long as you keep it professional. "I've seen men and women discuss their personal lives as if salaries are to be based on need," says Kathleen Myers, president of Advanced Practical Thinking Training, an executive-consulting firm in Des Moines, Iowa. "Salaries are based on the value the person brings to the company, not on who needs money."

But salary isn't the whole story; perks count, too. Many companies today reward employees with other incentives: extra vacation days, flextime, or even a new laptop. Beverly Kaye, Ed.D., co-author of the new book *Love it, Don't Leave It: 26 Ways to Get What You Want at Work*, calls these nonmonetary benefits "elegant currencies." "Employees often have too small an idea of what will make them feel compensated," Kaye says. If more money isn't possible, maybe an hour at the local spa, compliments of your company, will at least make you feel more appreciated.

With that in mind, we hope you're ready to march into your boss's office and start negotiating. And just in case you don't get the answer you want, try some of these comebacks from the experts. ■

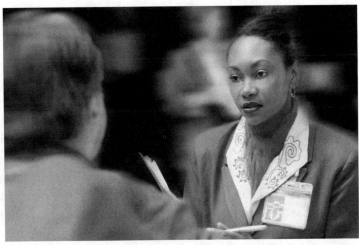

Money-Making Comebacks

Your boss says ...	"You're already at the top of your pay range."	"You're lucky just to be working here."	"With the shape our budget is in? Ha!"	"I guess we probably do need to talk about your salary—sometime."
You say ...	"Then let's talk about the skills I need to develop so I can move on to the next level."	"You're right; we're all fortunate to have jobs these days. Now let me show you what I've done above and beyond my regular responsibilities."	"This is important to me. If a raise isn't possible right now, then I'd like to discuss some incentives in lieu of money."	"Great. How about this coming Friday at 10?"

Tales from the **Testosterone** Zone

Real women reveal what they've learned about relationships from working in male-dominated fields.

BY LIZ KRIEGER

Turn on the television, and you'll probably catch a feisty female cracking a murder mystery, treating a trauma patient, or delivering a court ruling. These examples take their cues from reality: Women make up 49 percent of managers and professionals in the American workplace, according to the U.S. Bureau of Labor Statistics. However, in trade vocations, such as carpentry and cosmetology, a gender bias still exists. A new study published by the National Women's Law Center (NWLC) in Washington, D.C., found that high school girls are still being prepped to work in traditionally female fields. Girls make up 96 percent of the students in cosmetology classes and 86 percent of those in health-careers courses, while more than 90 percent of carpentry, automotive, and plumbing students are boys. "Since the balance of boys and girls in high school shop classes these days is by no means equal, there are fewer women on construction sites, in cockpits, and in auto-body shops," says Leslie Annexstein, NWLC senior counsel.

We asked three women to share their insights on men and relationships gained from working in the testosterone zone. Who knows? Maybe the next hit TV series will star Alex Kingston as a plumber.

DIANA COOPERSMITH, 34, SAN FRANCISCO
IRONWORKER

<u>How I got my start:</u>
I earned a degree from the San Francisco Art Institute; afterward, I was doing set construction for a local perform- ance art group. That inspired me to get my welding certification. This was in the early '90s, when the field was booming; there was just so much work, and they

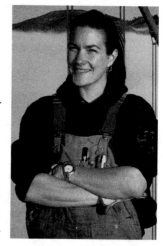

were pretty much begging women to join the ranks.
<u>Job perks:</u> I am strong from lifting, and I've learned how to carry heavy things. My job's a blast. Building high-rises or hanging on the Golden Gate Bridge is great. It's like being on top of a roller coaster.
<u>Occupational hazards:</u> It's a real bummer to be wearing the standard 40-pound tool belt and have cramps. It's also a huge pain to be 300 feet up in a sky- scraper and watch the men simply relieve them- selves off the side of it, while I have to descend all those flights just to go to the rest room.

Lessons about relationships: The men I work with can be very closed-minded and quick to judge. As a result, I've become more sensitive to others and more patient.

The female edge: Being 5 feet 4, I can easily squeeze into spaces that men can't. Sometimes that means I end up welding a column that's right against a wall, which is not exactly the most comfortable spot. But it's something I can do that a man can't.

The ultimate payoff: I have gained a lot of self-confidence, and I believe I can do anything a man can do. I look at men as equals.

CLAIRE WOAKES, 43, BERKELEY, CALIFORNIA
GENERAL CONTRACTOR

How I got my start: My first job was 25 years ago in Brooklyn, New York, and there were 200 men and me. I didn't know which end of the hammer was up. Eventually, I got paired up with a great guy, and he taught me so much.

Job perks: I never have to worry about working out because my job keeps me so active.

Occupational hazards: Some guys have tried to do things for me rather than letting me do them myself. Also, every time I start a new job, I feel like I have to work twice as hard as the others in order to prove myself.

Lessons about relationships: Men are horrible communicators. They might not call and keep in touch or do what you would expect them to—or do what a woman probably would. I used to take it more personally, but now I know that's just the way they are.

The female edge: I believe that I'm much better at dealing with people than guys are. That's especially important when you're remodeling people's houses and the situation can be chaotic.

The ultimate payoff: The other day, I was playing with my 2-year-old and showing her my drill when it occurred to me how cool it is that she will grow up being comfortable around tools—and with a mom who is, too.

MICHELLE LORCH, 35, MINNEAPOLIS/ST. PAUL
COMMERCIAL AIRLINE PILOT

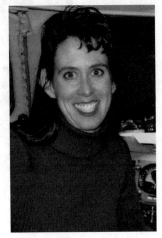

How I got my start: My dad flew private planes, so I was exposed to aviation early on. When I was a teenager, my parents asked me what I wanted to be, and I said a pilot. I went through Ohio State's aviation program, and my career took off from there.

Job perks: I can travel anywhere in the continental United States for almost nothing—$25 a leg—to see family and friends. One time, I set a friend up on a blind date, and I flew to Michigan to tag along and see how the evening went.

Occupational hazards: It's difficult for my family because I'm away from home for long stretches of time and can't be reached easily. Also, the things pilots are required to wear basically make me look like a man: the necktie, the man's hat, the plain-toed loafers. The female pilots look masculine, while the female flight attendants are encouraged to look feminine.

Lessons about relationships: I think women feel more of a need for social interaction. Sitting in a cockpit with men for hours, I've come to realize that men don't think it's necessary to talk all the time; now I'm a lot more comfortable in silence.

The female edge: When you're flying, you have to juggle several tasks all at once. I don't know if there is any proof or not, but I think women are better at multitasking than men.

The ultimate payoff: I really enjoy the interaction with passengers. After just about every flight, someone will come up to me and say that if they'd known a woman was flying, they would've felt more comfortable. I'm really happy to let girls know they can be pilots, too. ■

Change Your Words, Change Your Life

Look at everyday situations in a new light with this easy trick.

BY AVIVA PATZ

You probably don't think you need a vocabulary lesson. But research shows that your words have the power to change your perceptions of yourself and those around you. "The words we use to describe other people's behavior affect how we feel about them," says study author Ellen Langer, Ph.D., a psychology professor at Harvard University. "For example, you can be irritated by your husband's 'impulsiveness' or choose to admire his 'spontaneity' instead." Consider these examples to learn how you can adjust your attitude and give your relationships a boost.

Your mother calls several times a day to ask how the kitchen renovations are coming, whether you've written that thank-you note to Aunt Joan, and if you're voting in next week's elections.
The word that comes to mind …
Nagging. You've got a job, a mortgage, and a family of your own, and she still insists on treating you like a child.
Try calling it …
Connecting. "Recognize that your mother probably misses you and wants to have contact with you," Langer says. "If you find it annoying, try calling her instead and initiating the kind of conversation you'd like to have."

Your husband just lost his job and has spent the last week parked in front of the TV.
The word that comes to mind …
Moping. He's wallowing in failure.
Try calling it …
Coping. It implies he's nurturing himself. "If he looked for new work given his current feelings, he probably wouldn't present his best self," Langer says. "He may need to get distance from the blow to his ego in order to regain his confidence."

Your friend keeps you on the phone for an hour complaining about her boyfriend, your cousin asks you to plan the family reunion again this year, and your neighbor wants you to dog-sit when she goes on vacation.
The word that comes to mind …
Using. Why do people try to take advantage of you?
Try calling it …
Relying. "Instead of feeling resentful, you should feel good about yourself, because obviously your friends consider you dependable, open, and trustworthy," Penney says. "And if you really don't want to do something," she adds, "you can always say 'no.'" That's not being unkind; it's just taking care of yourself.

A co-worker dictates every detail on a team project, right down to the color of envelopes you should use.

The word that comes to mind ...

Pushy. Who put her in charge?

Try calling it ...

Direct. "Here you have someone with definite ideas who's going to work really hard, and it will benefit you in the end," says Alexandra Penney, co-author of *Magic Words: 101 Ways to Talk Your Way Through Life's Challenges.* "To get on equal footing, you might say, 'I like your directness; I'll be equally so.'" Then present your ideas in the same straight-forward way. ▧

Aviva Patz is a Health *contributing editor. She chooses to see "deadlines" as "guidelines" in order to keep her peace of mind.*

Is Overthinking Hurting Your Relationships?
Take our quiz to find out if your brain works overtime.

Even the most mellow people worry now and then. But women are especially prone to overthinking or rehashing events for no real gain. Susan Nolen-Hoeksema, Ph.D., a psychology professor at the University of Michigan, offers help in her book *Women Who Think Too Much: How to Break Free of Overthinking and Reclaim Your Life.* "When you overthink, you ruminate over what went wrong in the past and obsess over current concerns," she says. "You think all this analysis will lead to tremendous insight, but the quality of your solutions actually becomes worse." It's no wonder that such behavior contributes to anxiety, depression, and alcoholism. In fact, one recent study found that over-thinkers are three times as likely to have drinking problems as folks who know when to quit worrying.

1. Your boss makes a vague comment about one of your projects. You replay your bungled response so many times that you end up missing a deadline.
A. No, that's not me.
B. That's sometimes me.
C. Yes, that's me.

2. You're choosing a birthday gift for your new boyfriend. You decide on a shower radio, then return it for a sweater—then go back and get a gift certificate instead.
A. No, that's not me.
B. That's sometimes me.
C. Yes, that's me.

3. At the height of a temper tantrum, your child screams, "I hate you!" You spend the rest of the night moping about where you went wrong as a parent.
A. No, that's not me.
B. That's sometimes me.
C. Yes, that's me.

4. Finances look bleak. Instead of brain-storming ways to get out of debt, you pick the same old money fight with your mate.
A. No, that's not me.
B. That's sometimes me.
C. Yes, that's me.

5. "You look great for a woman your age," your husband says. Your translation, two hours later: "You're getting old, dear."
A. No, that's not me.
B. That's sometimes me.
C. Yes, that's me.

If you answered ...
Mostly As: Congrats—you're avoiding the overthinking trap.
Mostly Bs: You're middle-of-the-road. When you catch yourself starting to overanalyze, you usually find ways to break your mind-set.
Mostly Cs: You obsess like a pro. First, try to stop your thoughts. Read a book or watch TV to get your mind off the subject, then solve the problem at hand: If your boss is being vague, ask for clarification; if you've had a spat with your spouse, talk about it. To squash overthinking long-term, consider broadening your base of interests and friends; playing more roles in life can keep you from zeroing in on one aspect.

vital *stats*

85
Percentage of Americans who drink CAFFEINATED beverages

32
Percent caffeine INCREASES ADRENALINE levels (read: your perception of stress) throughout the day

60
Percent more likely five-cup-a-day java drinkers are to develop HIGH BLOOD PRESSURE than non-coffee drinkers

2
Times higher the number of people who die from INFECTIONS caught in hospitals as compared with deaths from traffic accidents

90,000
Estimated number of DEATHS each year caused by infections caught in hospitals

75,000
Number of those infections that resulted from UNSANITARY conditions

50
Percent of doctors and nurses who REGULARLY wash their hands

---

16 POUNDS
Weight of an average shovelful of WET SNOW

2,000 POUNDS
Weight of snow the average person SHOVELS in 10 minutes

50.5 MILLION
Number of FAKE CHRISTMAS TREES sold in the United States each year

33 MILLION
Number of LIVE Christmas trees sold

1
Number of acres of a Christmas tree farm that provide the daily OXYGEN SUPPLY for 18 people

9:1
Likelihood that a RESIDENTIAL FIRE will begin with the drapes versus with a live Christmas tree

150 POUNDS
Weight at which a woman on the Pill increases her RISK of pregnancy

152 POUNDS
AVERAGE weight of the American woman

56
Percentage of people who are bothered "a lot" by hearing "bad" or "rude" LANGUAGE in public

36
Percentage who ADMIT they've used such language in public themselves

140
Times per year that an even-tempered person DRIVES RECKLESSLY because of road rage

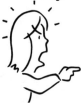

604
Times per year that HOTHEADS do the same

174
Average number of Americans who die annually from EXTREME HEAT

699
Average number of Americans who die annually from EXTREME COLD

34
Percentage of people who say they OVERSPEND "to be fair to everyone"

42
Percentage of households on the brink of BANKRUPTCY

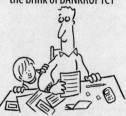

55
Percentage of people who say MONEY PROBLEMS are a cause of stress

$150 BILLION
Amount STRESS-RELATED illnesses cost American corporations annually

9
Percentage of people who'd give up their RIGHT TO SUE a drug company if that company would give them a pill to make any body part either bigger or smaller

---

Sources: Public Agenda, Colorado State University, National Mental Health Association, ABC News, MSN Money Central, SMR Research Corp., HealthWorks, Columbia University, National Association of Counties, Urban Programs Resource Network, National Christmas Tree Association, *Detroit Free Press,* Federal Emergency Management Agency, Centers for Disease Control and Prevention, RhoadesDev, ClassActionAmerica.com, MSNBC, Reuters Health —Reported by Amy Keyishian

chapter 8

mind & spirit

**improve stress management
and find more inner peace**

Make Over
Your Mood
in Minutes

Try these strategies for turning a bad day into a good one, in less than an hour.

BY CHRISTINA FRANK

Lots of things can turn your day dark while it's still bright and early: You and your husband bicker over breakfast, your pants won't button, the car won't start. Since no one wants to spend the whole day brooding, we scoured the latest research to find the quickest, most effective mood makeovers. We recruited people in funks to put these remedies to the test; the results may leave you singing.

SING, SING A SONG

Solo or in a chorus, singing can lower tension levels and improve your outlook, according to the British journal *Psychology and Psychotherapy*. **Why:** "One theory is that music transports you to another realm—it takes you out of your everyday existence," explains study co-author Elizabeth Valentine, Ph.D., professor of psychology at the University of London. Research shows that the most effective tunes are fast, relatively high-pitched, staccato, consonant, and in a major key, Valentine says. Songs that fit this description include "Soak Up the Sun" by Sheryl Crow,

"Good Day Sunshine" by The Beatles, or the "Hallelujah!" chorus from Handel's *Messiah*.
  Does it work? Like a charm, assuming you can find an embarrassment-free zone. Bummed out about an argument with a friend, our tester grabbed her Discman and sang along to "Good Day Sunshine." "It was almost impossible to feel mad," she says.

PUT YOUR GRIPES IN WRITING

You might think that fixating on someone's faults would only increase your ire, but research by psychologist Robin Kowalski, Ph.D., professor of psychology at Clemson University in South Carolina, suggests otherwise. In a recent study published in *Representative Research in Social Psychology*, Kowalski asked annoyed people to vent on paper, either directly to the person who offended them or to a third party. Another group wrote about random events. Those who wrote to the people they were angry with, regardless of whether the mad memo was actually sent, felt significantly happier afterward compared with the other two groups.

Why: "Unloading grievances can be cathartic," Kowalski says. "It allows you to get frustrations off your chest instead of stewing over them."

Does it work? Yes, says our tester, whose unemployed brother called to ask if he could live with her until he got on his feet. She typed him an E-mail, but she didn't hit "send."

EAT FEEL-GOOD FOODS

Mac and cheese doesn't have a lock on the comfort category. Foods that soothe vary from person to person. In a survey of 1,005 people, Brian Wansink, Ph.D., a nutritional-science professor at the University of Illinois, found that positive past associations stood out as the number-one factor behind the foods they chose. (Ice cream, chocolate, and cookies rated tops among women—no surprise there.) You might yearn for potato chips because they remind you of summer vacations or for chocolate cake because you always ate it on your birthday.

Why: Whether it's the ingredients in comfort foods or the happy recollections that provide the mood boost is hard to tell. But nutritionist Joy Short, R.D., of St. Louis University, believes expectations play a big role. "If you expect a certain food to lift your mood, it probably will, even if the effect is more psychological than physical," Short says.

Does it work? Yep. When our tester felt anxious about a looming deadline at work, she reached for plain M&M's—and they did the trick. (She has fond memories of snacking on frozen M&M's while studying for junior high exams.) However, the guilt over polishing off a king-size bag somewhat diminished the positive effect.

ASK FOR AMINOS

To banish the blues, try taking the supplement 5-HTP (5-hydroxytryptophan), suggests psychotherapist Julia Ross, executive director of Recovery Systems, a San Francisco clinic that has been using this and other amino acids to treat mood problems since the 1980s. Based on evidence she's seen in her clinic, Ross, who is also author of the book

The Mood Cure, believes the substance's antidepressant effects may improve your outlook in as few as 10 minutes. She says it has worked well for 85 of her depressed clients who take it regularly.

Why: Although clinical evidence to back up her claims is scant, Ross suggests that the amino acid increases production of the mood-elevating brain chemical serotonin. "My guess is that 5-HTP may work, but there's just no methodology to back it up," says Andrew Stoll, M.D., assistant professor of psychiatry at Harvard Medical School and director of the pharmacology-research laboratory at the university's McLean Hospital. One study by the pharmaceutical company Eli Lilly did show that combining 5-HTP with Prozac significantly promoted serotonin activity in the brain, compared with taking Prozac alone. "There is a benefit," says Vincent Morelli, M.D., assistant professor of family medicine at Louisiana State University School of Medicine in New Orleans, who has published research on alternative therapies for depression. "Some studies have shown that 5-HTP alone is just as effective as some of the older varieties of antidepressants."

Consult your doctor before trying 5-HTP if you already take a prescription antidepressant: You could be at risk for serotonin syndrome, a potentially dangerous condition that can cause fever, rapid heartbeat, nausea, and other serious problems. Even if you're not taking antidepressants, queasiness is another possible side effect. Ross recommends starting with a 50-milligram pill once daily, gradually increasing the dose to the optimal amount that relieves your symptoms. "It can take up to a week to get the right dose." Doctors say you can safely take up to 300 milligrams a day, but they strongly recommend that anyone taking 5-HTP do so under a physician's care.

Does it work? Our tester says that she felt brighter and more upbeat within a few minutes of taking one 50-milligram pill on a down day. But she admits that her experience could have been just wishful thinking. ∎

Turn Your Flaws into fine points

Make those personality quirks work for you.

BY VICTORIA CLAYTON

Your co-workers say you're a perfectionist, or your spouse calls you a control freak. Hey, nobody's perfect. But such personality flaws can actually become assets, says Marti Olsen Laney, Psy.D., author of *The Introvert Advantage*. Here, we discuss challenging traits, with advice on using the hidden strengths of each.

CONTROL FREAKS

You know you're one if: You're not comfortable unless you're calling all the shots.

Your challenge: Control freaks take on too much responsibility and give themselves too much credit, because the unpredictability of life makes them anxious. But much of what people think they control is often a matter of chance or luck, says Suzanne C. Thompson, Ph.D., professor of psychology at Pomona College in Claremont, California. "We overestimate how much influence we have. When good things happen, we give ourselves credit because it's satisfying to think we were the architect," explains Thompson, who has studied the "illusion of control."

When outcomes aren't so good, control freaks find it easier to blame themselves than chalk it up to random bad luck. The trouble is, they don't know where to stop. They micromanage their co-workers' jobs, their spouses' eating habits, their children's schedules, their friends' love lives. As a result, they often come across as bossy, self-serving, and manipulative, and they burn themselves out to boot.

Make it work for you: You're a born leader with an ability to size things up and act on them. The trick is learning to balance your desire for control with acceptance. "It's not just you in charge," Thompson

Nobody's perfect. But, fortunately, you can find hidden strengths in each type of challenging trait.

says. If you don't like what someone's doing, you can speak up about it, but you need to be willing to hear the other person's point of view, too. You also need to learn what's worth controlling and what isn't, Thompson adds. Before you insist that your husband change shirts, ask yourself if your life would be significantly different if he wore what he wanted. Chances are, it wouldn't. If you're remodeling your bathroom, though, you may decide that weighing in on the color of the grout and the style of the drawer pulls is indeed worth your time. But even then, you can't control how fast the tile layer works. Anticipate the details that will be out of your hands and let them go.

PERFECTIONISTS

You know you're one if: You work hard to reach goals, but your painstaking efforts sometimes get in your way. When you do succeed, you feel little satisfaction.

Your challenge: You crave approval and are terrified of rejection, says researcher Paul Hewitt, Ph.D., associate professor of psychology at the University of British Columbia in Vancouver and a specialist in the condition. According to Hewitt, many perfectionists become that way in part because they didn't receive clear guidelines from their parents when they were children. Having never been taught which behaviors would be rewarded and which would be punished, they grow up trying to do everything right.

Unfortunately, unbridled perfectionism has a serious downside. Numerous studies have linked it to depression, eating disorders, and suicide. Even in its milder forms, the trait can cause problems. "Perfectionism is associated with procrastination and a lack of satisfaction," Hewitt says. If you feel a job must be done perfectly, it's hard to start and even harder to finish. And since few things in life are truly perfect, you find enjoying your accomplishments nearly impossible. You might also experience trouble with relationships—you're tough not only on yourself, but also on family, friends, and co-workers.

Make it work for you: With your high standards, you have an enormous ability to achieve. The key is aiming for excellence, not perfection, Hewitt says. When you do something well, reward yourself. "Perfectionists think, 'OK, that's done. What's next?' They don't savor their victories." So take

a day off, get a massage, or find another way to congratulate yourself. Also, look at why you push yourself so hard and stop trying to buy love and respect through accomplishments.

INTROVERTS

You know you're one if: You begin to wilt long before the party ends.

Your challenge: If you're an introvert, interactions with others tend to zap your energy, whereas extroverts thrive on them, says Laney, a marriage and family therapist. Blame it on brain chemistry, which researchers have found differs between these personality types. When engaged in conversation, extroverts process information through short-term memory, a quick-access area of the brain that enables them to respond quickly. Introverts rely on long-term memory, a part of the brain with more-complex pathways. Because of this extra work, you may feel drained as you search for the right word or simply think things through.

A study published in the *American Journal of Psychiatry* points out another disadvantage: PET scans have shown that introverts tend to have more activity in the parts of the brain linked to planning, remembering, and problem solving. Extroverts buzz more in the sensory regions, so while they feed off the sights and sounds of the outside world, introverts focus on their own thoughts. Others may find you unexpressive or even a tad unfriendly, when you're merely busy thinking.

Make it work for you: Introverts can be respected as intellects with a knack for creative ideas, and they shine when addressing topics they care about. Laney advises leaving witty repartee to the extroverts and concentrating on subjects that mean a lot to you. Try to control the amount of stimulation around you. At parties, Laney recommends "staging," or starting at the edges of the gathering and working your way in. In everyday situations, take breaks when you can: Just five minutes alone in the bathroom at work can help you get your bearings. ■

Change Bad Habits for GOOD

Real women's strategies for achieving healthy goals—and expert advice on making those solutions work for you

BY STEPHANIE JO KLEIN

When you're faced with a challenge, such as losing weight or trying to quit smoking, setting up a system of rules and rewards can be key to staying motivated. "If I go to the gym five times a week," you might tell yourself, "then I can eat my favorite dessert on the weekend." When they work, rules stoke your willpower and provide the structure you need to keep you on track. But sometimes they can backfire. "Having a goal and a way to track it is helpful if you want to change your behavior," says Saul Shiffman, Ph.D., a University of Pittsburgh psychology professor who researches the ways that people break bad habits. "But if you're not flexible, you are more likely to collapse when things go wrong. Rigid plans are brittle plans."

We spoke to four women who set themselves self-imposed rules about health, fitness, and relationships. We then asked Shiffman and other leading experts for tips on rewriting those rules to work for—rather than against—you.

THE RULE: EAT COOKIES (ALMOST) NAKED
When Melissa Master, 27, started on the Weight Watchers program two years ago, her sweet tooth frequently sent her searching for snacks. "I decided that I had to be aware of the consequences if I was going to eat something," says the New York City magazine editor. Her rule? If she's craving something sugary or fattening, she can eat it, but only in front of her mirror—in her bikini. Although the nearly-nude-and-noshing rule has quashed a few cookie binges and at times encouraged her to hit the gym, Master wound up keeping off only 10 of the 40 pounds she had originally lost.

The Ruling: Master has the right idea by being realistic about the consequences of her food choices, but the rule won't get her very far when she eats away from the privacy of her home, says obesity expert Ruth Kava, Ph.D., R.D., director of nutrition for the American Council on Science and Health in New York City. "You have to figure out how to change your lifestyle long-term," Kava says. "You're not going to put on a bikini in the middle of a party to have a sweet, so this doesn't do much good." Instead, Kava recommends using different strategies for different situations. If you're out with friends, for instance, try putting on snug-fitting clothes so you'll be less likely to overeat.

THE RULE: WATER FOR COFFEE

Rachel Knighton, a 23-year-old public relations representative in Atlanta, discovered at a recent checkup that she was at risk for fibrocystic breast disease. Her doctor advised her to cut back on caffeine and fill up on water, a tough feat for someone who was used to drinking two cups of coffee and up to three 20-ounce bottles of cola a day. Her plan: If she drank a liter of water before lunch and another one after, she would reward herself with a cup of coffee in the morning and a soda at lunch. After one month, she'd curbed her extreme caffeine habits.

The Ruling: Knighton's success is all in the planning, says Gail Frank, R.D., a spokeswoman for the American Dietetic Association and also professor of nutrition at California State University, Long Beach. "For any change, you have to zoom in on the culprit; she's identified it and created a practical plan with a reward at the end." But Frank points out that you can't cure all your body's ills just by drinking 2 liters of water—and that's a difficult target anyway. "She should not set her goals so high that she sabotages her efforts," Frank says. "Besides, you can get water from many different foods, like fruits, salads, and vegetables."

THE RULE: ISSUE-FREE DINNER

Niki Elenbaas likes to talk about family matters as soon as her spouse walks in the door after work. He prefers to wait until he has had some time to eat and relax. Elenbaas, a 42-year-old communications executive in Seattle, and husband Jamie agreed that she would refrain from diving into issues until the end of dinner. As incentive, they made a bet with their friends: If Elenbaas could last a whole month without jumping the gun, the couple's pals would treat them to dinner at a favorite restaurant. The Elenbaases lost the friendly wager but say they've gained a new appreciation of their communication styles.

The Ruling: It's a smart move for couples to devise systems of talking about things that concern them,

says Michael S. Broder, Ph.D., author of *Can Your Relationship Be Saved? How to Know Whether to Stay or Go.* Instead of Elenbaas simply agreeing to remain silent so her husband can have his quiet time, Broder suggests that they come up with a plan that meets her needs as well as his. "If her husband asks for more

> If you're not flexible, you are more likely to collapse when things go wrong. Rigid plans are brittle plans.
> —Saul Shiffman, Ph.D.

transition time when he comes home from work, he also needs to ask how he can be more attentive to her," Broder says. "Perhaps they can talk briefly during lunch and then enjoy a relaxing dinner together." The best part of the couple's rule was the bet, Broder says. "Anything done in fun like this is great, and friends can give you incredible perspective."

THE RULE: SOCIAL SMOKING

Angela Bak, 24, was training for a half-marathon when she realized her half-pack-a-day smoking habit had to go. Rather than quit cold turkey, Bak, a marketing coordinator in Toronto, tapered her way down to social smoking. Her guidelines: no smoking 9 to 5; never carry cigarettes (you're less inclined to smoke if you have to bum from someone else); light up only one cigarette for every three or four a friend smokes. Bak says she now has more energy when she runs. She still smokes a few cigarettes when she goes out with friends on weekends.

The Ruling: Bak's success is unusual—and she could easily relapse to serious smoking, Shiffman says. "She should just quit. For cardiovascular disease, the risk is incurred at pretty low levels of smoking," he says. "Plus, very few people can smoke occasionally without being addicted. The risk of going back to high-level smoking is around 90 percent." His advice: Change your patterns. If you know that drinking makes you want to smoke, don't go to bars, or go but don't drink. "Instead of following your own rules, follow the rules on the box of nicotine gum or patches," he says. ■

5 STEPS TO STOP PROCRASTINATING

Learn what makes you put things off and what you can do about it.

BY ALICE LESCH KELLY

Even if you don't think of yourself as a procrastinator, you probably are. "Almost everyone procrastinates in certain situations," says Regina Conti, Ph.D., an associate professor in the department of psychology at Colgate University. For example, many people put off tasks they find difficult or boring, such as paying taxes or cleaning out the basement. According to one study, some 25 percent of people confessed that such behavior was a serious problem in their lives, and 40 percent admitted that procrastination had caused them to lose money at one time or another.

Not only does procrastination waste valuable time and raise your stress levels, but "it keeps you from attaining your goals and fulfilling your dreams," says Rita Emmett, a time-management consultant and author of *The Procrastinator's Handbook: Mastering the Art of Doing It Now.*

People who put things off may think it's a personality trait, but they've simply learned bad habits. To break them, you need to identify the ways you waste time—and why. Our program incorporates successful strategies from time-management gurus, organizational experts, and behavioral psychologists to help you do everything on your resolution list now.

1 FIGURE OUT YOUR PROCRASTINATION PROFILE.

When, how, and why do you procrastinate? You may do so in only some parts of your life. For example, many women perform efficiently at work and at home but put off workouts, diets, and routine medical checkups. "Women are so other-focused that they often neglect their own needs," explains Gail McMeekin, a career coach and author of *The 12 Secrets of Highly Creative Women.*

To pinpoint your profile, look back at some instances over the past six months when you have procrastinated. Which tasks did you put off—those related to your job, social life, financial matters, or housecleaning? Was it out of fear, perfectionism, boredom, or fatigue? And did you procrastinate by playing solitaire, organizing and reorganizing your closet, or watching *The Anna Nicole Show?* Identifying patterns will help you find ways to become more efficient.

2 PRACTICE "SELECTIVE PERFECTIONISM."

If you always expect to do things perfectly, you might put off certain tasks because you don't want to mess them up. But you can stop procrastinating without abandoning your high standards, explains Julie Morgenstern, author of *Time Management from the Inside Out* and the founder of Task Masters, a professional organizing company in New York City. "It's not about letting go of perfectionism; it's learning how to apply selective perfectionism," she says. Only 10 to 20 percent of most people's tasks really need to be perfect, Morgenstern says. For the remaining 80 to 90 percent, a less thorough job is adequate.

"At work, for example, interoffice E-mail doesn't have to be perfect, but proposals should be flawless," Morgenstern says. "Meetings with clients require extra thought; some staff meetings may not."

Perfectionists tend to strive for excellence without even thinking about it. If this describes you, break the habit by beginning each task with a question: Does this need to be done perfectly, or will "good enough" suffice? Going easier in some areas, Morgenstern says, will free you to invest your time where it really counts.

3 FIND A BETTER WAY.

Often, it's how you approach a task, rather than the task itself, that makes you procrastinate. You may put off paying the bills because you always do it at 10 p.m., when you're too exhausted to think clearly. Or you often skip workouts because spending 45 minutes on the treadmill bores you.

If you keep delaying things, change the way you do them. Pay your bills on Saturday morning instead of Tuesday night, with jazz playing in the background and a vanilla latte at your side. Hike a nature trail with your best friend instead of treading solo in the gym. Whatever the chore, look for ways to make it

How to Build a Better List

To be effective, a daily to-do list must be more than a catalog of all the things you'd really love to get done today but probably won't. The following tips, from time-management consultants Julie Morgenstern and Rita Emmett, can help you put together a list that really works.

- Set aside time each morning to write it. Use a notebook and don't rip out used pages. "There's an exhilarating feeling when you flip back through and realize all that you've accomplished," Emmett says.

- Set realistic goals. If you list 45 and only accomplish 8, you'll feel discouraged.

- Plan for downtime. Yes, doing nothing has its place in learning to be more productive. If you don't allot yourself any relaxation time, you may steal it at work in the form of procrastination.

- Schedule a specific day and time for each item. Don't just write down "exercise" on a list; instead, pencil in a 30-minute workout on Thursday from 5:45 to 6:15 p.m.

- If a task feels overwhelming, break it down into three to five steps and spread them out over the course of a week or month to make it feel less intimidating.

- Devote different parts of your day to such activities as calling, reading, or writing, and schedule accordingly. This way, you will spend less time moving from one task to the next.

- Record only what you plan to do today. If you know you won't have time to write that thank-you note to Aunt Edna, jot it down in your notebook for next Tuesday.

fun, interesting, or educational. If that doesn't work, delegate it or hire someone else to do it for you. Or just accept that sometimes you're stuck with distasteful obligations. Also, keep in mind that dreading your responsibilities can use up more time and energy than fulfilling them.

Is Fear Making You Procrastinate?

Whether you want to write a novel or lose those extra 20 pounds, fear of failure, uncertainty, disapproval, responsibility, the unknown—even success—can all keep you from trying.

If fear is holding you back, first identify what you're afraid of. Do you worry that if you write a novel, it will be lousy? Or that if you lose weight, your chubby family will resent you? Next, think about ways to defuse your fears. Talk with your family about your weight-loss goals; perhaps instead of resenting you, they'll offer to join you in your effort. And reword the reproaches that accompany your fears. Instead of telling yourself, "Everyone will think I'm an awful writer if I don't produce a best-seller," restructure the thought: "I am going to try my best and enjoy the process rather than worry about pleasing everyone."

You may also fear that if you fail, people will believe all of your previous successes have been unearned. "You are afraid of being found out, that people will discover you're a fraud," says Ellen Ostrow, Ph.D., a clinical psychologist and founder of Midlife Mentor, a coaching company in Washington, D.C. "When you succeed, you think of it as a fluke." This often happens to people who expect too much of themselves. "When you set impossibly high standards for yourself, you assume that everyone else will judge you by those same high standards," Ostrow says.

If you think fear is keeping you from succeeding, confide in a friend or a therapist. Discussing a problem with an objective outsider often brings underlying causes to light.

4 DOUBLE YOUR DRIVE.

There are two kinds of motivation: intrinsic, which comes from within, and extrinsic, which comes from outside. Each by itself can compel you to do something, but Conti has found that together they greatly increase your chances of success.

For instance, someone who loves painting may be intrinsically motivated to create a masterpiece that she can hang over her sofa. Other things may get in the way, though—parenting responsibilities, her job, fatigue. By adding an extrinsic motivator, such as a painting class, she is more likely to succeed. Likewise, if your garage is so full of junk that the car no longer fits (intrinsic), turn cleaning into a pleasurable

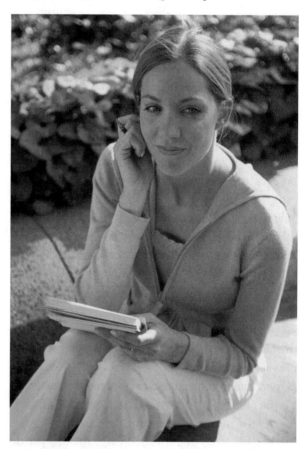

People who put things off may think it's a personality trait, but they've simply learned bad habits. To break them, you need to identify the ways you waste time—and why.

How Much Do You Procrastinate?

1. The last time you had an important report due at work, you:

A. Did it first thing. (0 points)

B. Spent the morning on other important job-related tasks, then did the report after lunch. (1 point)

C. Answered E-mail, took a long lunch, and reorganized your files. Then you panicked, rushed through the report, and handed it to your boss as she ran for the 5:45 train. (2 points)

D. Called in sick. (3 points)

2. Your daily to-do list usually has:

A. Fewer than 10 tasks. (0 points)

B. 10 to 20 tasks. (1 point)

C. 20 to 50 tasks—some of which have remained undone since 1989. (2 points)

D. What to-do list? (3 points)

3. Do you write things down on your list after you've done them just for the pleasure of crossing them off?

If so, give yourself 2 points.

4. Which scenario best describes your use of the Internet on the job?

A. You use it primarily for work-related research and E-mail (which you check only once or twice a day, not continuously) and occasionally for personal business. (0 points)

B. You sometimes browse online catalogs or forward particularly clever E-mail jokes. (1 point)

C. You use E-mail to stay in touch with most of your family and friends, sending and receiving E-mails and instant messages both at work and at home. (2 points)

D. Your co-workers refer to you as "The Clickster." (3 points)

5. Your garage needs cleaning. You:

A. Spend an entire Saturday throwing out junk. (0 points)

B. Put it off for a few weeks and then finally push yourself to do it. (1 point)

C. Hire a neighborhood teen to start on the job but never get around to finishing it. (2 points)

D. Ignore the mess and park in your driveway instead. (3 points)

6. Do you clean your house only when company is coming?

If so, give yourself 2 points.

7. What is your usual strategy for paying bills?

A. At least once or twice each month, you write out checks for all the bills that have come in since the last cycle. (0 points)

B. You're slightly disorganized, but you never pay late. (1 point)

C. You pay them shortly before they're due and are charged an occasional late fee. (2 points)

D. You frequently receive overdue notices and have to pay late fees. (3 points)

8. You're reading this article right now because you:

A. Are taking a well-deserved break after having accomplished everything on your to-do list. (0 points)

B. Couldn't help taking a peek when you noticed this book on the table. But you intend to get back to whatever you were doing as soon as you're finished reading. (1 point)

C. Have a huge, important project due in less than three hours and came across the book while you were rearranging your living-room furniture. (2 points)

D. A friend gave it to you and said, "Boy, do you need to read this!" (3 points)

KEY

0–5 points: You don't procrastinate often (but there's always room for improvement).

6–10 points: You occasionally postpone tasks that you find boring or unpleasant.

11–16 points: You procrastinate a lot. Your self-image, work performance, and personal relationships are probably suffering because of it.

17–21 points: Don't just read this article—memorize it.

occasion (extrinsic): Invite a friend to help, play great music while you work, and plan a feast of barbe-cued shrimp with plenty of crisp Chardonnay to cele-brate when you finish.

5 CONNECT TO THE "WHY."

Let's say your closets are filled with five years' worth of family photos. You're dreading sorting them, putting them in chronological order, and placing them in albums. How can you muster the effort to take on such a tedious job?

"Ask yourself, 'Why do I want to do this? What big-picture goal is this going to help me accom-plish?'" Morgenstern says. Thinking of photo organizing as a gift to your kids rather than a duty may make it more palatable. Sure, you need to clean up the area where the photos are stored. But more importantly, you want to give your children a solid sense of who they are and where they come from; you also want to look back easily at the important memo-ries of their lives—a vacation with their cousins, a visit from Grandma, a cherished friend who has moved away. Connecting a bothersome undertaking with a great "why" can help you get the job done. ▪

Alice Lesch Kelly is the co-author of Conquering Infertility: Dr. Alice Domar's Mind/Body Guide to Enhancing Fertility and Coping with Infertility.

Men's Pheromones Actually Reduce Stress!

To tame tension, hang out at the gym—preferably by the men's locker room—and inhale deeply. A new study shows that pheromones in men's sweat can reduce stress.

Researchers at the Monell Chemical Senses Center, a nonprofit research group in Philadelphia, and the University of Pennsylvania used cotton pads to collect perspiration from the underarms of male volunteers who hadn't used deodorant or scented soaps for four weeks. They blended the sweat samples into an extract and applied it to the upper lips of women ages 25 to 45. (The substance was masked by a fra-grance, so the women didn't know they were smelling sweat. Some thought they were involved in a study of alcohol, perfume, or even lemon-scented floor wax.)

Then the women filled out question-naires that were used to rate their mood. The results? Tension dropped 20 to 25 percent compared with a control group sniff-ing only ethanol. "You won't see male underarm sweat marketed as an anti-depressant anytime soon," says the study's co-author George Preti, Ph.D. "But our results suggest that there may be even more going on during social interactions than meets the eye."

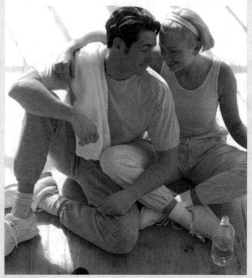

Yoga More Calming Than Simple Rest

Even if you're a novice, a single session of yoga may help lower blood levels of cortisol, a hormone that signals stress. During

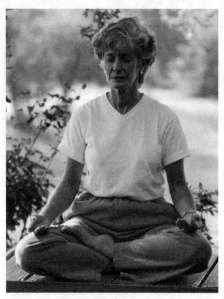

a recent eight-day trial, researchers at Thomas Jefferson University in Philadelphia measured levels of the chemical in men and women before and after they practiced yoga, then again before and after they sat quietly while reading or writing. After the yoga, cortisol levels dropped significantly, the scientists say, but not after the resting period. The study confirms earlier findings and points to yoga as a possible therapeutic tool.

How Guilt Can Hurt Your Wallet

Looking to save money? Quit being so nice. A recent study from the University of British Columbia in Canada found that shoppers often buy from friendly salesclerks to avoid feeling guilty. According to the researchers, many consumers think walking away empty-handed after someone has hauled out 15 pairs of size-8 sandals seems just plain rude. The secret to keeping your cash stashed: no chitchat. Engaging in pleasant banter is the first step toward plunking down your debit card.

Rest Better with Jasmine

If you toss and turn all night, try taking a jasmine-scented bath before bedtime. In a recent study, participants said the flowery aroma made them sleep well and feel alert the following day. Working on a grant from the National Science Foundation, the researchers had subjects sleep in rooms scented with jasmine, lavender, or nothing at all. The subjects, who tried all three air samples, reported feeling the least anxious the next morning after smelling jasmine; they also performed the best on cognitive tests given at several points throughout the day. The scientists observed the sleepers for only three nights, though, so you might want to take the results with a grain of (bath) salt.

Boost Your Willpower

Don't feel too bad if you quit your workout early or have a second slice of cake—your resolve is bound to run out sometime. But the good news is that it's easy to replenish. People tend to view willpower as a mental muscle, and failing to use it can make you feel like a wimp. But new research shows that willpower is an energy source, like fuel; when your supply hits bottom, you're more vulnerable to impulsive behavior. In one of several experiments, psychologists from Florida State University showed people a disturbing video and asked some of them to control their emotional response to it by stifling or amplifying their reactions. They then gauged the participants' physical stamina by testing how long they could squeeze a handgrip. The subjects who reined in their emotions during the video gave up on the squeeze test faster than those who didn't. Study author Roy Baumeister, Ph.D., believes they were worn out from exercising self-control. The best way to recharge? Sleep, Baumeister says. "When you're well-rested, you can resist temptation more easily."

Harmless Habits or Time Traps?

Four true confessions show you how to find greater satisfaction with your free time.

BY AVIVA PATZ

If you could design a perfect evening, would it involve three hours of TV, an hour perusing catalogs, and countless minutes checking your E-mail? Probably not. While these activities are fine in moderation, devoting too much effort to them burns through your leisure time without enriching your life. "If you reduce the energy and resources you spend on these habits, you're free to do things that have more meaning and lead to greater satisfaction," says Judith Wright, educator and author of *There Must Be More Than This: Finding More Life, Love, and Meaning by Overcoming Your Soft Addictions*.

The problem is not what you're doing per se, but why you're doing it and how often. "It's perfectly OK to E-mail back and forth with your sister for an hour after an emotional day or to flip through the Pottery Barn catalog to decompress," says psychologist Martin E.P. Seligman, Ph.D., author of *Authentic Happiness: Using the New Positive Psychology to Realize Your Potential for Lasting Fulfillment*. "These activities become problematic when they are the only way you know how to connect with people, relax, or otherwise fill your spiritual needs."

Four women speak out about what Wright says rank among women's top self-defeating behaviors, and experts weigh in on how to kick the habits.

NET ADDICT

I check E-mail when I wake up, after breakfast, every 10 minutes at work, after dinner, and again before I go to bed, even if I'm not expecting any messages.
—*Miriam Reynolds, 32, Montclair, New Jersey*

People tend to overuse the Internet, including checking E-mail, reading news, or joining chat rooms, to manage stress, procrastinate, and interact with other people, according to a recent study at York University in Toronto. While it's certainly fine to E-mail friends, typed missives should not replace human contact. "When the Web becomes your only source of social activity, that's a problem," says study co-author Richard Davis. "Women in particular are guilty of depending on the Web for social comfort." Try taking Internet "holidays" once every few hours, he suggests. Visit co-workers in person or talk on the phone at home. Break away from the keyboard more and more until you feel comfortable logging off whenever you want.

TOO-BUSY BEE

I wake up at 6 a.m. to run, then begin my daily activities: I'm working toward a master's degree, appearing on TV as a political commentator, and working with a

women's political action committee I co-founded. I spend time with my husband at night, and when I can, I make jewelry, knit, or do crossword puzzles.
— *Daedre Levine, 32, New York City, New York*

Why do women book themselves solid? "They may be compulsive and want to avoid anxiety or uncertainty, they may have trouble saying no to requests, or they may feel guilty just doing nothing," says psychologist G. Alan Marlatt, Ph.D., professor of psychology and director of the Addictive Behaviors Research Center at the University of Washington in Seattle. Regardless of why you overplan, the solution is the same: Balance the duties you must do with the pastimes you find personally fulfilling. "Schedule personal time twice a week, but don't fill it up in advance," Marlatt says. Instead, when the time comes, allow yourself to choose from a menu of favorite options, such as soaking in the tub or riding a bike. To free up more time, gradually drop low-priority activities until your want-to-dos are better aligned with your should-dos.

SEX KITTEN

I fantasize about sex a lot, maybe several times an hour. I also spend a lot of time at the gym—I get a sexual charge from it.
— *Tania Evans, 34, Colorado Springs, Colorado*

Flirting with friends, co-workers, or strangers and daydreaming about romantic or sexual encounters are perfectly fine if they enrich existing relationships, says sex therapist Sharon G. Nathan, Ph.D. But fantasy can escalate into mindless dating or loveless sex, often betraying a deeper need. "Many women are not really looking for men but for validation," she points out. "They want to feel desirable, to have something a man wants and be able to give or withhold it." Nathan suggests exploring the reasons you crave attention. If you feel you're not getting enough in your relationship, you may need to work on shoring up your self-esteem. "Give some thought to what messages or experiences you might have had that could be making you feel bad about yourself," Nathan says.

MATERIAL GIRL

You can't get Manolo Blahniks where I live, so anyplace I vacation has to have good shopping. When I go, I always pack my huge red duffel bag, and it's full by the time I get home.
— *Mary Hilowitz, 42, Anchorage, Alaska*

People who doubt themselves tend to define personal success by what they own, according to a recent study by Robert Arkin, Ph.D., professor of psychology at Ohio State University. "The quest is not for the things themselves, but for the status they convey," he says. For example, you might want a handbag because it's only available in Milan. "The bag then indicates that you have had an experience others have not, which may offset your feelings of self-doubt," Arkin says. The cure? Don't spend so much time evaluating yourself. Use this stop-and-go technique: If you're at a restaurant ogling the 3-carat diamond ring on a woman's finger and you think, "I would love that; too bad I'm stuck with this measly pebble," say "stop" to interrupt the self-doubting cycle. Then say "go" to shift your focus, in this case to your dinner conversation or the dessert menu. ▪

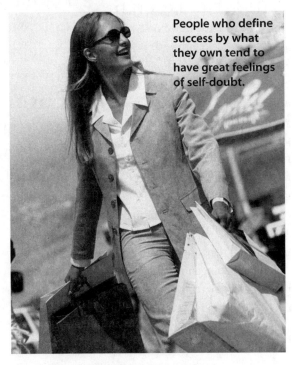

People who define success by what they own tend to have great feelings of self-doubt.

Make Your Anger Work for You

Go ahead—get mad. New research reveals healthy ways to let your frustrations rip.

BY AVIVA PATZ

You know your sister's mad when she breaks out in hives. You can tell your mother's irked by her snippy tone. You know your husband's angry ... because he says so.

Why can't women express anger as directly as men? "We get the message early that if we do, people won't love us," says psychologist Deborah Cox, Ph.D., who co-wrote the new book *The Anger Advantage* with Karin H. Bruckner and Sally D. Stabb. "So we hide it and feel guilty about it." For many women, repression can lead to depression. But properly harnessed, Cox says, negative emotions can be powerful agents of growth and change. "When you're consciously aware of your anger, you're able to make deliberate, responsible choices," she says. "For example, you might realize that you're not getting a say on a committee or that you're doing more than your share of work in a relationship. Getting mad about it gives you an impetus to fix it or move on. It puts you in control."

To learn how your rage can work for you, take a look at these "mad makeovers."

> For many women, repression can lead to depression. But properly harnessed, negative emotions can be powerful agents of growth and change.

YOUR $!#X@ BOSS

Your manager asks you to work late, *again*, to help finish a project your colleague fumbled. You're getting peeved about putting in overtime without extra pay—or at least a little appreciation.

Old reaction: Say nothing and simply complete the assignment like a dutiful worker. Anger is an ugly, unattractive feeling that gets you nowhere.

Why it's bad: Bottled-up bitterness leaves the problem unsolved and can leak out in other ways: You might screw up the project or "accidentally" lose the computer file, both of which will hurt you in the end. On the other hand, if you do your usual good job, you'll just get more work dumped on you.

New reaction: If your boss is easy to approach, be assertive about your needs. You might say, "Of course, I'll help out in a crisis, but I'd also like to talk about long-term solutions." If you're worried that you might sound resentful, focus on the facts—in this case, the long hours you've been working. "That will give your boss an opportunity to respond to your needs without putting him on the defensive or forcing him to deal directly with your emotions, which he may find uncomfortable," Cox says.

YOUR **BLABBERMOUTH** BUDDY

You learn that everyone in your circle knows the secret you told your girlfriend. She not only betrayed your trust, but also put you in an embarrassing position.

Old reaction: Complain to your other friends about her behavior and, to retaliate, let slip that she's had work done on her eyes.

Why it's bad: You may blow off some steam in the short term, but this kind of petty tit for tat can permanently damage your relationship with your girlfriend, not to mention with the rest of the group. After all, you've proven that you can't be trusted.

New reaction: Talk to the friend—not about what she did, but about how it made you feel. You might say, "When I heard ___, I felt hurt and, frankly, a little puzzled." Give her a chance to explain the circumstances. There may be a piece of the story that would help you understand how the secret got out. If she denies any wrongdoing, though, she might not be able to work through this with you, now or ever. "In that case, you may decide to stay friends, but on a different level," Cox says.

YOUR **LAZY** SPOUSE

It's a Sunday afternoon, you've been watching the kids all weekend, and you really need some time for yourself. Meanwhile, your husband is glued to a documentary on World War II submarines.

Old reaction: Lash out at him, yelling, "You're not the only one around here who works all week, you know. Do you think the kids take care of themselves? I feel like a single parent!"

Why it's bad: Yelling may provide instant gratification, but putting him on the defensive hurts your chances of getting what you want.

New reaction: Make eye contact and tell him you need to talk as soon as he can take a break. "When you have his attention, skip the 'you're a lousy father' talk, and frame your needs in terms that show you value him," Cox says. "You might say, 'I know you can be a great dad. The kids love to spend time with you, and I want you to spend time with them.' " Emphasizing your need for an equal partnership rather than exploding will be better for both the situation and your romantic life, Cox says.

THE **MOM** FROM HELL

Your mother, who's visiting for the week, criticizes your hairstyle ("I always liked it shorter"), your cooking ("You have so many lovely spices you could use"), even your parenting skills ("She's lucky you're her mother—most people wouldn't let a 5-year-old get away with that").

Old reaction: Take her comments to heart and begin blaming yourself for your failings: Maybe your hair has gotten too long and maybe you are too lenient with your children.

Why it's bad: What starts out as admirable openness to constructive criticism ends with your self-esteem in the toilet.

New reaction: Be honest in a loving, respectful way. "It's important to say something like, 'I'm an adult now, and I'm doing the best I can. Maybe I do things differently than you did, but I still need your support,' " Cox says. What if your mother blows up or says she never wants to speak to you again? "Let her know that you want her to stay in your life and that you want to stay in hers," Cox says. The confrontation might drive a wedge between you temporarily, but being truthful with each other may improve your relationship in the long run. ■

> It's important to be honest, but in a loving, respectful way.

HIGH
Expectations:
Don't Let Them Bring You Down

Everyone wants a perfect life. But when you force others to fit your dreams, the result is anything but.

BY KIMBERLY GOAD

W e all have expectations of the people in our lives. You go on a date with great hopes that he'll be fun and smart. You take a new job, optimistic that you'll be intellectually fulfilled by your co-workers. You have children and believe they will see the world pretty much as you do. In this goal-oriented society, the expectations you have of others are, let's face it, to be expected.

But are they healthy?

Experts warn that, often, they aren't. Women are especially prone to letting their expectations—of husbands, bosses, mothers, and friends—set them up for disappointment. New York City psychotherapist

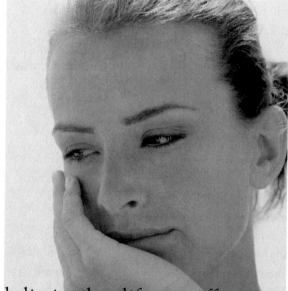

Expectations that are too high limit what life can offer you.

Faith Bethelard, Psy.D., co-author of *Cherishment: A Psychology of the Heart,* says that's a very limited way to live. "When your happiness is contingent on others being a certain way—'My husband has to be this kind of man,' 'I have to work with these kinds of people in this kind of job'—you aren't opening yourself to what life has to offer. Ninety-nine percent of the time, people aren't going to do things exactly the way you want." Rather than having narrowly defined expectations, Bethelard suggests, "have the intention to surround yourself with helpful, supportive people."

The following three women learned how to let go of their high expectations regarding people and circumstances. In doing so, they became happier and more contented with their lives than they could ever have imagined.

I could grow from the pain or grow bitter.
—Rosa White, 36

The Expectation: Rosa White had always dreamed of having a house full of kids. One of seven children raised in a close-knit family, she was still in high school when she created a collage of what she wanted her life to look like: Interspersed with the photographs of the bride, the groom, and the big house were pictures of babies. Lots of them. In the summer of 1991, she knew she'd met her future husband when Art White told her on their third date that he, too, dreamed of having several children. Two months later, they got married; right away, they began trying to get pregnant.

The Reality: Time passed, but White did not have any luck conceiving. After enduring eight years of fertility treatments, four miscarriages, and one failed adoption, her frustration turned to anger, then resentment, and, eventually, depression. "For 11 years, I had put my life on hold," White says. "I wanted to go back to college to become a psychologist, but I kept thinking, 'Any day now, I'm going to be pregnant.' I could have had my master's degree by now."

The Lesson: "I had to redefine what it means to be a mother; I had to consciously separate pregnancy from motherhood," says White, the adoptive mother of a baby girl. "After one of Itzhak Perlman's violin strings broke during a performance, he said, 'Sometimes it's the artist's task to see how much music you can make with how much you have left.' That's how I felt. I could grow from the pain or grow bitter." As president of the Nevada chapter of RESOLVE: The National Infertility Association, White uses her experience to help others battling the same problems. "I understand the pain of infertility," she says.

My hope overrode my experience.
—Julie Powers, 43

The Expectation: When she moved to Colorado, Julie Powers was fired up about her new career selling posh resort real estate. The market was booming, and the company she worked for was growing. Powers' expectations of her new supervisor were equally high. Though she suspected from their initial meetings that her boss was going to demand a lot, Powers also assumed she'd be an advocate. "I thought she would be supportive of a new employee. Because I was going to be generating money for her, I thought she'd want me to do well and maybe even throw some business my way," Powers recalls.

The Reality: Instead of being a mentor and teaching Powers the intricacies of the local housing market, her boss did just the opposite. "She told me it would be trial by fire," Powers says. Then things got worse: Rather than giving her new employee leads, the boss began to take Powers' hard-won clients for herself. "I thought that of all people, she'd treat me fairly," Powers says. As she found out, though, "it was all about making money."

The Lesson: Powers quit the job and went to work for another agency. But she learned an important lesson about what had happened: "My hope overrode my experience." She had anticipated that her boss would be supportive, and when she wasn't, Powers felt cheated and professionally lost. At the new company, she has learned to be more realistic. "I think good people still expect to find goodness in others. But I try to be more wary." Powers' tempered expectations have led to success; she's on good terms with her boss, and sales are climbing.

I learned that I have the power to be happy no matter what the circumstances.
—Carol Tuttle, 45

The Expectation: Carol Tuttle picked up everything she knew about marriage from her parents. Her father, a successful self-employed engineer, was the breadwinner, her mother the homemaker. For Tuttle, the underlying message was that she "had to be married to feel whole," she says. In 1980, at 23, she married her college sweetheart, Jon, and projected all her expectations onto him.

The Reality: Seven years into the marriage, Tuttle's vision of a happy life began to fray. Her husband quit his job and went back to college to earn an MBA. Tuttle, meanwhile, had just given birth to their fourth child in six years. Her husband's career change, coupled with the family's growing need for money, "tipped me over the edge," she admits. "I needed him to fulfill the role of caretaker, and there was almost no income." Realizing that she was living her parents' marriage, Tuttle slipped into depression.

The Lesson: "I realized the situation would not change until I learned that I have the power to be happy no matter what the circumstances of my life," says Tuttle, now a therapist in Salt Lake City and the author of *Remembering Wholeness: A Personal Handbook for Thriving in the 21st Century.* Unsurprisingly, once she released her expectations of her husband, he was free to succeed. And so was she. ▓

Do You Expect Too Much?

Circle the statements below that are most like you.

1. When I tell my mate I love him, I want to hear him say it back right away, with feeling.
2. When I give a friend a gift, I like to receive a note of thanks (E-mails don't count).
3. I get upset when I need highlights and my hairstylist is booked solid.
4. I'm frustrated when my child doesn't like the same things I did at her age.
5. Slow salespeople drive me nuts.
6. "Nothing is ever enough for you" is a phrase I've heard more than once in my life.
7. I don't like caring for my mate when he's sick. Can't he get his own orange juice?
8. I wish my parents would stop asking me when I plan to:

   A) get a better job   D) have a baby
   B) get married   E) start saving money
   C) lose weight   F) all of these.
9. My boss and I are friends, so I expect her to understand if I miss a deadline now and then.
10. Sometimes my family and friends bug the heck out of me, and I don't know why.

If you circled more than five statements, you may need to shift your expectations in a healthier direction. "When we drop our expectations completely, we walk away in defeat," says Janice G. Yamins, Ph.D., a clinical psychologist in New York City. Instead, make sure that what you expect includes, as Yamins says, "the other person's moment in life."

By making your expectations more realistic, you allow others to actually meet them. "It's not just about something you want," Yamins explains. "It's an expectation in a relationship." Your boyfriend forgot your six-month anniversary? Before you get mad, remember that he had a big project due at work. Mark your next milestone on the calendar, make plans together, and then expect him to follow through. (You may want to call and remind him.) Your expectations will be more reasonable, and your relationship will be better for it.

Poetry Slamming:
The Latest Way to Boost Your Self-Esteem

BY EVA MARER

I'm no Madonna, but the second I stepped onstage, I felt the power. A halo of light glowed over me, blotting out the faces of the crowd. I led off with my ode to a New York City brownstone: "In gray splendor, metal blooms/A green lawn scattered with brown leaves...." My own voice startled and energized me. When my two minutes of fame were up, the crowd erupted in cheers and whistles. Reluctantly (and a little sheepishly), I stepped down. My heart seemed to slosh around in my chest like a boat on a sea of goodwill. Now it was my turn to clap and tap my beer on the table in appreciation of the rest of the audience as, one by one, they shared their musings on everything from a father's lost love to how hard it is to hold on to a woman when you're 3 feet tall.

Believe it or not, I was on assignment. And only minutes before, I had been shaking in my chair and silently cursing my editor, whose idea it was for me to test the age-old theory that poetry—writing, reading, and performing it—is a healing art. In the past 15 years, poetry open-mikes and their cousins, competitive slams, have become a national phenomenon at hundreds of venues, such as the Cornelia Street Café in New York City's Greenwich Village, where I tested my mettle. Open-mike nights are like kids' talent shows (the audience even rallies behind clunkers), unlike poetry slams, whose heckling spirit makes them seem more like *The Gong Show* channeled through a decade of rap.

The stress of stage fright—and the pressure to compose a poem for the occasion—nearly canceled out any foreseeable therapeutic benefits. But later I basked in that loopy glow that comes only to those who risk making fools of themselves. The verdict: Despite its initial bends, my adventure left me feeling inspired and confident for days. ∎

Eva Marer is a Manhattan-based writer who regularly contributes to Health.

Get Slammin'

"When you share your poetry, you also share a part of yourself, and that can help you work through difficult emotions, overcome loss, and build self-esteem and confidence," explains Nicholas Mazza, Ph.D., a professor of social work at Florida State University and also editor of the *Journal of Poetry Therapy*. Or poetry slamming can be just plain fun. As one slammer puts it, "Before you get onstage, you feel like you're going to throw up, but afterwards, you suddenly feel like you are the life of the party."

Tap into the healing power of poetry at the following Web sites.
- Find time to rhyme with the Academy of American Poets (www.poets.org), which sponsors National Poetry Month each April. Click on "Events Calendars" to search by state.
- Visit Poetry Slam Inc. (www.poetryslam.com/venues.htm), which lists events by state.
- Learn about the history and philosophy of slam from Marc Kelly Smith, who invented the form, at www.slampapi.com.

Laugh Stress Away

New clubs aimed to make you giggle are popping up across the country. Could they be your ticket to better health?

BY MAUREEN KENNEDY

I'm no spoilsport, but having to cluck like a chicken in a public park was enough to test my mettle.

You're probably wondering what business a grown woman has acting like a farm animal. I'd like to claim the subterfuge of playing with my nieces, but actually I did it because I was curious about the Hollister, California, laughter club, a group of about 10 adults who meet twice a week to chuckle and chortle. They believe that laughing regularly strengthens their immune systems, lowers their blood pressure, and combats stress. In the past three years alone, as many as 60 of these clubs have popped up around the country, and hundreds of people, from school-age kids to senior citizens, are taking silliness seriously.

Madan Kataria, M.D., an Indian physician who prescribed laughing to his patients in Bombay, founded the first club in 1995. Three years later, Steve Wilson, an Ohio psychologist, brought the idea to the United States after participating in one of Kataria's laugh-ins. It may sound wacky, but don't snicker too quickly: Studies have shown that merely smiling can prompt the brain to release endorphins, the natural painkillers many experts think reduce stress and boost the body's immune activity.

I arrived early on a Saturday morning and met Dave Bulman, Sr., and Dave Bulman, Jr.,

a father-and-son duo who belong to the Hollister club. Robin Pollard, who leads the group, and her husband, also named Dave, soon joined us.

"Ha, ha, ha," Pollard and her husband called out in greeting.

"Ho, ho, ho," the two Bulmans cheerily responded.

"Oh my God," I mumbled.

Pollard, who trained with Wilson to become a club leader, started us off with the Texas laugh. We stood in a circle and pretended to tip a hat (presumably 10-gallon) while saying, "How-dee, ha, ha, ha." After a few other warm-up laughs, we moved on to animal variations, including the lion and the chicken (complete with hands under armpits and clucking noises). It was so ridiculous, I couldn't help but join in.

"It doesn't matter why you laugh," explains Jodi Deluca, Ph.D., a neuroscientist at Embry-Riddle Aeronautical University in Daytona Beach, Florida. "Even in small doses, it improves our overall quality of life. You can condition people to feel more positive."

So will I become a member of the laughter club? Probably not. Yes, I did laugh. At the same time, though, I felt weird and kind of self-conscious, which stressed me out. The next time I get the urge to behave like a barnyard bird, I think I'll go find my nieces instead. ■

New Rx: A Laugh Track CD

Sure, they look fab in a pair of diamond studs, but your lovable lobes are much more than just jewelry hangers. Experts now say that simply hearing laughter—even if you don't feel like chuckling yourself—can help lift a black mood.

Researchers in Austria recently produced a CD filled with the giggles, chortles, and guffaws of celebrities. Depressed patients who listened to it in addition to taking medication showed significant improvement compared to those who went without the laugh track. Fortunately, you don't need it to feel better (the disc is available only in Europe, anyway): Pop in Austin Powers, sit back, and help yourself to a little mood medicine.

How to Handle a Summertime Slump

And you thought you only had to deal with the winter blues.

You've heard of seasonal affective disorder (SAD), the malaise that makes you want to hibernate through winter. A less common version can strike in summer. In both cases, the funk may be connected to a change in light, says Norman E. Rosenthal, M.D., clinical professor of psychiatry at Georgetown University Medical School in Washington, D.C., and author of *The Emotional Revolution: How the New Science of Feelings Can Transform Your Life*. The symptoms play out in very different ways: In winter, lack of light can cause people to feel glum, weepy, and sluggish; in summer, long stretches of daylight and intense heat can produce severe anxiety and irritability. "People with summer SAD may find it hard to eat or sleep and have difficulty concentrating on work or relationships," Rosenthal says. While no one knows what causes seasonal swings, researchers suspect there is a genetic component, since two-thirds of sufferers have family histories of major mood disorders. Summer SAD strikes fewer than 1 percent of the population, most often women of childbearing age. If you suspect you have it, small lifestyle changes may help: Crank up the air-conditioning, take cold showers, keep the shades drawn to limit your exposure to light, and wear sunglasses outside. If symptoms persist, see your doctor. She might recommend antidepressants, Rosenthal says.

Learn to Be Lucky

So you've never won the lottery, and someone always beats you to that primo parking space. Is it bad karma or something else? In his book *The Luck Factor*, Richard Wiseman, Ph.D., a psychologist at the University of Hertfordshire in England, examines the personality differences between people who consider themselves fortunate and those who don't. His conclusion: You can learn to be lucky. Below is our Cliff's Notes synopsis of the book's four key concepts.

1. Make the most of chance opportunities. You stumble upon a hot job lead, or maybe you meet an even hotter guy. Follow up. Lucky people tend to notice and act upon good things that seem to come out of nowhere.
2. Trust your hunches. They usually won't steer you wrong. When Wiseman asked his lucky subjects how they make decisions, they said they "simply knew" when a choice was right.
3. Forecast good fortune. Expectations are often self-fulfilling prophecies, Wiseman says. Believe that good things will happen, and voilà! Your predictions are much more likely to come true than if you convince yourself that you're doomed.
4. Turn bad luck into good. OK, so the rose-colored glasses don't always work, and sometimes bad things happen anyway. But even in the face of misfortune, lucky people tend to look on the bright side: A job layoff, for instance, becomes a chance to discover a more exciting career. Rather than dwell on the negative, lucky ducks are quick to let go—and move on.

Take a Sabbatical
from STRESS

An extended respite from reality is a wonderful way to find new energy and focus.

BY SHARON GOLDMAN EDRY

Kelly Brown was in a rut. An attorney in Washington, D.C., she was unfulfilled at work, depressed by the recent death of her grandmother, and in need of a challenge to jump-start her motivation. "I just felt stuck," says Brown, now 39. She talked to her husband about taking some time off. The two pooled their savings and went on an eight-month adventure, which included several weeks of language study in Guatemala and travel throughout South America. "It was so exciting to feel like I wasn't on a lockstep track," Brown says. "I returned with a real sense of accomplishment."

The Browns weren't independently wealthy, nor did they have to abandon their careers. The two were able to negotiate enough time from their bosses to take a sabbatical. According to a survey by Mercer Human Resource Consulting, 15 percent of employers offered paid sabbaticals in 2002, up from 11 percent in 1998.

Jumping off life's endless treadmill may sound like an unrealistic fantasy, but an extended break for travel, study, or reflection is no longer a luxury for tenured professors or well-financed Wall Street types. More and more people—among them women, both single and with families—are doing whatever it takes to break out of their routines. "A vacation is like conjuring up the perfect artificial

day, while a sabbatical is about getting off the path you're on and finding new meaning in life," says Hope Dlugozima, co-author of *Six Months Off: How to Plan, Negotiate, and Take the Break You Need Without Burning Bridges or Going Broke*.

One of the most compelling reasons to take a significant chunk of time off is the lasting benefit to your overall well-being. "Going on a sabbatical can be very good for your health," says Arnold Spokane, Ph.D., a work/stress expert and professor of counseling psychology at Lehigh University in Bethlehem, Pennsylvania. "Stress that builds up over time from work and family can lead to everything from weight gain to anxiety; any break has significant benefits." But the typical American vacation, Spokane says, may not be long enough to relieve the tension and

While a vacation affords an idealized vision of your life, a sabbatical can help you discover practical ways to change it.

may actually compound it. Even so, it's easier, and more accepted, to book a week in the Bahamas.

Guilt, which often accompanies the desire for a longer getaway, stops many women from packing their bags, says Cheryl Jarvis, author of *The Marriage Sabbatical: The Journey That Brings You Home*. "If a woman leaves home for six weeks to take care of a dying parent, she's a saint. But if she leaves for the same amount of time to take care of herself, all of a sudden she's negligent and selfish," says Jarvis, who asked 55 women to recount their educational and creative quests. "Our culture still elevates selfless women. Nonetheless, it's essential to have time to rediscover your strength and gather your own energies."

Alexandra Sheldon, 46, has been going on regular pilgrimages to art colonies for up to two months at a stretch since before her sons, now 9 and 13, were born. "Logistically, it's very hard for me to leave," says the professional artist and homemaker, whose husband, Christophe Peter, runs their household in Boston while she's out of town. "I have a lot of anxiety about how things will go without me. It's never perfect—there's always a pull in the other direction. But I know I have to do this for myself."

Of course, the pack-up-and-go impulse might not be realistic during some stages in life: if you're caring for an infant, looking after an elderly parent, or just starting a new job, for example. Even if the only responsibility you have is finding a temporary home for your cat, for most there's still the question of funds. According to Lori Simon Gordon, author of *Rest Assured: A Sabbatical Solution for Lawyers*, planning and patience are necessities. "It might take a year or two to save money and decide what you'll do and how to do it," says Gordon, who took a yearlong photography and jewelry-designing sabbatical in 1995. A variety of possibilities exist to finance your respite, including fellowships, scholarships, and volunteer programs.

To get the greatest benefit from your time away, Spokane encourages women to strike a balance between doing too much and doing too little. Make sure you have some specific goals, but don't overdo it. "I have a hard time sitting around, so I definitely fell into overscheduling myself," says Stephanie Braun, 33, who took a year off to do volunteer work thanks to a generous sabbatical program offered by her consulting firm, Accenture. "When I first left work, I was so excited about having time that I signed up for lots of classes and volunteer work. After a while I said,

'Whoa, pull back a little bit.' It's not just about cramming things in; it's also about thinking over your priorities and what you want to accomplish."

Returning from your sabbatical may require some planning, too. "We had such high expectations that our lives would be drastically different when we came back, we were actually depressed when they weren't," Kelly Brown says. "You come back to the same life, so you need time to adjust." To fend off post-sabbatical blues, Dlugozima recommends building in a transition period (from three days to do your laundry to two weeks if you need to reset your internal clock, depending on how long you've been gone) and marking the end of your journey with a special event, such as a dinner with friends and family.

While many women change their careers, relationships, or residences after a leave of absence, others, like Braun, pick up where they left off, but with a new perspective. "A sabbatical is a great chance to focus on finding the right balance," she says. "It allows you to think about what you want out of life." ■

Short on Time?

According to Pamela Ammondson, author of *Clarity Quest: How to Take a Sabbatical Without Taking More Than a Week Off*, you can enjoy the benefits of a prolonged break in just a week or two if you prepare. "Lay the groundwork by renewing your energy: Pare down your schedule and practice relaxing," she says. That means simplifying your life, getting enough rest, and exercising. Spending a short period away may give you all the stress relief you need. "A couple of weeks worked for me," says Jennifer Houle, 31, who manages the Shelby Cullom Davis Center for Historical Studies at Princeton University. She says the time she spent at Kripalu, a yoga center in Massachusetts, left her feeling rejuvenated. "There was no TV and no E-mail; I ate right and exercised," she says. "In addition, I brought some skills back home—I do yoga or meditate almost every day now." Next year, she might try a longer retreat. "I got so much out of two weeks, who knows what a month will do?"

How to Tap Your Intuition

Try this step-by-step plan to help you make better decisions.

BY DOROTHY FOLTZ-GRAY

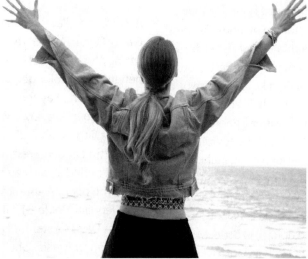

Two years ago, I walked into a house and knew I was home. "If you're ever going to sell," I told its startled owner, "please let me know." Six months later, he called to tell us that he had accepted a job in Utah. Two days after that, my husband and I made an offer on the property. Some people might call our actions impulsive; I call them intuitive.

Almost anyone could match my story with her own: the seemingly good job you turn down because you sense something's amiss, the person you don't trust despite her pleasant smile, the medical test you insist on because you just know that something's wrong. These flashes of instinct are what scientists call intuition, an essential knowledge that arises independent of rational thought.

Intuition seems to turn up out of nowhere, but that doesn't mean it's magically plucked from the sky. In fact, most experts agree that it is a product of life lessons and that much of it is tucked beyond our consciousness. "Intuitive wisdom is born of experience," says David Myers, Ph.D., a professor of psychology at Hope College in Holland, Michigan, and author of *Intuition: Its Powers and Perils.* "Often it represents learned expertise that's instantly accessible. For example, a chess master can look at a board and intuitively know the right move. But most of this knowledge is not articulated or directly taught."

Of course, not all hunches can be explained by experience: the mother who senses when her child is in danger or the decision you make to take a different route home that ends up avoiding a huge traffic jam, for instance. Some researchers slide such incidents into the category of coincidence; others shrug them off as inexplicable.

Most experts agree, however, that your inner voice possesses the potential to enrich your life. When combined with careful factual analysis, it can help you make better decisions. The following sections give you insight into your own intuitive powers, proposing ways to channel them into sound choices and offering ways to avoid the pitfalls of relying on gut feelings alone.

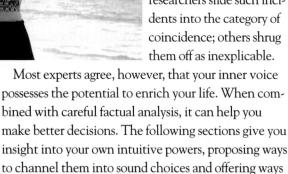

STEP 1
REVIEW YOUR DECISION-MAKING STYLE

Before you can use your gut to guide you, you must recognize its signals. For example, when you meet someone for the first time, do you feel a fluttering in your stomach? When you are puzzling over a decision, do you hear an inner voice or see images in a dream? The way we receive intuitive messages is as individual as our fingerprints, says Laurie Nadel, Ph.D., author of the book *Sixth Sense: The Whole-Brain Book of Inhibition, Hunches, Gut Feelings, and Their Place in Your Everyday Life.* Examine whether and how you use your intuition to help you make choices.

Let's say, for instance, that one of your job duties is hiring people. What factors do you consider? The way a person looks, a list of skills, personality? Finally, take stock of your past decisions. Which judgments proved to be right or wrong, and why? Which factors misguided or confirmed them? By evaluating how you face decisions, you will avoid repeating mistakes and be more apt to choose wisely in the future. The review process in work situations or relationships augments the knowledge that eventually informs our intuitions, explains Gary Klein, Ph.D., a research psychologist and author of the new book *Intuition at Work: Why Developing Your Gut Instinct Will Make You Better at What You Do.*

"It's a matter of testing your intuition, listening to it, following it, and then seeing what the results are," says Ellen Hall, co-author of *Listen to Your Inner Voice.* "If the results are good, follow it again."

STEP 2
CONSIDER THE FACTS

Back up your intuition with knowledge. When my husband and I made that speedy home offer, we had years of discussing and looking at houses behind us; it's a kind of running hobby of ours. We had the place inspected, talked to our financial counselor, and reviewed the prices of comparable properties nearby. We imagined ourselves living there: Is there enough space to create a study? How will we like living in this part of town? Not all these questions had ideal answers, but the positive responses were sufficient to give us the green light. In fact, all of our hunches have been vindicated: The house is wonderful—though we don't have room for a study.

"Intuition won't tell you where your guests will sleep or where you'll put the washer and dryer," Klein says. "If you don't have a large base of experience, it's just too dangerous to trust your intuition only. Start with that, but then check it out more rationally. Imagining the reality can protect you from misguided intuition."

STEP 3
DON'T OVERANALYZE

Yes, there's a need for reason, but don't let facts snuff out feelings. Intuitive reactions are subtle, complex, and easily overruled by analytical rigor. Let your initial perceptions develop without trying to explain why you feel the way you do.

Studies by psychologist Timothy D. Wilson, Ph.D., a professor of psychology at the University of Virginia and author of *Strangers to Ourselves: Discovering the Adaptive Unconscious,* found that people who depended on instincts alone made more reliable predictions of their relationships' futures than those who overthought their feelings.

"It can be difficult to get to the bottom of gut feelings and know where they come from," Wilson explains. "Trying to dissect them is like trying to analyze how we perform a skill we're really good at, like dancing or serving a tennis ball. It can make things worse." For one thing, individual points rarely make up the whole story.

In the words of the 18th-century philosopher Immanuel Kant: "We can never, even by the strictest examination, get completely behind the secret springs of action."

AVOID THOSE INTUITIVE PITFALLS

Intuition is not infallible. The knowledge you've stored over a lifetime may contain stereotypes and biases that influence you without your realizing it. Even if a hunch is strong, you could be missing some subtle but important clues. Below are tips on when to listen to your inner voice—and when to tune it out.

Don't confuse intuition with anxiety or wishful thinking. Pay attention to what you're feeling, but weigh that against the facts, says psychologist Timothy D. Wilson, Ph.D. "For example, if you shy away from something repeatedly that other people don't, your reaction may be anxiety, not intuition." If that's the case, you need to deal with what is behind your fears.

Another test is to imagine the aftermath of following your emotional pulls. Let's say you buy a purple dress you think is perfect for you, despite its high price and a slightly snug fit. How will you feel when the bill comes in? Will you be excited about wearing it to your class reunion? Imagining your future reality could illuminate—and override—wishful thinking, which often poses as intuition.

Shelve intuition when only the rational will do. "There are certain arenas in life, like relationships, where using intuition is most appropriate," says intuition expert Ellen Hall, while other

> There's a need for reason, but don't let facts snuff out feelings. Let your initial perceptions develop without trying to explain why you feel the way you do.

decisions—primarily medical, financial, educational, and professional ones—need facts and figures to shore them up. A doctor may have a nice bedside manner, but check out his credentials. Deciding which credit card to choose is another example of a rational decision.

Don't make snap judgments. You may have a negative reaction to a new colleague, but is that response relevant? First, find out how well you work with this person. Don't bury the negative feeling, but let it rest until you see what she brings to your work experience. "There are times, such as at work, when how we feel isn't necessarily the most critical issue," Wilson says.

Let your intuition speak. It's easy to crowd out intuition with mental chatter: shoulds and shouldn'ts, worries, day-to-day demands, and deadlines. Give your intuition a chance to breathe. Go for a walk, meditate, or simply sit quietly and see if your feelings are consistent. "There is great wisdom in the body," Hall says. "If you pay attention, you will learn a lot." ▪

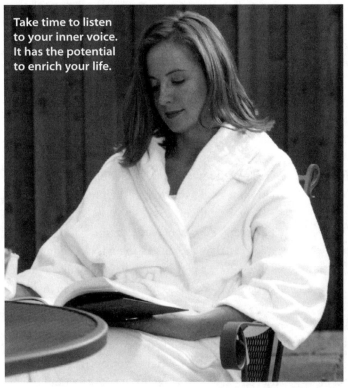

Take time to listen to your inner voice. It has the potential to enrich your life.

How Intuitive Are You?

Take this test to see how instinct plays out in your life.

1. When I'm faced with a decision:
A. I follow my inner compass.
B. I analyze the issues systematically.

2. When I have a nagging feeling that something is wrong:
A. I heed my suspicions vigilantly.
B. I do nothing without obtaining firm evidence first.

3. When I face a new environment, situation, or person:
A. I often have a physical reaction, such as rapid breathing or stomach tightening.
B. I often have an intellectual response, such as making lists, checking maps, or reviewing names.

4. I view the past as:
A. A learning opportunity.
B. Spilled milk.

5. When I describe events to my friends:
A. I prefer to fill them in on the big picture before giving them the story in detail.
B. I like to present a blow-by-blow account of the facts as they happened.

6. I generally make decisions:
A. On my own.
B. With the input of others.

7. At meetings, I love to:
A. Brainstorm ideas.
B. Analyze strategies and options.

8. My work strength is:
A. Embracing new concepts.
B. Sticking to the proven path and organizing goals.

9. When I observe people, I notice:
A. Subtle body language.
B. The specifics of what they say.

10. When I meet people:
A. I come away knowing whether I like them or not.
B. I withhold judgment until I've observed them in several different circumstances.

KEY

8–10 As: You are an intuitive wizard who could benefit from getting in touch with your rational self.

5–7 As: You have natural intuitive skills that could be even sharper.

2–4 As: You're likely ignoring your perceptive talents in favor of your rational side.

0–2 As: Rational thinking is your forte, but tuning in to instinct more often could help bolster even your most practical decisions.

How to Read People

By paying attention to what psychologist Lillian Glass, Ph.D., author of *I Know What You're Thinking: Using the Four Codes of Reading People to Improve Your Life,* calls the four communication codes—bodies, faces, voices, and words—you can hone your intuitive sense of others. Use these three basic pointers to read what's plain to see.

Observe body language. Bodies reveal what words may hide. "If a person is slumped over, she may have a poor self-image," Glass says. "If she's standing with her head high, she probably feels good. If her body is rigid, that tells you she's uptight."

Watch the face. Psychologist Paul Ekman, Ph.D., director of the Human Interaction Laboratory at the University of California, San Francisco, says the human face reveals basic emotions. "One of the first signs of anger is thinning lips," Ekman says. A sign of sadness is an upward angle at the inner corners of the eyebrows. "When you learn to recognize the signs, you expand your intuition."

Listen to vocal cues. The person in the restaurant who insists on talking at the top of her voice probably wants attention, Glass says. If someone uses an overly sweet voice, she may be sitting on a mound of anger. If another speaks inaudibly, she likely lacks self-esteem.

Renew! Recharge!
Redecorate?

Forget feng shui. Vastu is the latest way to arrange your space for optimal well-being.

BY ABIGAIL GREEN

Stressed? Sluggish? Scatterbrained? A quick fix could be as easy as putting your bed in a different corner of the room or buying a new rug. Vastu, an ancient Indian philosophy similar to feng shui, maintains that all things, including your body, are composed of five elements: space, air, fire, water, and earth. Too much of any one component can throw your body and mood out of whack. For a healthy balance, make sure that your surroundings complement your dosha, or personality. "It makes us feel better when we live in a space that reflects who we are and what we love," says Kathleen Cox, author of *The Power of Vastu Living.*

Here's how you can determine your dosha. Find the characteristics that best describe you and follow the cues to create the healthiest space for your type. Will vastu change your life? Probably not. But we thought it would be fun to try.

DOSHA: VATA

Associated element: Air
You tend to be: Energetic, creative, and slender
You struggle with: Decision making, staying focused, and sleeping soundly through the night
Vastu solutions: Strengthen your ability to concentrate by sleeping and working in the southwest corner of your room, where earth steadies and strengthens flighty vatas. Or seek out water's calming powers in the northeast corner. Soothe nervous energy with mellow colors, such as green, light blue, and white. To nurture your reflective side, place a bowl of water filled with floating flower petals on your desk.

DOSHA: PITTA

Associated element: Fire
You tend to be: Intense, outspoken, and athletic
You struggle with: Losing your temper, controlling competitive urges, and relaxing
Vastu solutions: The grounding powers in earth's domain (the southwest corner) can temper your impulsive ways; consider sleeping and working under the influence of water (the northeast corner) to douse your hotheaded tendencies. Cool down by surrounding yourself with blues, greens, and whites, or tickle your toes with earth-tone natural-fiber rugs that balance fire's intensity.

DOSHA: KAPHA

Associated element: Water
You tend to be: Calm, forgiving, and curvy
You struggle with: Inactivity, lack of drive, and resistance to change
Vastu solutions: For a surge of fiery energy, sleep or work in the southeast corner of a room. To jump-start your motivation, get a push from air's movement in the northwest area. Counteract listlessness by painting the walls red, yellow, or orange; curling up with a brightly patterned bedspread; or arranging colorful fresh flowers.

Ease Your Pain with Aromatherapy

Get a whiff of this: A University of Quebec study in the journal *Physiology & Behavior* found that women's pain receptors responded favorably to pleasing smells. Twenty females held their hands in uncomfortably hot water longer when they inhaled pleasant fragrances, such as baby oil, vanilla, or citrus. Funky odors, such as vinegar or perm solution, threw the women subjects over their pain thresholds. The reason may lie in the link between the olfactory system and the limbic system, a part of the brain that is responsible for emotions and associated with pain perception.

Conducting my own experiment, I pitted vinegar, baby oil, and vanilla against a real-life challenge that many women face: body-hair removal. I shaved and waxed my bikini area, then plucked my brows, while my bewildered boyfriend took turns holding the three scents under my nose. The verdict follows.

Shaving: While good smells had little effect, vinegar made this relatively painless process slightly uncomfortable.

Waxing: Nothing could turn this harrowing chore into a spalike experience, but vanilla and baby oil made it less painful than a *Baywatch* marathon.

Plucking: Oddly, tweezing while smelling baby oil hurt more than plucking without a scent. The vanilla candle, however, seemed to soothe the sting.

Freshen Your Mood with the Right Fragrance

If you love the smell that dryer sheets leave on just-washed clothes but wish there were a more natural way to get it, try this: Place three to five drops of your favorite essential oil (available at health-food stores or from some bath-and-body lines) on a clean, dry washcloth and toss it in the dryer along with your laundry. The fragrance will gently infuse your clothes and linger for a few days.

The beauty of this method is that you can tailor the scent to match your mood. Emilie Davidson Hoyt, founder of the bath-and-body product company Lather, suggests lavender to relax, citrus to rejuvenate, and eucalyptus to ease fatigue. You won't reduce static this way, but then again, dryer sheets won't change your state of mind.

Hands-Free Massage Helps You Find Balance

Reiki, the ancient Tibetan healing art that aims to get your energy flowing so you feel balanced and calm, is becoming a common offering on spa menus around the country. But there's a new twist on this thousand-year-old practice: The Centre for Well-Being at the Phoenician resort in Arizona claims to increase the impact by combining chakra balancing with Reiki. "There are seven chakras, or energy points, on the body," explains Leonie Rosenberg, the spa's Reiki master and creator of the new treatment. "When any one of them is out of balance, your mind, body, or spirit may be ill or out of balance, too." During the procedure, the therapist drizzles essential oils on each chakra; then she places her hands above and below it. Meanwhile, the client is asked to visualize a color and listen to a positive affirmation related to each chakra. "It's more effective than Reiki alone because it brings in several senses, not just touch," Rosenberg says. "It incorporates smell with the essential oil, sight with the color, and sound with the affirmations." While the Phoenician's spa is the first to offer this treatment (at $115), it will no doubt be making its way to a spa near you soon.

Get the Most from Your
THERAPIST

Follow these six steps to find the help you need.

BY WAYNE KALYN

Tony Soprano isn't the only one who's anxious these days. With the threat of terrorism up and the economy down, many Americans have tough issues of their own to negotiate. The good news is that, like the beleaguered mob boss, increasing numbers of people are seeking therapy to resolve them.

Research shows that talking with a therapist is often just what the doctor ordered for depression and generalized anxiety disorder, not to mention those mental speed bumps caused by ever-changing roles at home and at work.

So if you or a loved one is thinking about getting help for the first time or you've had a less-than-successful experience in the past, this guide can help make the next one productive and healing. Toward that end, we have talked with psychiatrists, psychologists, pastoral counselors, and senior experts at national mental-health associations to get you the inside scoop.

"People see a Woody Allen movie and think that's what therapy is all about," says Kathy HoganBruen, Ph.D., senior director of prevention at the National Mental Health Association in Alexandria, Virginia. "In fact, many therapists don't care about exploring the kind of relationship you had with your mother. For almost everyone, there is a therapist and a therapy that will help you get well."

These six steps will help you find the right combination.

> When you sit down together, see yourself as an educated consumer, not a passive patient.
> —Kathy HoganBruen, Ph.D.

1 INTERVIEW THREE THERAPISTS

Why three? "Because, like a consumer of any service, you want to compare and contrast the therapists' manners, personalities, and answers when you first talk with them," explains Harriet Braiker, Ph.D., author of *The Disease to Please* and a psychologist with private practices in Beverly Hills and Pasadena, California. "The ultimate goal is to narrow the field to one person you would actually like to see."

Before you ask around for recommendations, figure out your hot-button issues. Do you think you could benefit from antidepressants or antianxiety medicines, or are you dead set against taking them? Many talk therapists have referral arrangements with psychiatrists, who can prescribe medication. Also, would you be more comfortable with a therapist of the same sex? Studies show that gender and race have little influence on a client's success in counseling, but if talking with an opposite-sex practitioner is out of the question for you, consider that when you're looking for potential prospects.

A call to your insurance company is also a smart move. "If your plan authorizes only 10 sessions, then you want to ask about therapists who offer short-term treatment," HoganBruen says.

Now, assemble your shortlist of candidates. The most helpful recommendations, experts say, come from friends with similar value systems. "The best referral sources are people who have been in therapy with the person they are recommending," says Nancy McWilliams, Ph.D., professor of applied and professional psychology at Rutgers University in New Jersey. Admittedly, this approach might not be for everyone. If you'd rather not divulge that you're seeking help, the idea that a potential counselor has seen (or is seeing) someone you know might make you uncomfortable.

If you prefer a more professional approach, sit down with a physician you trust, explain the nature of the problem, and ask for a referral.

If talking face-to-face about your problem just adds to your anxiety, call your state mental-health association or the 1-800-THERAPIST referral service (800-843-7274) for names; or visit the Web site of the American Mental Health Alliance (www.americanmentalhealth.com).

When you finally call the offices of your three choices, ask what they specialize in—depression, marital problems, phobias—and their credentials. When you meet with them, listen objectively to their answers and take notes. If a candidate balks at questions about academic qualifications or licensing, cross him or her off the list. Listening to

your instincts is crucial. Is there rapport between you and the therapists you have chosen? Sleep on your options for a day or two before you make your final decision.

GO FOR A TRIAL SESSION

"Many, but not all, therapists will allow you to have a low-cost or abbreviated first session to see if the arrangement will work," HoganBruen explains. "When you sit down together, see yourself as an educated consumer, not a passive patient."

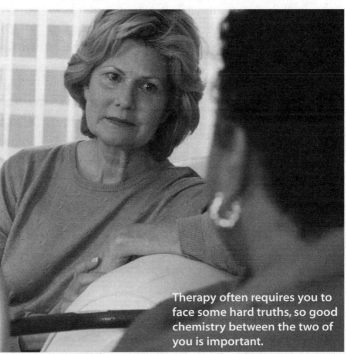

Therapy often requires you to face some hard truths, so good chemistry between the two of you is important.

During the trial run, gauge your comfort level. Is the office environment inviting? Is this a person you feel you could talk with as openly as you need to?

"If therapy is a game of hiding from a therapist or misrepresenting yourself, it's not going to be effective," Braiker says. That's exactly what it could become, however, if you choose a treatment provider or program that doesn't mesh with your needs.

To prevent a mistake, find out how a typical session will play out. Will you do most of the talking, or will the therapist interact with you?

How often will she want to see you? And probe the therapist's view of your problem—does it jibe with yours?

"Some therapists believe that anxiety and depression primarily have genetic or biological roots," HoganBruen says. "As such, they will likely recommend medication. Others believe that problems spring more from environmental factors, such as relationship dysfunction or job stress, and they will be more likely to recommend talk therapy."

Try to determine whether the therapist's approach is a good match with your temperament. Cognitive-behavioral therapy, for instance, teaches clients to challenge their thought patterns. You'll be asked to complete weekly homework assignments, and you'll receive a timetable for success. Psychodynamic therapy, Freud's brainchild, sometimes requires you to plumb your past for answers to your problems; in other instances, you might focus on the here and now. "Some clients do wonderfully well when they lie on a couch and explore past relationships," McWilliams says. "Others prefer the problem-specific, more focused treatments that cognitive-behavioral therapists offer."

CREATE A PLAN OF ACTION

After you've spent two or three sessions outlining your problem, the therapist should offer more than a cursory, "Very good. I'll see you next Tuesday at 4." She should provide a modus operandi for future sessions. A realistic scenario might be: "This is what I'm thinking. We will meet for 10 sessions and re-evaluate. Now let's create an action plan together; you will let me know your goals for therapy and what you want to accomplish, and I can provide some guidance on how to do that." If she doesn't, ask.

"The action plan will be more precise or vague depending on the type of therapy you are participating in," HoganBruen says. "Cognitive-behavioral therapists, for instance, typically create a step-by-step plan that supplies guideposts about where you may be month by month and specific steps on how to get there. It can be long or short, depending on the type of problem you are trying to solve. Depression and anxiety may require longer action plans—sometimes up to a year—than marital problems or workplace issues."

When outlining the course of action, tell the therapist how many sessions are covered by your insurance and request that she evaluate your progress halfway through. Treatment plans aren't one-size-fits-all, though: You might not resolve your issue in the time frame allowed by your policy. If that's the case, ask about sliding scale fees once your coverage runs out. You may end up being charged less, because cost is sometimes tied to your ability to pay.

You and Therapy: Perfect Together?

Is everyday life becoming a series of increasingly higher and joyless hurdles? Answering no to several of the following questions from the National Mental Health Association indicates you may have a problem that therapy could help.

1. Do you look forward to the future and plan ahead for it?

2. Do you find joy in everyday life?

3. Are you able to trust and love other people?

4. Do you feel reasonably energetic throughout the day?

5. Do you sleep and eat well?

6. Can you accept and laugh about your mistakes and weaknesses?

7. Are you realistic about your abilities and goals?

8. Are you able to face life's challenges and responsibilities?

9. Do you handle minor inconveniences with ease?

WORK IN TANDEM

4

"Most therapists these days view the client as a collaborator, not a helpless patient who wants the all-knowing therapist to fix the problem," HoganBruen says. "The client should have input and shouldn't blindly follow what the therapist says."

Although it is normal to quake in your Freudian boots when you first enter therapy, your nerves will usually stop jangling by the end of the initial session. In fact, a good therapist will help put you at ease.

"Remember to distinguish between your feelings for the therapist as a person and for the process itself, which is not pleasant chitchat but hard work requiring you to face some hard truths," says Jeremy Safran, Ph.D., professor of psychology at New School University in New York City, who has studied the effectiveness of different therapies. "It is normal to veer between like and dislike of the therapist, depending on what you're discussing. In the end, though, it is the chemistry between the two of you that will often make the therapy bearable."

Several sessions should let you know whether the relationship has legs. Do you feel respected and listened to? Do you trust that this person will do his or her best to help you feel better?

"Most clients have a little internal alarm system that tells them when a therapist is stepping over the line," says Rev. C. Roy Woodruff, executive director of the American Association of Pastoral Counselors in Fairfax, Virginia, which has certified 2,000 pastoral counselors throughout the United States. If a therapist shows disrespect or distaste for you as a person or for the nature of your problem, aggressively pushes for answers to questions you have refused to talk about, judges you harshly, or shares his or her problems with you instead of dealing with yours, you should probably issue a pink slip.

> As difficult as it can be to find a new therapist and tell your story from scratch, it's preferable to continuing with someone you don't click with. —Diana L. Dell, M.D.

CHECK YOUR PROGRESS

5

You know a cold or headache is getting better when your runny nose starts to dry up or your temples stop pounding. Therapy, though, usually works in inches, not 10-yard leaps. A client should see counseling as a two-stage process: improving the acute symptoms that first brought you into the office and then addressing the larger problem that caused them. Symptoms often clear up quicker than their source.

"Sure, people can have an 'aha' experience, but for most of the work in therapy, recognition about a problem—whether a fear of spiders or difficulty in a relationship—comes in stages," says Diana L. Dell, M.D., a reproductive psychiatrist at Duke University Medical Center in Durham, North Carolina. "That said, statistics indicate that on average, most people are in therapy for three months or less. They get back to where they can function, and they move on."

Feeling better by degrees is a sign that treatment is working, but you may also see more tangible evidence. "If you had trouble socializing and now you find yourself going out with a friend once a month, you can say you're making progress," HoganBruen says.

"With focused problems, such as a phobia or a panic attack in a crowded elevator, you should see a mild shift in your thinking in three months or so," Safran says. "With more chronic, diffuse problems—if you've never been happy, say, or if you have had a series of self-destructive relationships—it can take six months to two years or longer before you see any daylight."

Even though the therapist maintains a certain position of power in the relationship, you still need to recognize the clout you have as a consumer. If you ever have any concerns about the progress of therapy, it's a good idea to spend a session talking it over. If solutions prove elusive, you should find a new partner.

"As difficult as it can be to find a new therapist and tell your story again from scratch, it is preferable to continuing with someone you no longer click with," Dell says.

KNOW WHEN TO CALL IT QUITS

When do you terminate the relationship? The short answer is when you feel better, say the experts with a chuckle. It ultimately depends on the nature of your problem and the therapist's approach. Some will help you recognize the endgame of treatment by asking you to write down what you'll feel like when you're better. In general, though, most therapists won't suddenly rise up from their chairs one Tuesday and say, "Ta-da, you're better!" Rather, you will have to arrive at that realization yourself.

According to Braiker, you'll know to break things off when the reasons that brought you into therapy are resolved and your initial goals have been met. "You'll notice that you've gained back function in areas of your life where there was dysfunction, whether it be in school, work, or your family," HoganBruen says. "Success with problems like getting along with your mother is easier to measure than feeling vaguely unhappy. You know you're better because you didn't argue with Mom over Thanksgiving dinner, or you can now talk on the phone with her for more than five minutes. How do you measure happiness, exactly?"

If you have doubts, then slowly phase out your visits—from once a week to once a month, for instance—and see how you feel. You might say, "I'd like to aim toward winding this down in the next couple of months" instead of abruptly announcing, "I ran out of money, and this is my last visit."

"The gradual approach gives you a chance to use the skills you have learned to counter negative cognitions and fears on your own," HoganBruen says. And it gives the therapist an opportunity to reinforce those skills and perspectives during your last several sessions.

"I always tell my clients that if anything comes up in three days, three months, or three years, they can come back for a couple of booster sessions or for a whole new round of therapy," Braiker says. "And many of them do. I let people know that it isn't good-bye so much as the door is always open." ▪

Resolution of the problem that brought you into therapy is a good sign it's time to move on.

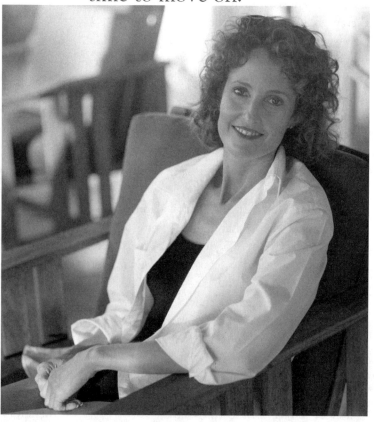

What the Degrees Mean

Anybody can hang out a shingle that reads "psychotherapist," a profession that in many states isn't regulated by law. That's why you need to get details about a potential therapist's degree and license. Credentials, however, are only one component of your choice before you commit.

"As long as you're seeing a licensed mental-health professional, one kind of therapist isn't necessarily better than another," says *Health* columnist and psychologist Ali Domar, Ph.D. "What's most important is that you feel comfortable with the therapist and that you are making progress." That said, here's a quick rundown of what to look for in each type.

Psychiatrist

If you need medication for severe depression, an anxiety disorder, or a phobia, see a psychiatrist, the only mental-health professional who has an M.D. and can prescribe medication. Not all psychiatrists, however, regularly use talk therapy. Ask about this when you call to make an appointment.

Psychologist

If you have marital or family problems, mild depression, or anxiety, a psychologist might be the answer. These professionals specialize in talking with clients about their problems but can't prescribe medication. Ask your prospect if he or she is licensed as a psychologist; certification requires five to seven years of postgraduate training in psychology. Many therapists with "Ph.D." after their names are licensed not as psychologists but as marriage counselors or family therapists. If you have rapport with a candidate, this doesn't really matter.

Social Worker

This kind of therapist is equipped to handle the same issues as psychologists, but he or she has only two years of postgraduate training. The title "licensed independent clinical social worker" (LICSW) assures you that the therapist has ample experience with patients.

Pastoral Counselor

A certified pastoral counselor is trained in psychology and theology. Ask if the practitioner is certified by the American Association of Pastoral Counselors (AAPC) at the Fellow or Diplomate level, which means that he or she has master's degrees in both theological and counseling/psychotherapy studies, or the academic equivalent, from accredited institutions.

Why Women Are Wired for Worry

If you worry a lot, you can probably blame your genes—and your sex. Scientists have found that estrogen lowers levels of a stress-tempering brain enzyme known as COMT, which may explain why women tend to be more high-strung than men. Some women have it particularly bad. According to new research from the National Institute on Alcohol Abuse and Alcoholism (NIAAA), one in six people have as much as 75 percent less COMT than the general population, leaving people who are deficient more vulnerable to anxiety.

Don't fret too much over this news, says NIAAA research physician Mary-Anne Enoch, M.D. "It can be advantageous to have an anxious temperament," she says, noting that low COMT levels won't cause the kind of extreme agitation that leads to panic attacks and phobias. In fact, they can even be beneficial. "You might be a bit more aware of your surroundings, you can often concentrate better, or you may have a superior memory," she says. But pay attention to your signs of stress: If anxiety is making you miserable, take measures to chill out.

Survivor Lessons

Repress, deny, avoid—some experts say these strategies may be the ticket to dealing with grief.

BY SUZ REDFEARN

Mary Fetchet is on a very tight schedule. If she's not meeting with the mayor of New York City, she's talking with the governor or traveling to Washington, D.C., to campaign on behalf of the families of September 11 victims. Her days are usually 12 hours long, and she likes them that way.

Being this busy would wear some people down, but not Fetchet, who says her hectic pace has gone a long way toward helping her cope with the loss of her 24-year-old son, Brad, who was on the 89th floor of Tower Two when it collapsed two years ago. Following the terrorist attack, Fetchet spent weeks searching for information about her son and then, finally, planning his memorial service. After that, instead of resuming her life as a 30-hour-a-week social worker, Fetchet quit her job and began gathering other relatives of the victims in her living room, where she passionately shared her newfound skills in dealing with the bureaucracy of tragedy. Together, she and the families discussed how to file death certificates, collect from the victims' compensation fund, and air their opinions about a suitable memorial. In October 2001, Fetchet formalized her efforts. She named the group Voices of September 11th and began devoting 80 to 100 hours a week to aiding the survivors of 9/11 victims. And she's glad she has. "I do much better if I have something to immerse myself in," Fetchet says.

Some might expect Fetchet to head straight for a therapist after suffering such a devastating loss. But according to controversial new studies, Fetchet's coping style—which some people might label avoidance or denial—can actually be more beneficial than opening up about a trauma, especially in its immediate wake.

"The idea has been that people should seek professional help when they've gone through something upsetting," says George Bonanno, Ph.D., an associate professor of psychology at Columbia University Teachers College who has done research on trauma survivors. "But we now know that unless people are having tremendous difficulty, therapists should leave them alone." In other words, many experts now believe that survivors should be able to deal with their pain as they wish. That might mean choosing to repress or avoid their feelings until a later point. Or they might channel the loss into something positive, as Fetchet did with her activism.

This school of thought, which has been developing for years, has gained new ground in the aftermath of September 11. Following the tragedy, hordes of well-meaning psychologists and grief counselors encouraged survivors to discuss their feelings—and then discuss them some more. Indeed, over the last 20 years, a huge disaster-recovery industry has sprung up based on the idea that talking through trauma is the way to heal. Companies struck by devastating events pay therapists to flock to the sites and, within 24 to 72 hours, funnel all victims through individual or group counseling, sometimes whether the victims want it or not. The hope is that people will find reliving the event cathartic, thus warding off post-traumatic stress disorder (PTSD), a condition that typically causes flashbacks, sleeplessness, and agitation. Long-term effects can include problems with jobs and relationships, as well as substance abuse.

But only recently have psychologists begun studying the results of such on-site therapy, and the evidence isn't looking good. At worst, it can actually retraumatize a person. "People should not be forced to face their emotions right after something tragic has occurred," explains Richard Gist, Ph.D., a trauma researcher at the University of Missouri-Kansas City. Gist was called upon to help survivors of the 1981 collapse of the Hyatt Regency pedestrian skywalks in Kansas City, Missouri, which killed 114 people. He was also on hand at the 1989 United Airlines crash in Sioux City, Iowa, in which 111 people died. After that disaster, Gist and his colleagues began tracking the survivors and rescue workers who had been counseled. He found that, in most cases, immediate therapy following a disaster didn't seem to help and, in some instances, might have hurt. According to Gist, those who went through debriefing were more likely to experience PTSD symptoms than those who went without therapy. These results don't just apply to plane crashes. Separate studies involving earthquake survivors, soldiers in the 1991 Gulf War, and victims of car accidents have shown the same thing.

Other researchers have looked beyond disaster intervention to study responses to other kinds of painful events, focusing on the effects of repressing pain or minimizing loss. One study in Tel Aviv, Israel, compared heart-attack survivors who tended to bottle their emotions with those who didn't. Nineteen percent of the nonrepressors developed PTSD, versus just 7 percent of the repressors. While the study authors point out that the latter group might simply have been better at handling stress than the former, they suggest nonetheless that repression may indeed be a useful coping tool.

Not surprisingly, some people, especially those who run debriefing companies, are critical of these new theories, and many psychologists agree that there are times when people should not wall off their feelings, as in cases of sexual abuse. But increasingly, mainstream therapists like Patricia Berliner, Ph.D., a New York City psychologist whose clients include family members of 9/11 victims, think distancing one's self from negative events has its place. "It's inappropriate to open up a painful topic with someone before they're ready," Berliner says.

While you don't want to avoid your problems forever, giving yourself some time to heal makes sense.

Thankfully, most people don't personally experience horrific incidents like 9/11. But nearly everyone has their own nightmares—the loss of a job, the death of a loved one, a serious injury—to live through. So what's the best way to cope? When should you hash things out, and when should you try to just ignore your pain? Trust your instincts, the experts say. While you don't want to avoid your problems forever, "it makes sense to give yourself time to react in whatever way feels natural, and that might mean stepping back from the situation until you're ready to handle it," Gist says. He adds that people often experience anxiety or sleeplessness for up to six weeks following a traumatic event. After that, if you're still having such problems, you should see a professional. (To find a therapist in your area who deals with PTSD, call the American Psychological Association at 800-964-2000 and ask for a referral.)

Other experts agree. If you want to talk to a therapist soon after a painful occurrence, you should, says Richard J. McNally, Ph.D., professor of psychology at Harvard University and author of the new book *Remembering Trauma*. However, you might first want to turn to the comfort of friends and family, he says. And if you would rather cope on your own, losing yourself in work or a project you value can help. Volunteer, plant a garden, spend more time with your family—anything to get outside yourself.

That strategy is working for Fetchet. "I will always live with the loss of my son," she says. "But focusing on helping other families has allowed me to heal." ■

When War Hits Home

Take a glimpse into how the fighting in Iraq affected one journalist's family, with lessons for us all on love, friendship, grief, and coping in uncertain times.

BY LEE WOODRUFF

When ABC news reporter Bob Woodruff left the United States in early 2003 to cover the war in Iraq, his wife, Lee, began sending mass E-mails to concerned family and friends. Her letters included regular "Bob updates," as well as thoughts from the home front while she tried to maintain a normal routine for their children. Lee shares some of those messages here.

TUESDAY, MARCH 25

I just had the longest conversation in many weeks with Bob. He and his Marine division are on their way to Baghdad, and, as you may have seen on the news, caught in a horrific sandstorm. In the early days of the campaign, when he was in Kuwait, he said the storms made everyone look the way the workmen at our house did after they sanded our wood floors. Thank God for that analogy, I told him, because if he didn't put it in the context of the household, I'd never be able to understand it. (Sarcasm often comes in handy—gotta keep your sense of humor through all this.)

> **What is this war going to do to Bob and the other journalists covering it? I fear he'll come back having witnessed too much.**

But today, all humor was gone. There was fatigue and frustration in his voice. I could hear wind and sand blowing around him. He was on TV this morning in full garb, and last night I saw him riding atop a tank in the convoy. While they have seen minimal combat, the conditions are grueling. Bob said he has sand in every orifice: under his eyelids, toenails, and other places you'd rather not know.

The kids can see Dad on TV, though letting them watch his reports is hard when you consider what the pictures and stories are telling. Cathryn has had many tough nights. Mack has this great theory that Dad is safe because the Marines are protecting him. I happen to like that theory very much.

As for me, I have my moments—in the car when a song comes on the radio, when I read your heartfelt E-mails. Tears come at the oddest moments. Fortunately, I have great support here. One of my dearest friends, Melanie Bloom, is just a few towns away. Her husband, David, is embedded with NBC, so it helps to compare emotions.

Enough for now.—*Lee*

MONDAY, MARCH 31

Bob says he hasn't taken a shower since they moved into the Kuwaiti desert 23 days ago. Water is scarce, so they need to save all they can for drinking. He even shaves dry most days with a battery-operated razor. Most everyone sleeps on the ground by the vehicle's wheels, but when there is a fear of snipers, they sleep in the tank, packed with men, knees to chests, heads on their knees.

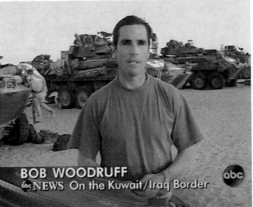

BOB WOODRUFF
NEWS On the Kuwait/Iraq Border

The contrast to our lives here at home is sobering. The other day, I was walking down a Manhattan street, talking to him on the cell phone (which is bizarre enough in itself), telling him about a bill that had come in. I was trying to figure out how to handle it, and obviously the annoyance was creeping into my voice when Bob cut me off. "Lee, I'm sitting here in a tank with a bunch of guys who are making barely more than minimum wage and putting their lives on the line every single day," he said in a hushed, exhausted tone. "It just isn't important."

And then there was the day last week when his division had to face its first casualty. It was a young man whom Bob had spent some time with, hanging out, chatting up. He stepped on an unexploded artillery shell, not far from where Bob had been earlier. Bob told me how he and some of the Marines helped him into the ambulance, but the young soldier—in his early 20s, with a 1-year-old son—died in the medic chopper.

What is this war going to do to Bob and the other journalists covering it? One of my biggest fears is that he may come back as some sort of Stanley Kubrick character, having witnessed too much. After Bob was in Afghanistan, there was a dullness in the back of his eyes that took weeks and lots of hugs, story times, and multiplication drills with the kids to erase. I think that a person can see too much hate.

Some days, I just can't make him laugh. That scares me. It's hard to fight back images of our last night together. After we tucked the last kid into bed, we fell into a viselike hug, the unspoken thought connecting us as heavy as a rope: *What if I never see you again?* "Well, of course I will," you tell yourself, but it's a surreal thing to pack your husband off for war: "Do you have your sunscreen? Socks? Oh, and what about that last anthrax shot?"

By now, each of us here at home has our coping mechanisms firmly in place. Mine is to write. Cathryn's is to create pictures, notes, and stories for her dad that sit in a pile for his return home. Mack's personal theory of the cloak of military protection is still holding. One morning, as he watched an image of his father riding on a tank in full gear and helmet, he turned to me as he poured the milk over his cereal. "Was Dad just riding on a tank?" he asked casually. "I think so," I replied, as if such a sight were perfectly normal. "Cool," he said, and took a bite of Cap'n Crunch. Maybe I am getting something right after all.—*Lee*

THURSDAY, APRIL 3

Bob's company name is Delta. I like to imagine it as a big Brownie troop, minus the crafts and rug squares. Right now they can see smoke in the distance and POWs guarded by Marines on the side of the road. Last night there was heavy artillery fire overhead. Most of it was us firing at the Iraqis, but at one point they fired back, and everyone in Bob's division had to put on gas masks for three hours—and try to sleep that way.

Things at home are the same. The twins will turn 3 this weekend, and we will sing "Happy Birthday" when Bob calls. This is their second birthday that he's missed, but luckily, they're too young to know the difference. They have learned to reply that

Daddy is "in a rock" when you ask them. Both Nora and Claire absorb my stress like two dry sponges on a wet counter, so for their sakes, I'm trying to stay rested, and I remind myself to do things like burst into spontaneous songs when I'm with them.

At times, though, I feel pangs of guilt. The other day, for instance, Bob called when his division had stopped on the side of the road long enough for him to try to get a line out. "Tell me something that takes my head completely out of the desert for a moment," he said. "What are you going to do today?"

"I'm not sure you really want to know," I cautioned.

"Why not?"

"Well, actually, I'm going to get a massage in about an hour," I said. For days, my shoulders had been hunched up so close to my ears from tension that I was beginning to resemble SpongeBob SquarePants.

"That's great," he said halfheartedly. "You really deserve it—you must be very stressed."

Well, we both are.—*Lee*

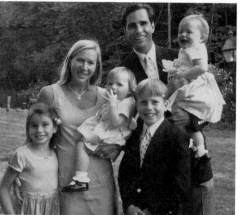

Lee and Bob Woodruff with their kids, Cathryn, Mack, and twins Clair (in Lee's arms) and Nora

MONDAY, APRIL 14

The phone call in the middle of the night is almost a cliché. But when it happens to you, it is very real, very sudden, like the wind slamming a door shut. A part of me had been waiting for that call since the war began. But what you realize, when the call comes, is that you are never ready. Not even one tiny bit. I got that call because my friend Melanie's phone was turned off, as I knew it often was at night. And so it was me they reached. The gentle instructions I got were to get in the car and start driving to her. They wanted me to be there when she got the worst news of her life.

It seems egregiously unfair that so many important decisions need to be made at the moment of a person's deepest sorrow. And the grooves of grief are ground much deeper by the unexpected shock of it all, by the lack of preparation. I never knew how many little things went into someone's death. Choosing the right black patent leather shoes for the little girls to wear; finding out what day, exactly, someone's paycheck stops; seeing a row of suits and shirts, still in their dry cleaning bags, hanging in the deceased's closet. There is the smell of too many flowers in the house; the prescription to "take the edge off" your friend's grief as she grapples with the shocking news that her life and the lives of her girls have changed forever. Then there is the sheer amount of food and drinks required to keep a house full of family fed when everyone is too numb to even think about cooking.

Let me tell you about David Bloom the way I knew him. He loved breakfast: big plates of pancakes and bacon and sausage, bowls of fruit, but no coffee. Caffeine, for him, would have been redundant. I remember warm summer days with the top down in the Blooms' Jeep, the four of us singing like fools at the top of our lungs on our way to play tennis.

My children loved him like an uncle—the hockey games, the piggyback rides. He never lost his sense of wonder.

So Bob is back, though his homecoming was not the joyous occasion I had envisioned. Instead, he was airlifted out of Iraq to give the eulogy at his friend's funeral. All this makes Bob's return bittersweet, intertwined with grief. But he is home, and we have learned to live for the moment, to snuggle when we can, let the dishes sit in the sink, worry about the dust bunnies under the dresser later. That's what David would have done. If he'd made it home. For us, the war is over.—*Lee* ▪

Lee Woodruff is a freelance writer who lives in New York with her family.

51

Percentage of Americans who GRILL on Labor Day

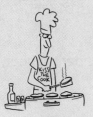

57

Percentage of grillers who say they are CONCERNED with food safety

14

Percentage who say they regularly use MEAT THERMOMETERS

39

Percentage of women who believe a woman in her 40s can CONCEIVE as easily as a woman in her 20s

33

Percent chance women ages 19 to 26 have of conceiving each month they try

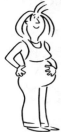

5

Percent chance for women AGE 40

90

Percentage of OVERWEIGHT women who've tried to lose weight on their own

2.9 POUNDS

Average WEIGHT LOSS after one year among people who've tried to lose weight on their own

9.5 POUNDS

Average weight loss after a year among people who joined a dieting SUPPORT GROUP

46

Percentage of women who say REGULAR SEX is important to their fitness and health

60

Percentage who say VITAMINS are

67

Percentage of mothers who correctly identify an OVERWEIGHT CHILD as such

32

Percentage who classify an overweight child as "about the RIGHT weight"

46

Percentage of patients who feel they've been kept WAITING too long in a doctor's office

13

Percentage who have CHANGED DOCTORS because of the wait

34

Percentage who feel their doctors don't spend enough TIME with them

17

Percentage who have changed doctors because of their physicians' PERSONALITY or manner

$1.7 BILLION

Sales of SOY-BASED foods in 2002

55

Percentage of women who say they EAT soy-based products regularly

41

Percentage of Americans who can name specific HEALTH BENEFITS associated with soy consumption

13

Percentage of Americans who feel they or members of their immediate families will be SOMEWHAT LIKELY to contract SARS in the next year

37

Percentage who think that one quarter or more of people with SARS die from the disease

9.6

Actual percentage of FATAL SARS cases worldwide (as of September 2003)

82

Percentage of women who say they'd keep an embarrassing health CONDITION (such as an STD) a secret from their boyfriends or husbands

28

Percentage who wouldn't mention it to their DOCTORS

20

Percentage of Americans who believe an HIV vaccine exists and is being kept a SECRET

Sources: Hearth, Patio & Barbecue Association, Opinion Research Corp./Roche/www.talkingweight loss.com, *The Journal of the American Medical Association*/New York Obesity Research Center, Drugstore.com, Vagisil Women's Health Center, National Institute of Environmental Health Sciences, Advanced Fertility Associates Medical Group, Centers for Disease Control and Prevention, Harvard School of Public Health, World Health Organization, Mintel Consumer Intelligence, United Soybean Board, Opinion Research Corp./Gynecare, National Institutes of Health, *The Wall Street Journal* Online/Harris Interactive Health-Care Poll —Reported by Laura Gilbert

Index

Contributors

Karen J. Bannan
Beth Bernstein
Michael Castleman
Sheree Crute
Lynne Cusack
Michelle Dally
Nancy Davidson
Sharon Edry
Daryn Eller
Christine Fellingham
Christina Frank
Susan Freinkel
Donna Freydkin
Kim Goad
Abigail Green
Catherine Guthrie
Marticia Heaner

Lambeth Hochwald
Patricia Jacobs
Nancy Kalish
Wayne Kalyn
Diana Kapp
Alice Lesch Kelly
Maureen Kennedy
Stephanie Jo Klein
Liz Krieger
Lynda Liu
Eva Marer
Jennifer Matlack
Kathleen McAuliffe
Michele J. Morris
Joe Mullich
Marty Munson
Judith Newman

Patty O'Conner
Peggy Orenstein
Lauren Picker
Jennifer Pirtle
Ben Raines
Sarah Schmidt
Alyssa Shaffer
Fran Smith
Lori Seto
Kimberly Conniff Taber
Ayelet Waldman
Tracy Teare
Linda Villarosa
Liz Welch
Lee Woodruff
Grace Young
Eilene Zimmerman

Editorial Advisory Board

Contributing Editors

Christie Aschwanden
Michele Bender
Kerri Conan
Alice D. Domar, Ph.D.
Dorothy Foltz-Gray
Timothy Gower
Brett Hill
Peter Jaret
Alexis Jetter
Petra Kolber
Dimity McDowell
Aviva Patz
Nancy Ross-Flannigan
Robin Vitetta-Miller
Liz Weiss